TAKE
CONTROL *of*
pain

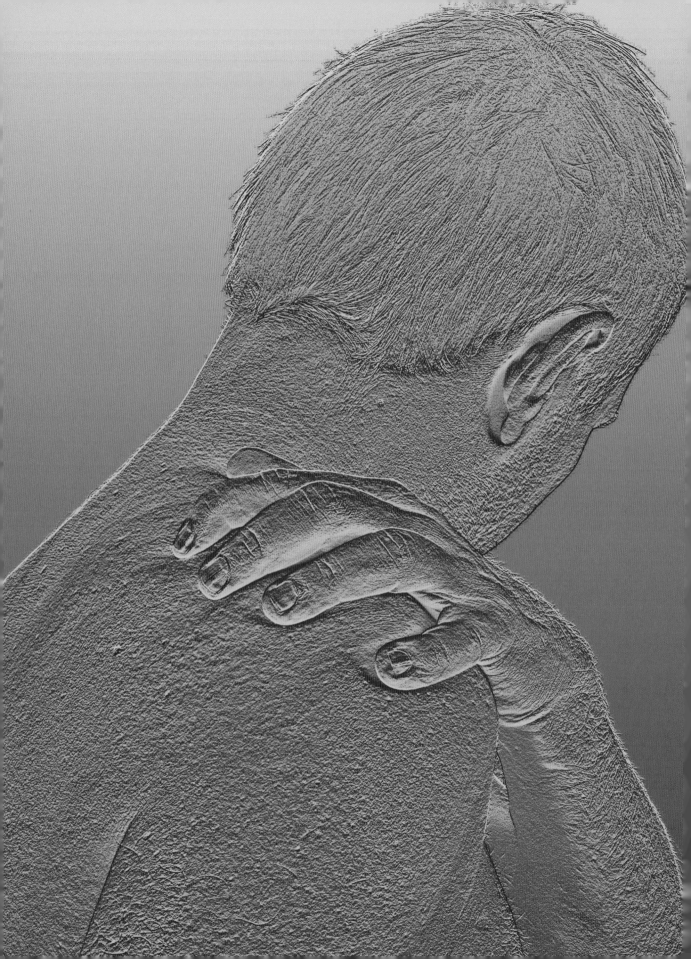

TAKE
CONTROL *of*
pain

**Hundreds of ways to manage
your pain and start living again**

Reader's
Digest

Project Editor
Helen Bateman

Designer
Joanne Buckley

Proofreader
Susan McCreery

Fitness Photography
© Jill Wachter
All other pictures are Shutterstock

Illustrations
Chuck Rekow

Indexer
Diane Harriman

Reader's Digest General Books

Editorial Director
Lynn Lewis

Managing Editor
Rosemary McDonald

Art Director
Carole Orbell

Take Control of Pain is published by Reader's Digest (Australia) Pty Ltd, 80 Bay Street, Ultimo, NSW 2007
www.readersdigest.com.au; www.readersdigest.co.nz; www.readerdigest.co.za; www.rdasia.com

This book is adapted from *Make Pain Disappear*, published by The Reader's Digest Association, Inc, USA, in 2010

National Library of Australia Cataloguing-in-Publication entry

Title: Take control of pain: new and proven ways to relieve joint pain, backaches, headaches and more.
ISBN: 978-1-922083-27-2 (hbk.)
ISBN: 978-1-922083-28-9 (pbk.)
Notes: Includes index.
Subjects: Pain–Diagnosis. Pain–Treatment. Backache–Treatment. Headache–Treatment.
Dewey Number: 616.0472

Prepress by Sinnott Bros, Sydney
Printed and bound by Leo Paper Products, China

We are interested in receiving your comments on the content of this book. Write to: The Editor, General Books Editorial, Reader's Digest (Australia) Pty Limited, GPO Box 4353, Sydney, NSW 2001, or email us at: bookeditors.au@readersdigest.com

To order additional copies of *Take Control of Pain*, please contact us at:
www.readersdigest.com.au or phone 1300 300 030 (Australia)
www.readersdigest.co.nz or phone 0800 400 060 (New Zealand)
www.readersigest.co.za or phone 0800 980 572 (South Africa) or email us at customerservice@readersdigest.com.au

Medical consultants for *Take Control of Pain*

CHIEF MEDICAL CONSULTANT
Will Howard, FFPM (ANZCA)
MBBS, Dip Med (Pain management)
Director, Pain Service, Austin Health,
Melbourne, VIC; Fellow of the
Faculty of Pain Medicine (ANZCA),
Fellow of the Australian and New
Zealand College of Anaesthetists

CONSULTANTS
Mina Borromeo, BDSc, PhD
Associate Professor, Convener and
Specialist, Special Needs Dentistry,
Melbourne Dental School, University
of Melbourne, Melbourne, VIC

Rochelle Cairns, BAppSc (Psych),
GradDip (Psych), PhD (Psych)
Senior Health and Clinical
Psychologist, Pain Service, Austin
Health, Melbourne, VIC

Angela Chia, MBBS FANZCA
Head of Chronic Pelvic Pain Clinic,
The Royal Women's Hospital,
Melbourne, VIC

Anne Daly, D Clin Physio, M Manip
Physio, BAppSc (Physio)
Musculoskeletal Physiotherapist,
Pain Service, Austin Health,
Melbourne, VIC

Suzie Ferrie, BSc, BA Phil (Hons),
GradDip (Food Tech), MNutrDiet
Accredited Practising Dietitian,
Sydney, NSW

Kathy Kramer, BA, MBBS, BSc
(Med) (Hons)
General Practitioner, Sydney, NSW

Rodger Laurent, MD, ChB,
MMedEd, FRACP
Rheumatologist, Head of
Rheumatology, Royal North Shore
Hospital, Sydney, NSW

Juli Moran, MBBS, FRACP
PGDipPalMed
Director, Palliative Care Services
Austin Health, Melbourne, VIC

John Quintner, FFPM (ANZCA)
Consultant Physician in
Rheumatology and Pain Medicine,
Pain Medicine Unit, Fremantle
Hospital, Fremantle, WA

Paul Rolan, MBBS MD FRACP FFPM
DCPSA
Professor, Pain Management Unit,
Royal Adelaide Hospital,
Professor of Clinical Pharmacology,
University of Adelaide,
Adelaide, SA

Daniel Stiel AM MD MSc FRACP
Gastroenterologist and Executive
Clinical Director, Royal North Shore
Hospital, Sydney, NSW

THE AUSTRALIAN PAIN SOCIETY

These days, there are many organisations whose purpose is to help people with pain. Australia is well served by having organisations such as Painaustralia, the Australian Pain Management Association, Chronic Pain Australia, the Australian Pain Society and the Faculty of Pain Medicine.

Take Control of Pain has been written by experts. Many of them are members of the Australian Pain Society, a society of health professionals from the many disciplines involved in treating pain, including dentists, doctors, laboratory researchers, nurses, occupational therapists, pharmacists, physiotherapists and psychologists.

I extend my thanks to all my colleagues who assisted in its production.

CHIEF MEDICAL CONSULTANT
Will Howard

OTHER CONSULTANTS AND CONTRIBUTORS

Gary Ansel, MD, FAAC
James Banks, MD
Mark Berner, MD
Steven Berney, MD
Scott L Blumenthal, MD
Felicia Busch, MPH, RD, FADA
Mehul J Desai, MD, MPH
Ragi Doggweiler, MD

Dermot R Fitzgibbon, MD
Kimberly Harms, DDS
Steven Hickman, PsyD
Christine Keating, MD
Oanh Lauring, MD
David N Maine, MD
Beth Minzter, MD, MS
Theodore W Parsons III, MD, FACS

Glenn B Pfeffer, MD
Eamonn Quigley, MD
Andrea Rapkin, MD
Barbara Soltes, MD
Jacob Teitelbaum, MD
Mara Vucich, DO

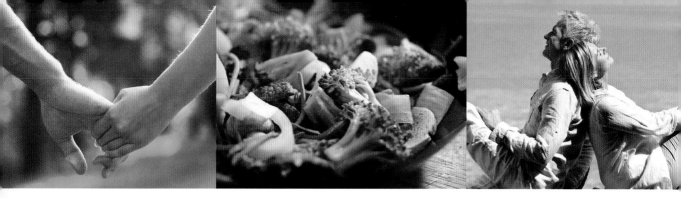

Contents

8   Introduction: Take charge of pain

PART ONE

About pain

12   **Chapter 1** Understanding pain

20   **Chapter 2** Change your thinking, change your pain

28   **Chapter 3** Some facts about pain pills

PART TWO

Six steps to taking charge of pain

40   **Step 1** Adopt pain-managing attitudes

46   **Step 2** Get the right help

58   **Step 3** Move more, ache less

76   **Step 4** Laugh it away ... and other mind–body solutions

88   **Step 5** Sidestep your pain triggers

96   **Step 6** Pain-proof your diet

PART THREE

Being in charge

Back, neck and shoulder pain

108   Back pain

114   Neck pain

118   Shoulder pain

Body pain

121   Chronic fatigue syndrome

126   Fibromyalgia

131   Lupus

Cancer pain

135   Cancer pain

Face and mouth pain

140   Burning mouth syndrome

143   Dental pain

147   Sinusitis

150   Temporomandibular disorder (TMD)

Gastrointestinal pain

154   Diverticulitis

157   Haemorrhoids

160   Heartburn and GORD

164   Inflammatory bowel disease

169   Irritable bowel syndrome

173   Ulcers

Head pain

177   Cluster headaches

181   Migraines

186   Tension headaches

Joint pain

188   Bursitis

192   Gout

196   Knee pain

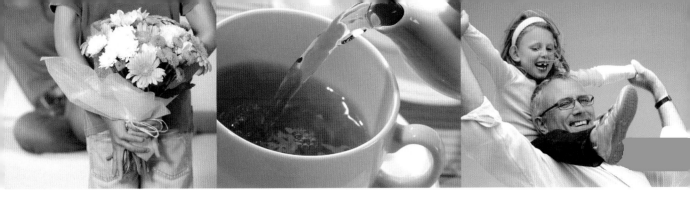

200 Osteoarthritis
206 Rheumatoid arthritis
211 Tendon pain

Leg and foot pain

214 Achilles tendon pain
217 Bunions
220 Foot and ankle arthritis
223 Peripheral vascular disease
227 Plantar fasciitis

Mystery pain

230 Mystery pain

Nerve pain

234 Complex regional pain syndrome
239 Diabetic neuropathy
244 Shingles
247 Trigeminal neuralgia

Overuse injuries

251 Carpal tunnel syndrome
254 Muscle and tendon soreness
258 Repetitive stress injury

Pelvic pain

261 Endometriosis
266 Interstitial cystitis
271 Menstrual cramps
275 Premenstrual syndrome
279 Vulvodynia

Skin pain

282 Burns
286 Psoriasis

PART FOUR

Exercises for pain relief

292 Ease your pain with exercise
294 Back pain
302 Carpal tunnel syndrome
304 Elbow pain
306 Foot and ankle pain
312 Hand osteoarthritis
316 Hip and knee pain
324 Neck pain and temporomandibular disorder (TMD)
329 Shoulder pain

PART FIVE

Useful resources

336 Help yourself to manage your pain
337 My self-care contract
338 Pain diary
339 Pain-trigger log
340 Exercise record
341 Medication log
341 Management log
342 Stress diary
343 Index

Take charge of pain

What was your life like before pain entered the picture? Chances are, you could take a morning walk, play a good game of tennis or golf or swing your grandchildren around and around without thinking about how long it was going to take you to recover. You could work hard, never miss watching a football game, eat two slices of pizza or plant a bed of daffodil bulbs in your garden, without worrying about triggering a nagging, lasting pain flare-up.

But then pain *did* enter the picture. Not short-term pain, the type that hurts for a few hours or a day, then goes away. That's called acute pain, and is part of the bumps, bruises and bangs of everyday life. Everyone has the occasional hurt, whether it be a tension headache, sore muscles from an overly strenuous day or something heavy dropped on your toe. These types of pain go away in short order, and life goes on.

Rather, we're talking *chronic* pain, the type that lasts. The type with names and diagnoses, such as arthritis, migraines, bursitis, sciatica, chronic back pain. The type that makes you want to do less because you're worried that activity and movement might cause yet another flare-up. Estimates are that one out of five adults today lives with chronic pain. Some of it is related to age; the older you get, the more the wear on your joints, bones, muscles and indeed all of your organs.

Some people with chronic pain get overwhelmed by it and give up the many activities that had given their life meaning. Others keep fighting a battle they continually lose, a never-ending cycle of excessive activity that causes their pain to flare up followed by lots of rest and recovery, getting demoralised and depressed by these recurrent defeats.

That's why we created *Take Control of Pain.* This book may not be able to take all your pain away, but it can help give you your life back. We scrutinised countless studies and interviewed dozens of pain management experts to find the approaches that have given millions of people the strategies to do again the things they once loved.

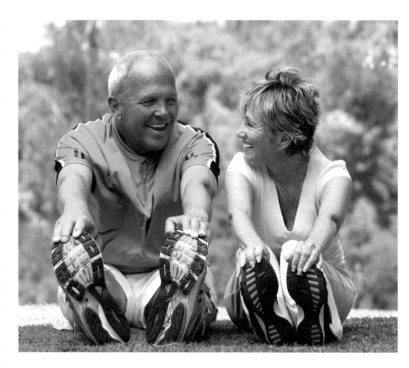

In these pages, you'll find just about every effective option for managing and easing minor aches and serious pains (from headaches and stomach cramps to nerve pain and cancer pain, and even so-called mystery pain), so that you can mix and match different strategies and find a formula that suits you.

You'll learn, for example, how your attitude towards pain can substantially relieve not only the hurt, but also the suffering (and you'll learn the difference between the two). How even short-term use of certain combinations of drugs—say, nonprescription ibuprofen and an antidepressant—can bring improved pain relief. How a low-level electrical charge can reset nerves that are still sending pain signals long after the initial injury has healed.

You may be surprised to find how much the little things you do yourself—from applying ice, soaking in Epsom salts, listening to your favourite music, laughing, eating chocolate, having a cup of tea or doing laps at the pool—can reduce your pain and boost your energy, restoring your zest for life.

Often chronic pain cannot be taken away, but there's a great deal that you, with assistance and guidance from your doctors and therapists, can do to ensure that you can do the things that make your life worthwhile.

The Editors

PART ONE

About
pain

CHAPTER 1

Understanding pain

No one should live in pain

Pain is a part of life, but we don't want it to rule our lives. *Take Control of Pain* gives you explanations and advice to help you understand and manage pain. Some of this advice is directed to situations with acute pain, such as a toothache, and some with how to best manage pain that lingers or recurs, such as lower back pain. Because chronic or recurrent pain tends to cause more people more problems, it receives more attention.

Acute and chronic pain

There's an essential difference between acute and chronic pain. Acute pain acts as a warning, letting us know that damage is about to occur or has just occurred; in acute situations our body usually needs the affected part to be rested so that the body can focus its resources on dealing with that challenge and recovery from it. But in persistent pain, the situation is completely different: the damage is completed, so rest or avoidance of an activity just means we miss out on participating in life. Sadly, many people become demoralised when pain fails to resolve and they stop their activities. This just compounds the negative consequences of having chronic pain.

The role of the central nervous system

Our central nervous system (CNS) shifts our pain levels up and down. The experience we call pain is the result of complex and rapidly adjusting neural mechanisms that process sensory signals from our body; the processing is profoundly influenced by neural states, including our emotions and thoughts. These adjusting mechanisms can turn pain up or down, like the volume control on a TV, changing the amount of pain we feel, or even whether we feel it at all.

The central nervous system is made up of our brain and our spinal cord; both regulate pain levels but the brain has by far the greater role. This doesn't mean the pain is imagined in our brain. It simply takes note of the biological fact that our brain changes the amount of pain we feel—and that's a fact.

That's why the histories of battles in war or in sport or in other challenging circumstances, such as dealing with an emergency, have an abundance of anecdotes where people have done amazing deeds despite severe injuries. (You may remember Manteo Mitchell running through the pain of a broken leg in the 400-metre relay in the London Olympic Games in 2012.) The brain turns off pain signalling until the challenge or crisis is over. But it doesn't have to be a crisis to shut down pain signalling: distraction by something as everyday as a joke will do the trick.

In studies of people who volunteered to plunge their hands into ice-cold water and hold them there, the study subjects reported feeling less pain when they were laughing at a funny video or listening to jokes than when they were just sitting there with their teeth chattering. Part of it is distraction—humour can take your mind off your troubles—but laughter also relaxes tense muscles and releases feel-good chemicals called endorphins, which act as the body's natural painkillers.

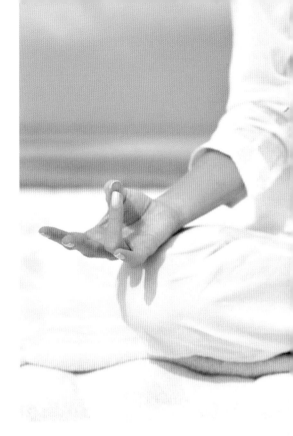

No matter what its cause, your pain can usually be better managed, often by you.

The high cost of persistent pain

Persistent pain is often associated with reducing our usual activities, such as work, sport and other recreation and times with family and friends. When we stop doing the things we enjoy, we can get irritable and become miserable. Jobs and relationships can be lost. Moderate to severe depression is common. The world can become a difficult and dark place. Even worse, pain gets ramped up by mental states such as depression or anxiety or when we are stressed. On the other hand, if you are doing things that you enjoy, and are reminding yourself that the pain flare-up will pass, you are more likely to feel calm and in control, and ultimately experience less pain.

You can learn to control and even change those unhelpful thoughts that may otherwise lead to depressed feelings. Interventions such as cognitive behavioural therapy (a psychological treatment that helps you learn to challenge unhelpful thoughts, beliefs and attitudes), meditation, yoga, relaxation and even antidepressants are new methods that can help people re-engage in their lives.

That's why clinics specialising in pain conditions combine both medical experts from a range of specialties able to provide a number of medications and procedures with psychologists and other professionals skilled at optimising psychological strategies. Psychological strategies are especially useful in situations when standard medical techniques such as medication or surgery have not been able to take away or reduce pain.

How staying active can help

It's very important that, despite pain, you continue to be active—mentally, physically, emotionally, socially. You may not be able to do things at the level you did before persistent pain turned up uninvited. But it's essential that you continue to participate in those things that give you satisfaction and your life meaning.

That may mean cutting back somewhat on the level of activity that you used to have, or adjusting how you do things. Sometimes it requires standing back and considering what your key aims are, and then planning to get there in achievable steps.

Pain is isolating. It can rob you of what you treasure most in life.

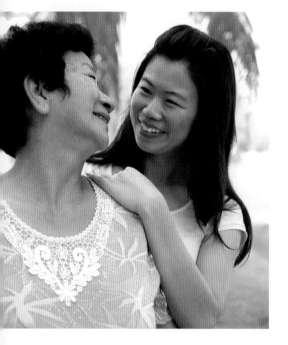

You may be able to sort these matters out for yourself. Or you may need some extra help from a therapist such as a physiotherapist—they're expert advisors in suitable types and amount of physical activity; or help from a psychologist—their expertise includes dealing with the negative emotions that can come with chronic pain and using non-drug methods to control pain. And your doctor(s) will be needed for advice about the role of tests, medications or procedures. But the most important person to take charge of pain will be you!

More is not better

Whether you have a pain from an acute or a chronic problem, beware the common pitfall of trying to 'push through' it. That's the domain of the elite athlete—and their bodies pay a price in the long term (often sooner). The smart way to manage pain is to do achievable amounts that don't cause a significant increase in your pain and to build gradually and steadily from that base. This is so important that it has a special name in the world of pain medicine and rehabilitation, where it's called 'pacing'. So ignore those stories in the media about the pro athlete who overcame the odds and came back early from injury. If you don't ignore them, you're not being respectful of your body and you're likely to make your pain worse.

Overcoming obstacles to better pain management

If your pain is persistent, the path to management may not always be smooth. Be prepared to be open to new ways of doing things, and to the idea that pain management does not necessarily mean pain reduction or pain cure.

Working with health professionals. You may find yourself dealing with a doctor whose favourite treatment strategy may not be the best one for you. Or one who simply doesn't know much about pain management. 'It's a hard situation for patients and for doctors, too', says Judith A Turner, PhD, a professor in the department of psychiatry and behavioural sciences at the University of Washington in Seattle. 'You're both frustrated that you're not getting better.'

But as Dr Will Howard, Director of the Pain Service at Austin Health, Melbourne, emphasises, 'The key problem is that patients and doctors are looking for a medical solution to a problem that can't be solved by a medical treatment. So patients visit more and more doctors, have more and more tests and X-rays, keep trying more unhelpful drugs or procedures—which can bring additional problems for the patient—and these things keep failing. There comes a time when we should say, "Sorry, we don't have the medical answer for your problem: it's time to change our approach".'

Enlist a team. That's when it's time to enlist a team of specialists to help you. A good physiotherapist who knows a lot about pain can help you become physically active again. A psychologist can make a big difference. Your general practitioner may be the coordinator of your therapists. Or your doctor may request extra assistance from a pain clinic. Another resource may be a sports clinic. Don't assume they are only for athletes—they are geared towards working with ordinary people in pain who just want to get back to their normal day-to-day activities.

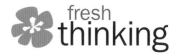

fresh thinking

'Why we hurt and why we suffer both have a strong psychological element. That doesn't mean our pain is in our heads, but that our minds affect how pain is received in the nervous system.'

—Grace Keenan, MD, founder and director of Nova Medical, a four-site integrative health facility in Ashburn, Virginia

Foster teamwork. You, your doctor and other health professionals need to be a team: they do their part, you do yours. 'Take responsibility for finding ways to deal with the pain', says Dr Judith Turner. 'It's like diabetes—it's up to the patient to maintain her diet. With pain, there are ways to keep it under control, but it takes active work.' Dr Will Howard explains, 'Our philosophy is that the patient should be working at least as hard as the therapist. That's what gets results for the patient.'

Evaluate and change your thinking. You may be thwarted by your own fears and attitudes. You may believe that acknowledging pain is a weakness, a sign that you're not coping. That's not surprising in a culture that coined the phrase 'suck it up'. Such an attitude may make you less likely to seek help. You may fear that your pain signals something serious, again robbing yourself of an opportunity for help. Some people are afraid that exploring pain management means rounds of painful tests or expensive procedures. Others may turn down helpful medications because they're afraid they'll become addicted.

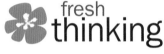

fresh
thinking

'The best approach to treating
pain is a multidisciplinary one.'

—Chris Criscuolo, medical director of
the Pain Management Program at The
University of Nebraska Medical Center

Relief is at hand

Fortunately, the solutions lie in your hands. Here are some strategies to help you to start to get on top of things.

Admit how you're feeling. If you have pain, acknowledge it and focus your energy on finding ways to better manage it. Dwelling on the changes and losses you have experienced and resting on the couch all day is a sure route to dissatisfaction and depression; or the opposite, refusing to admit to yourself (and the people around you) that you have significant pain often results in trying to do too much and making the pain even worse.

Address your depression. If you are down in the dumps and feeling depressed, if you're constantly irritable and struggling to find interest in family, friends, activities or work, tell your doctor. You may need some counselling or a course of antidepressant medication. There should be no embarrassment about this: we all have times like this in our lives. When depression is active, pain can feel much worse and it's difficult to take control of, so it's important that you get help quickly.

Talk to your doctor about opioids. It's smart to listen to what your doctor has to say about the benefits and risks of opioids. In persistent

Being a successful pain manager

You and your team of health professionals need to accept that medicine is yet to find the medications or procedures to cure some sorts of pains. Here are ways to help you manage your pain successfully.

Plan. Decide what your key goals are, then work out how they can be achieved. Just wishing it won't work. Identify the small steps that will get you to your goals.

Pace. You know your pain and you know what you can do without making your pain flare up. So aim to be active without exceeding that limit, whether for chores, exercise or recreation. Aim to consistently achieve about 70 per cent of your limit. As time goes by, your limit will usually steadily improve.

Set limits. To pace effectively, you've got to set limits, not just to yourself but to others too— your boss, family and friends.

Get moving. Exercise improves mood, improves sleep and often distracts us from pain. Regular exercise develops our stamina and strength, which allow us to do the things we want to do.

Manage your thoughts and emotions. Recognise your unhelpful thoughts and replace them with more helpful ones. This is a great way to better manage pain, improve your mood and reduce worrying.

Take appropriate medication. The purpose of medication is to help manage your pain so that you can get on with the things that are important to you rather than to reduce your pain.

Be persistent. If you're going to be in charge, you have to be as persistent as your pain.

pain, opioids, if used, should be regarded like any other therapy— that is, just one part of your management plan. Opioids should be combined with all the other aspects of your management. Your pain control strategies remain the key to being in charge of your pain. Sometimes your doctor will want a second opinion before commencing, or continuing, or increasing opioid medication. She may request assistance from a pain management centre (most larger hospitals have these centres) where they have more experience integrating opioid treatment with other pain control strategies.

Improve your communication. You may have a hard time describing your pain to your doctor or even articulating what it is you want her to do. You know you want your pain gone and your life back, but what does that mean? Are you okay with not jogging anymore but still determined to get back to bicycling? Explaining what you need can give both you and your doctor a better idea of how to manage your pain.

Plan the visit with your doctor. Your time with your doctor is short, so make the best possible use of the visit. Plan before you go by writing a list of what you want from the appointment. This may include questions you have, and inform the doctor of these at the start. Set the agenda—but be realistic. The doctor will want

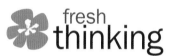
fresh thinking

'The key problem is that patients and doctors are looking for a medical solution to a problem that can't be solved by a medical treatment.'

—Will Howard, FFPM (ANZCA), Director, Pain Service, Austin Health, Melbourne

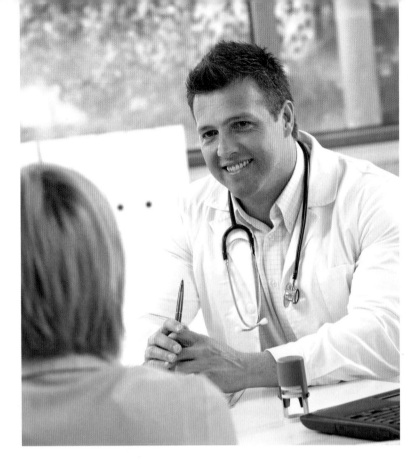

Chatting to your doctor and reminding yourself that you have options is key in better managing pain.

a summary of the overall effect of the pain: giving a rating out of 10 is often useful. If it's long-standing pain, the doctor will want to know the usual severity over weeks or months, not what it was yesterday afternoon. You might say, for example, 'Doctor, my pain is usually 4 out of 10 in the mornings but on a bad day it gets to 7 or 8. I have high pain that lasts for a day, on average, once a week'. If you want to discuss a new treatment, print out some of the research you found on the Internet to share with your doctor. But beware: a report of one or even a handful of successes is often shown to be excessively optimistic when a scientifically rigorous study is conducted. We all (doctors, too!) want treatment to be successful and that can unconsciously bias our interpretation of results. That's why we need science.

Overcoming setbacks

Everyone has difficult days, whether they have pain or not. Coping with a day of pain flare-ups calls for a few strategies to help you get back on track fast. Here's what works.

Stick to your routine. Tough as it sounds, get up and get moving. Even if you scale back your activities, sticking to the basic structure of your normal days will help you feel more in control of your pain and remember that even on these days you still have a life.

Turn anger to energy. When you wake up feeling lousy, it's tough not to get angry. But instead of feeding your fury, use that mental energy to make sure you're reliable with your pain management strategies. It might be because you overdid things yesterday, so if there's an obvious reason, learn from that mistake. But don't waste energy over-analysing what you did: sometimes pain just gets worse for no apparent reason. The important thing is to stay in control of your thoughts and emotions and to maintain your pain control strategies. Reminding yourself that the pain flare-up will settle and that you have plenty of options is the key to getting through.

Work with your pain. It's better than wasting your energy fighting it. Steven D Hickman, PsyD, director of the University of California, San Diego, Center for Mindfulness, tells this story to illustrate two ways of approaching pain. One windy day, you buy a sheet of posterboard and head out of the shop, the cardboard sheet facing the wind, and find yourself blown back into the shop by a sudden gust. If, instead, you angle the board sideways, you can easily get to your car. 'You allow what happens to pass through you instead of being buffeted', says Hickman. The point is that even on difficult days you can decide where to put your energy—you can fight your pain with anger and disappointment or you can accept it and walk with it. 'That doesn't make the situation go away', says Hickman, 'but how you move through it can change it significantly'.

Doctors' favourite remedies

Doctors know pain—and they've had lots of experience in seeing what works and what doesn't. We asked a few top doctors to share their favourite tricks for putting the kibosh on pain.

Go for a walk. Getting out of the house or the office for half an hour is great for your mood and for your body. If your pain is bothersome, make a deliberate effort to think of something other than the pain for that half hour. You can focus on the weather regardless of rain or sunshine, or make the opportunity to smile at a neighbour or passerby. —Will Howard, FFPM (ANZCA), Director, Pain Service, Austin Health, Melbourne

Sunlight. A deficiency of vitamin D, the sunshine vitamin, can contribute to pain. Ask your doctor to check your levels of this vitamin. If they're low, taking a supplement or spending a little more time in the sun can work wonders. —Ann Haiden, DO, osteopathic physician and integrative medicine internist in San Francisco

Bumper support. For people with aching backs, heaving groceries from the supermarket trolley into the car is a peril. Put your foot on the bumper of your car for support as you lift. At home, lift the bags to the boot lip, then lift them from there to your arms. —Ziya Gokaslan, MD, and Lee Hunter Riley III, MD, back surgeons at Johns Hopkins Hospital and authors of *The Back Book* (Johns Hopkins Press, 2008)

The green stuff. Surprisingly, diet can affect nerve pain. Try a vegan diet (no meat or dairy products), then slowly reintroduce other foods, one at a time. Monitor your pain through each change of diet. —Gordon Irving, MD, medical director of the Swedish Pain Center, Seattle

CHAPTER 2

Change your thinking, change your pain

As pain runs down your leg, pounds in your temple or stabs into your heel, the last thing on your mind is your thinking patterns. Why in the world would it matter whether you pay attention to your thoughts? In fact, it matters a lot, because pain, as you've seen, is not a simple, straightforward process. Everyone experiences it differently, and how much distress it causes varies from person to person, and even from day to day—and a lot of that depends on how you think.

When you knock your knee on the edge of the coffee table, your nerves send a message to your spinal cord, where specialised cells filter the message, either directing the sensation to your brain instantly or blocking it. If the pain is relatively minor and you were having the time of your life at a party when your knee encountered the table, you might not feel the pain until the party lights dim, or you may never feel it at all and wonder later how you got that ugly bruise. What gets felt and noticed shifts constantly, which helps to explain why we have individual differences in pain and even variations in our own reactions to pain. Your background may also shape your pain experiences. How you responded to pain as a child, or how your parents reacted to your bumps and bruises, can also affect how much pain you feel. If you noticed your parents went calmly about their routines even with an aching back or sore knee, you may do the same.

'We learn about pain from our earliest memories, and those memories are informed by all sorts of things', says Scott M Fishman, MD, chief of the Division of Pain Medicine at the University of California, Davis. 'In colder, stoic cultures, for example, people don't complain of pain as much as those in warmer cultures, where people may express pain in more physical terms. There's no right or wrong pain personality. Pain is what a patient says it is.'

The point is that pain doesn't happen in a vacuum. If we tend to be very frightened by it or certain that it means something dire is happening to our bodies, we're likely to feel more pain. If we feel that we always get the raw end of a deal in life, we may experience pain differently from if we tend to see obstacles as minor problems to be surmounted. If we've been raised to take pain in our stride, we may shrug it off and actually feel less of it.

You can use the fact that pain isn't straightforward to your advantage. Once you understand how your thinking style affects your pain—that is, how you perceive it, how you talk about it and the place you assign it in your life—you'll be on your way to learning how to better manage your pain.

The way you think about pain can have a really large impact on your experience of pain. If you are hopeful, optimistic and realistic in your thoughts, your pain level will seem lower. On the flip side, there are a number of different unhelpful thinking patterns that can contribute to increased pain. Some of these are listed below. See if you identify with any of them. The good news is that these patterns can be altered and lead to fewer fears, improvement in mood, a reduction in focus on pain and consequently, a better quality of life.

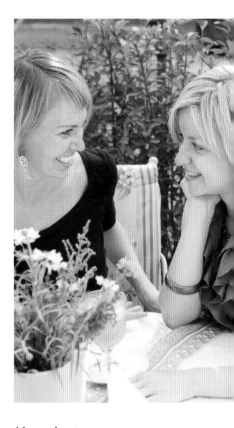

Keeping up pleasurable social activities will help keep the focus away from your pain.

Catastrophising (or the 'what ifs?')

You are someone who focuses on pain. You have an active imagination, envisioning pain as evil, certain that it is leading to further disease or disability. You ask yourself constantly 'What if … ?' Your easy access to medical information on the Internet, on television and in books feeds your fears. You read about a disease, even a rare one, and you're sure you have it. You may visit your doctors often, even for minor complaints. Your pain has unnerved you, and who can blame you for seeking the reassurance that you're not totally falling apart?

When pain strikes, you stay on the couch or head for bed. You're wary of doing anything that might make you feel worse. What if you do something that causes your pain to flare up? Slowly, you give up favourite activities—tennis, lunch dates, trips to the farmers' market—certain that rest is what you need. Somehow you got the message that, when you're in pain, inaction is the best prescription. There's real fear embedded in this stance: what if you do go out and enjoy a day of activity, only to have a flare-up the next day? Thus, you conclude it's best to stay put.

The problem with this thinking style is that it leads to a heightened focus on pain, increased muscle tension and avoidance of things that give you quality of life.

Shoulds

You keep going no matter what. After all, that's what you got praised for as a child: you were the one with the perfect attendance record, who never let a cold, a sports injury or a bad night's sleep interfere with duty because you 'should' be able to do it. Rackner calls such people 'strong stoics', people who are embarrassed or ashamed of admitting they're in pain. Some people take a global view: how can they complain about a little pain when other people are dealing with bigger issues, such as losing their home in a bushfire or dying of cancer? Or they may simply be proud of toughing it out. They'd rather suffer from pain than be seen as a wimp or complainer because they 'should' be able to manage.

When others do things that don't conform to how you think they should be done, you may find yourself becoming angry. When you don't do things the way that you think you should, you end up feeling guilty. These are two sure-fire ways to feel miserable and angry with the world, and ultimately to increase your pain and to alienate yourself from others.

All-or-nothing (or 'black and white') thinking

You view the world in absolutes, it's either a 'good' or a 'bad' day, things are great or they are terrible. The problem with this style of thinking is that it doesn't allow for shades of grey. When you colour your whole day as 'bad', you don't leave much room for recognising the okay or even good things that occurred. This is a great way to increase your pain. Yes, you may have experienced more pain for the day than previously, but you still managed to get up, to have a shower and to eat a meal. If you can manage to balance out your thinking in this way, pain doesn't seem to have quite so much control over your life.

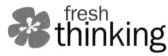

fresh
thinking

'Sensation is a nerve impulse going from one area to the brain, saying, "I feel stabbing pain". The emotional component, which is distress, is how upset, how fearful, how angry you are to have that feeling. Even if you can't do anything medically about the pain, you can do something about distress.'

—Steven D Hickman, PsyD, director, University of California, San Diego, Center for Mindfulness

Outsmart the emotion

Certain emotions, such as sadness and anger, often accompany ongoing pain. But there are ways to get around them so you can start to feel better both emotionally and physically.

A sense of loss. Pain can be perceived as a robber, taking away your ability to continue loved activities or even to be with people. Try refocusing your thoughts on what pain allows you instead. For example, if you were an avid gardener and now you are unable to do the heavy lifting because of a bad back, don't just give it up. Raise your flowerbeds, garden with pots only or hire someone to do the tough stuff. You may not be able to crawl on the floor with your children, but pain won't stop you from cuddling them on the couch while you read them a story.

Vulnerability. When pain is persistent, you can often believe that your life is not your own. You can start to think that pain is dictating what you can do and how you feel on any given day. It can give you the false notion that you're vulnerable to anything bad that comes your way. There's another way to think of your pain: as motivation to take better care of yourself, to try those new things you might not otherwise. Once you start taking more control of your own care, you'll feel less vulnerable.

Anger. Pain may make you think that you've been sideswiped by a hit-and-run driver. When you tell yourself that, you are like a victim. It's natural to be angry—at your circumstances, your doctors who can't make it all go away, even yourself. Start thinking of anger as energy and use it to find ways to manage your pain, rather than settling for life as its victim. Take control of those anger-producing thoughts and change them around.

Shame. Nobody wants to feel less than able, or dependent. But when someone is generously giving you a hand, remember how good you feel when you do something for someone else, says Rackner: 'Tap into that. You're doing a friend a favour by letting her bring a casserole over'. Accepting help is a strength.

Mental filter

You pay attention to all the difficult, sad or horrible things that occur, and ignore some of the other better things going on. It seems like tunnel vision, with all the 'not so great' things right in front of you. You pay more attention to these and forget about the good things. When someone asks you about your week, you forget about the days when you were able to do things easily and focus on the times when you experienced pain flare-ups. Thinking this way serves to drive your mood down, and drive up your pain level.

Overgeneralising

You take a single fact and think it applies to all situations. You go shopping and experience a pain flare-up and think that you 'always' get pain when you go out. The problem with this type of thinking is that you start to overinflate the frequency of a problem. This serves to focus only on the things you can't do, and to lower your mood.

Magnifying

You notice problems and turn up the size of them, making them loud and overwhelming. This thinking style takes everyday problems that we face and turns them into something huge to surmount. This can lead to a feeling of powerlessness and massive distress over the size of what you feel you have to overcome.

Personalising

You subconsciously want to hang on to your pain because it serves you in some way. When you think this way, you may try to seek attention for your 'suffering'. You may be afraid that once you're well, everyone who caters to you may vanish. It could be that once you have manageable pain, you will have to face other problems in your life, such as an unsatisfactory job or relationship. The problem with this thinking style is that it can catapult you into viewing yourself as disabled and lead to a spiral downwards of activity and mood.

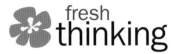
fresh thinking

'Once you open the subconscious and release suppressed emotions, they are gone. Most people almost immediately see changes: their pain is less, their anxiety and depression are less.'

—Larry Altshuler, MD, director of the Balanced Healing Medical Center in Oklahoma City

Changing thinking

One of the best ways to change your thinking is to write down your thoughts, feelings and behaviours. From there, you can evaluate whether your thoughts fit into one of the unhelpful thinking styles. The good news is that you can evaluate them and come up with a new thought that is more helpful, truthful and realistic. This is a great way to improve your mood, and help you take control over your wellbeing and pain.

Situation	Thought	Feeling	Behaviour	What's an alternative, more helpful thought?
What was happening at the time?	What was going through my mind?	What emotion did the thought cause?	What did I do?	
A friend invites me for dinner to their place	'Oh no. How can I get through that evening? It will cause a pain flare-up, and I won't be able to cope.'	Anxiety and fear	Stayed home	'I can go for a while, as it will give me a feeling that I am in control, not my pain, and it might even be enjoyable. Even if I do get a pain flare-up, I have had them before, and I know they pass.'

Other helpful ways to manage pain

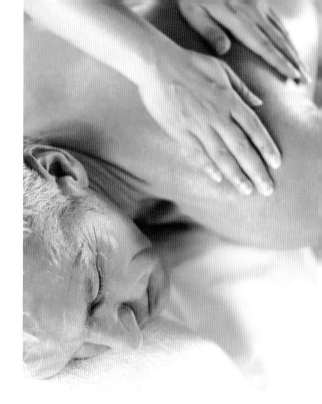

If your pain is persistent, the path to management may not always be smooth. Be prepared to be open to new ways of doing things, and to the idea that pain management does not necessarily mean a reduction of pain or pain cure.

Try hypnosis. Learning to be able to sit with pain may be helpful. Hypnosis, essentially a state of deep relaxation induced with the help of a therapist, can lower anxiety, helping you become less acutely attuned to every fear your pain arouses.

Seek reassurance. Instead of letting such worries nibble away at your wellbeing, exacerbating your pain, ask your doctor for a dose of reassurance.

Keep perspective. Sometimes what you fear may turn out to be exactly what's wrong with you. But it's more likely that your worry is only intensifying your pain and undermining your spirits. Remind yourself of the things you do to stay well: you eat a diet full of fruit, vegetables and whole grains; you exercise most days; you work at getting a good night's sleep. If you don't do those things, give them a try. They might just calm your nerves.

Recognise that to improve your self-management, you need to acknowledge your pain. No one's suggesting that you should harp on it. But acknowledging to yourself and your doctor that you have pain is the first step to getting on track to better management.

Be courageous in being active in managing pain. For you, it might take more bravery to address pain than to experience it in silence. Use that discipline you've cultivated to force yourself to try new approaches—such as stretching, or getting active—that may be outside your comfort zone.

Replace stoicism with realism. Being quiet about your pain doesn't mean your family and friends don't know about it. It may have changed how you act around them or caused you to withdraw from others, even stop going to social events, because you fear it will only exacerbate your condition. If you don't acknowledge that you're in pain, you won't take steps to get a new life for yourself—one that incorporates pain rather than ignores it.

Try a massage. It helps release tense muscles and increases the flow of blood and nutrients to inflamed parts of your body.

Switch to being active. It's good to look after yourself, but taking to your bed isn't the answer and usually doesn't help much. Instead, try going for a walk. Walking helps release tense muscles and increases the flow of blood and nutrients to your body. It brings a general sense of wellbeing and achievement. Walking is a sure-fire way to boost your mood.

Pace yourself. Keep a calendar of your activities and outings. If you notice that two events a day are going to tax you, spread the activities across the week. Or, if two outings are fine, don't do laundry beforehand, schedule laundry for a light day. Remember that pacing your activities may also mean planning on doing more.

Set small goals. Don't try to go from 0 to 60 all at once. Slowly begin to add back the things you've given up, or new things that you would like to try. Join a walking group and do a little more each time. Don't plan on overhauling your entire garden this year; instead, section it out and do a little at a time, and note your achievements. Adding activities slowly will let you find a pace that suits you.

Step outside your skin. Sometimes we're better at giving advice to others than we are at taking the same good advice ourselves. Ask yourself, 'How would I respond if my son or daughter or best friend

Reframing your pain

People tend to react to pain in ways that aren't always helpful. But for every thought like this that you have, there's a more truthful, realistic and helpful way to see the situation.

Take one: Things are never going to get better.
Take two: Having a pain flare-up today is not the same as forever.

Take one: I am a prisoner of my pain.
Take two: I know I can manage the pain because I have before.

Take one: I miss the things I used to do.
Take two: I can still do a lot of things I used to do and I can try to create some new goals for myself.

Take one: What's the use of trying to feel better?
Take two: I always feel more hopeful on days when I work to manage my pain.

Take one: I don't trust anything the doctor tells me.
Take two: I can share doubts with my doctor and we can work out a way to manage my pain as a team.

were handling pain this way?' Chances are you'd advise them to pace their activities and maybe see a psychologist to help them to manage their thoughts and feelings.

Acknowledge and learn to manage your anxiety. It may be helpful for you to see a psychologist who can help you address your stress. It is common to be fearful of talking about things that worry us. The problem with this is that avoiding fears can sometimes make them seem bigger than they actually are. A psychologist may be able to help you identify and address your worries so that you don't fear them as much.

Consider counselling. These are tough questions that you don't have to face alone. Consider seeing a psychologist to begin to address them.

Muse with meditation. Practising mindful meditation, for example, in which you sit quietly and notice how you respond to the thoughts that flow through your mind without reacting to them, may help you become more aware of your judgments and expectations and of your relationship with anxiety and pain.

Be informed. When it comes to pain, information is an ally. By understanding your therapies and treatments that have been recommended, you are taking responsibility for your pain management, which is the best possible route. One caveat: don't let your craving for knowledge consume you. You know well that your pain is only a part of your life, not its entirety.

Share what you learn with your doctor. 'People who do the best at managing pain are those who can see medical people as their partners, who don't think that the solution lies outside themselves', says Scott Fishman, MD, co-author of *The War on Pain*.

Use what you know. Being educated about your condition is a great start, but the key is to act on what you know. If you learn that increasing exercise may be effective for your back pain, give it a try. If several articles mention that swimming in a warm pool will help, join the YMCA, then get out your bathing suit. If taking nonprescription pain relievers will only lead to rebound headaches, pack up the pain relievers and talk to your doctor about alternatives. Make knowledge your springboard to action.

CHAPTER 3

Some facts about pain pills

How do you spell relief? Millions of people turn to pain medications, both prescription and nonprescription, to bring a fast end to their soreness, aches and, in some cases, agony. And let's face it: a couple of aspirin or a shot of a triptan medication can be a godsend when you have a migraine, and on days when your arthritis flares up, ibuprofen may be an important factor to keep you moving. We're lucky to have so many medications that help with pain. But pills come with trade-offs; they help with the pain, yet they also pose a risk of unwanted side effects. The twenty-first century thinking on painkillers is that they are a part of a pain management program in which self-care, physiotherapy and psychological techniques are just as important.

The use of medication should involve consideration of safety and of overall quality of life. Quality of life isn't a simple issue of pain relief: you have to take into account the influence of side effects and also what changes in function are brought about by the medication.

'I have cases where people rate their pain as a 10 out of 10, take medications and the rating goes down to one', says Scott M Fishman, MD, professor of anaesthesiology and pain medicine at the University of California, Davis. 'But they are sleepy all the time, and their life is worse. I also have patients who rate their pain as an eight. We get it down to a seven, and they can have their life back. The person who has little change in their pain score may be a treatment success. The key is improving quality of life.'

The fact is that medications on their own are unlikely to eradicate pain. But you can help them work more effectively by taking other steps to get relief—by changing your approach, regulating your activity, learning relaxation techniques, adjusting your diet and ensuring you have good sleep habits. 'We are a pill-focused society', says Fishman. 'We want to take pills to cure everything. But pills can only do so much. Pain medication treats only part of the problem. And there is always risk. In fact, there is no risk-free option, including doing nothing. The question is, how much risk do you want to take? You choose the therapy that's the most effective with the least amount of risk.'

Just read on to discover what you need to know about using common nonprescription and prescription pain relievers both safely and effectively.

Common pain relievers: what you need to know

When it comes to pain, most people want to take the simplest, fastest route to relief. Often that entails a trip to the shops for paracetamol or nonsteroidal anti-inflammatory drugs (NSAIDs), which are pain relievers such as ibuprofen and naproxen. Here are answers to some of the common questions about these commonly used pain medications.

Coming soon: his-and-her pain meds

Men and women differ in their responses to pain. Studies have found that women feel more pain than men. Even when men and women have the same ailments, women experience more intense pain. The genders also differ in how they think and feel about pain, probably because they experience it in different parts of the brain. MRIs show that women in pain have more activity in the limbic region of the brain, the centre of emotions; men have more activity in the cognitive centres. Sex hormones may play a part as well: women's pain threshold and pain tolerance vary depending on where they are in their menstrual cycle.

In response to these differences, researchers are working to develop gender-specific drugs. For example, morphine is being rethought in relation to gender: in some animal experiments, females required twice the dosage that males did to relieve pain. One reason is that males may have more of the receptors to which morphine binds itself in order to work. Researchers have also found that a class of painkillers called kappa-opioids, which includes nalbuphine and butorphanol, work better for women. They're now being used for labour pain as well as for short-term pain. Stay tuned for more his-and-her pain drugs.

How do NSAID and paracetamol painkillers work?

• Nonsteroidal anti-inflammatory drugs, NSAIDs, such as ibuprofen and naproxen, work by blocking production of prostaglandins. Prostaglandins cause inflammation, which increases the sensitivity of nerve endings and results in the generation and transmission of pain signals. Chemical variations among NSAIDs can affect how well you absorb them, how quickly they act and, to a minor extent, what side effects they have. If one doesn't work or bothers your stomach, try another.

• Paracetamol relieves pain but not inflammation. It is not an NSAID. It works by affecting the pain and temperature control centres of the brain. It's generally not as powerful as NSAIDs, especially for big pain. A review of 15 studies of people with osteoarthritis showed that pain decreased six more points on a scale of 100 in people who took NSAIDs than in patients who took paracetamol. But paracetamol tends to be gentler on the stomach and have fewer side effects than NSAIDs. But you must not exceed the recommended dosage (for adults, 4 grams per day) because excessive doses can cause fatal liver damage.

What to use?

NSAIDs are most effective for arthritis pain, muscle aches, headaches, toothaches, backaches, menstrual pain and neck pain. Paracetamol relieves mild to moderate pain of headaches, muscle aches, menstruation, colds and sore throats, toothaches, backaches and osteoarthritis, but it doesn't lessen inflammation. Pain relievers containing caffeine tend to work better when used for *occasional* headaches, because the caffeine temporarily constricts the swollen blood vessels that cause pain. But when the medication wears off, the blood vessels can swell even more, potentially causing rebound headaches. These medications should not be used frequently.

What are the dangers of long-term NSAID use?

NSAIDs block an enzyme that protects the stomach lining from the corrosive effects of stomach acid, which is why prolonged use can cause bleeding of the stomach lining or ulcers. In some cases, the bleeding is pronounced and even life threatening. About a quarter of people who take NSAIDs regularly will have a stomach reaction such

fresh thinking

'If you're going through your day and you suddenly have a headache, you reach for an aspirin. But your body is talking to you and it's not saying, "I'm low on aspirin". It's important to think about what's going on: did you have enough to drink today? Are you feeling muscle tension?'

—Steven D Hickman, PsyD, director, University of California, San Diego, Center for Mindfulness

as nausea or pain. Signs that your NSAID is causing stomach bleeding or an ulcer include stomach pain, black or bloody stools and vomiting blood (which often looks like coffee grounds). *Stop taking NSAIDs immediately and see your doctor.* Your doctor may prescribe another medication to take with NSAIDs to protect the stomach lining.

NSAIDs can cause kidney damage—ensure you don't get dehydrated when taking them. People who have diabetes or high blood pressure should be especially careful. NSAIDs have recently been linked with a higher risk of heart disease, particularly in people who are already at risk. NSAIDs impair blood clotting, so they're a bad idea for someone on blood thinners or who has poor clotting or anaemia.

No one should take these drugs lightly. The side effects of NSAIDs are pretty much the same whether they are obtained without a prescription or by prescription, but a prescription allows access to stronger formulations and longer use. It's uncommon for short-term use (a few days at a time) to cause problems; use greater than this should be discussed with your doctor.

Choose the therapy that's the most effective with the least amount of risk. Taking the lowest effective dose of pain relievers is always a smart idea.

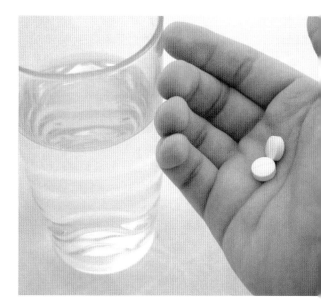

Are some pain relievers safer than others?

'The safest one is paracetamol', says Gordon Irving, MD, medical director of the Swedish Pain and Headache Center in Seattle. Guidelines from the American College of Rheumatology recommend paracetamol as the first choice for people with osteoarthritis. The Arthritis Society of Canada states that paracetamol is often prescribed for moderate pain due to its lower stomach impact. 'You have to think of them all as dangerous drugs and only take them if they are really helping', says Irving.

Antidepressants: not just for the blues

Though pain and depression often go hand in hand, you don't have to be depressed for antidepressants to lessen your pain. Here are five conditions for which antidepressants seem to be helpful.

Nerve damage (neuropathy). Among their actions, antidepressants increase the amount of noradrenaline in nerve junctions: this effect is known to lessen pain signalling. (Note: depression is not

Friendlier pain fighters

If you're discouraged about nonprescription anti-inflammatories or concerned about side effects, there are alternatives. Here are a few to try.

Ginger. Research has found ginger to be an effective anti-inflammatory. A recent study at the State University of New York found that 6-gingerol, the anti-inflammatory ingredient in ginger, prevents the production of pro-inflammatory cytokines, chemicals involved in inflammation. Ginger is available as a fresh or dried root, as a tea, and in powder, tablet, capsule or extract form. Take 1 to 5 grams in capsule form (to prevent stomach upset) daily, spread through the day in smaller doses.

Fish oil. Fatty fish, such as salmon, tuna and bluefish, contain omega-3 fatty acids, which have an anti-inflammatory effect. Although their heart benefits get the most press, studies have shown that this anti-inflammatory effect may reduce morning stiffness and joint tenderness in people with rheumatoid arthritis. Fish oil may also boost the painkilling benefits of NSAIDs. The American Heart Association recommends eating fatty fish at least twice a week, or you can take fish oil capsules, available in health and natural foods stores. A typical dose would be 1200 to 2400 milligrams twice a day of EPA and DHA, the fatty acids in fish oil. Check with your doctor before starting on fish oil because doses this high can impair blood clotting.

Capsaicin creams. Capsaicin is the fiery ingredient in chillies. Sixteen studies have found it more effective at temporarily reducing pain than a placebo. Wearing rubber gloves, apply a 0.025 per cent mixture (capsaicin in a cream base) on the painful spot four times a day. Do not apply on broken skin. You may have to use it for several weeks before getting relief.

Bromelain. Several studies have shown that bromelain, an enzyme found in the stem and juice of pineapples, can relieve pain and inflammation, particularly pain due to sprains, muscle strains and sinusitis. Some experts recommend 80 to 320 milligram tablets two to three times per day, though more (up to 2000 milligrams a day) may be used for certain conditions. Bromelain tablets are available in health and natural foods stores.

Willow bark. One study showed that four willow bark extract capsules per day, each containing 240 milligrams of the active ingredient salicin, was as effective as a COX-2 inhibitor in reducing lower back pain. Like NSAIDs, willow bark used for a month or more may cause stomach ulcers.

due to damaged nerves.) Antidepressants that feature this action are tricyclic antidepressants such as amitriptyline (Endep) and nortriptyline (Allegron). These drugs tend to be sedating, a side effect that can be utilised by taking the medication at night so that it promotes sleep as well as relieving pain. Antidepressants known as serotonin-noradrenaline reuptake inhibitors (SNRIs) are less sedating and are emerging as antidepressants of choice for nerve damage pain that can occur from diabetes, shingles, sciatica and stroke. Examples are duloxetine (Cymbalta), venlafaxine (Effexor) and desvenlafaxine (Pristiq).

Fibromyalgia. Duloxetine (Cymbalta) has been approved by the FDA (in the USA) for fibromyalgia. Studies also indicate that tricyclics and other antidepressants can help relieve pain, fatigue and sleeplessness in about 25 per cent of fibromyalgia patients. Tricyclics appear to work best for a combination of pain, depression and sleeplessness. The tricyclic most commonly used for fibromyalgia is amitriptyline (Endep), but it can become less effective over time; doses that are much lower than those used for depression are effective.

Studies on selective serotonin reuptake inhibitors (SSRIs), which include fluoxetine (Prozac, Lovan and generic formulations), sertraline (Zoloft and generic formulations), paroxetine (Aropax and generic formulations) and fluvoxamine (Luvox), suggest that they improve sleep and wellbeing and lessen fatigue in some people with fibromyalgia. Since sleep and pain seem to be linked in fibromyalgia, improved sleep is critical.

Rheumatoid arthritis. Depression is common in people with arthritis pain. Tricyclic antidepressants may help with depression and also with pain and sleeplessness.

Migraines. Tricyclics may also be helpful in preventing these nasty headaches.

Chronic pelvic pain. Tricyclics may help improve sleep and lessen the intensity and duration of pain in women with chronic pelvic pain. In some cases, particularly when depression accompanies the pelvic pain, a combination of tricyclics and SSRIs is used.

Anticonvulsants: not just for seizures

In some situations pain is generated by disorders of the neural system. Peripheral nerves can be damaged by pressure from a herniated disc in the spinal canal or by shingles infection or by metabolic abnormalities such as diabetes. The central nervous system can be damaged by a stroke. Anticonvulsants suppress some neural activity and this can result in less pain being generated. Unfortunately, suppression of neural activity results in side effects such as poor concentration, impaired memory, drowsiness and poor balance.

A relatively new class of anticonvulsants, the gabapentinoids, has been found to be particularly useful for neuropathic pain. The gabapentinoids comprise gabapentin (Gantin, Neurontin and other generic formulations) and pregabalin (Lyrica). In addition

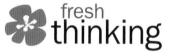
fresh thinking

'Medications work because you have receptors in your body on which they work. But the receptors were not given to you by pharmaceutical companies. You produce pain-relieving chemicals yourself. You can produce more of them using coping skills, by pacing yourself, by learning what your trigger points are and by just relaxing.'

—Gordon Irving, MD, medical director of the Swedish Pain and Headache Center, Seattle

A guide to nonprescription pain pills

Most of us have stood in front of rows of pills wondering what's best for us. Use this information to help you use painkillers safely and effectively.

Medication	Best use	How it works	Adult dosage	Side effects	Drug interactions
Paracetamol (Panadol and many generic formulations)	Relieves fever and mild to moderate pain from headaches, muscle aches, menstruation, colds, sore throats, toothaches, backaches and arthritis. Does not address inflammation.	Its precise mechanism is unclear. Reduces pain. Counteracts fever.	1000 mg every 4 to 6 hours but do not exceed. Maximum dose in adults is 4 g per day.	Side effects are uncommon; upper abdominal discomfort may occur at higher doses.	Drug interactions are uncommon.
Ibuprofen (Advil, Brufen, Nurofen and other generic formulations)	Relieves the pain and swelling of arthritis, shoulder pain from bursitis or tendinopathy, gout, menstruation, headaches, muscle aches, toothaches and backaches. Reduces fever.	Stops the production of prostaglandins, which cause pain, fever and inflammation.	For arthritis: 300 to 800 mg three to four times per day. For pain, menstrual cramps, fever: 200 to 400 mg every 4 to 6 hours. The maximum dose without a doctor's advice is 1200 mg daily. Take with food.	May increase the risk of heart attack or stroke, especially in people already at risk. Can cause pain, life-threatening bleeding or ulcers in the upper gastrointestinal tract.	It can reduce the effect of blood-pressure medications. It is a blood thinner and thus should not be used with warfarin (Coumadin). If you take lithium, ibuprofen can increase blood levels of lithium.
Naproxen (Naprosyn and other generic formulations)	Relieves the pain and swelling of arthritis, shoulder pain from bursitis or tendinopathy, gout, menstruation, headaches, muscle aches, toothaches and backaches. Reduces fever.	Stops the production of prostaglandins, which cause pain, fever and inflammation.	250 to 500 mg twice per day of regular naproxen, 750 to 1000 mg once per day of controlled-release tablets.	May increase the risk of heart attack or stroke, especially in people already at risk. Can cause pain, life-threatening bleeding or ulcers in the upper gastrointestinal tract.	It can reduce the effect of blood-pressure medications. It is a blood thinner and thus should not be used with warfarin (Coumadin). If you take lithium, ibuprofen can increase blood levels of lithium.

to gabapentinoids' role for neuropathic pain conditions, roles for other sorts of pain have been proposed.

When sleep medications help

Pain interferes with sleep, and sleep deprivation compounds pain. Sleeping pills are a quick fix but, if used frequently, they tend to lose their effectiveness. Worse, some types are habit forming: that means if you're not taking them all the time you'll feel anxious and irritable and have worse insomnia. So a sleeping pill is fine if you use it for an *occasional* need, for example your body clock disrupted by a change of time zone, a new routine or even the first week of a new job. You're better off minimising your use of sleeping pills by implementing good sleep habits: see 'Better sleep without medication' page 36.

Here are some medications that are suitable for short-term or occasional use:

Benzodiazepine hypnotics. Temazepam (Normison, Temaze and generic formulations) and oxazepam (Murelax, Serepax and generic formulations) are suitable. Beware: they can be habit forming. They should not be used for more than a week or two at most.

Non-benzodiazepine hypnotics. These include common prescription sleep medications: zolpidem (Stilnox and generic formulations) and zopiclone (Imovane, Imrest). These drugs also can be habit forming and should be limited to short-term use only, that is, 4 weeks or less.

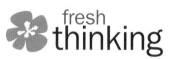

'When doctors suggest antidepressants for pain, they do not think the pain is in your head. The pain-relieving properties are different from the depression-lifting ones.'

—Scott M Fishman, MD, co-author of *The War on Pain*

Bringing in the big guns

If your pain is chronic and severe, your doctor may prescribe opioids. There are many opioids on the market: buprenorphine (Norspan), fentanyl (Durogesic), hydromorphone (Dilaudid, Jurnista), morphine (Anamorph, Kapanol, MS Contin) and oxycodone (Endone, OxyContin, OxyNorm).

Codeine, found in many preparations, is converted to morphine and this is considered the main way that codeine brings about pain relief. Using codeine preparations is commonly thought to avoid exposure to significant amounts of opioid but really it is a matter of dosage. For example, taking eight tablets of Panadeine Forte per day is approximately equivalent to 30 milligrams of morphine.

The long-term benefits and risks of opioids are uncertain. Although they have been shown to improve pain scores, they do not seem to improve function. In other words, you might feel better, but you might still find yourself sitting on the couch rather than getting up and about.

Better sleep without medication

Even if you do take sleeping pills temporarily, you should start practising good sleep habits. Here are a few tips.

Skip the naps. Often, taking the edge off with a catnap only makes it harder to fall asleep at night. If you need to rest your body during the day, or you undertake some relaxation therapy, ensure you stay awake.

Be boringly predictable. Go to sleep and get up at the same time every day, even on weekends. That helps set your body clock so your body will fall asleep when it's supposed to.

Dedicate your bedroom to sleep and sex. Don't learn to associate your bedroom with working, paying bills or watching TV. Do those things elsewhere.

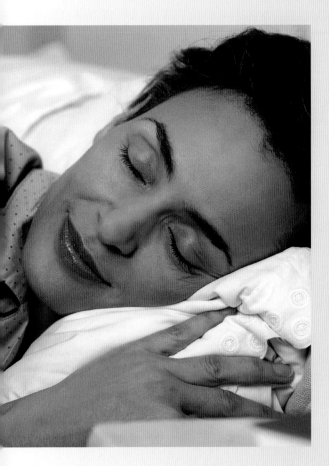

Catch the 'sleep wave'. When you notice yourself getting sleepy, you should get straight into bed. This means that your pre-bed sleep routine needs to be done earlier in the evening and it sets the scene for winding down.

Exercise. Want to fall asleep 15 minutes sooner and stay asleep 45 minutes longer? Get some exercise during the day. A Stanford University study of middle-aged and older adults found that four 30 to 40 minute sessions per week of aerobics, brisk walking or stationary cycling did the trick for most people if they kept at it. Of course, exercise can also help with pain. Try to exercise at least a few hours before bedtime. Exercise raises your core body temperature and your body needs a lower internal temperature to fall asleep.

Smoking and coffee. Quit smoking. Cut back on caffeine, or at least don't drink or eat anything with caffeine for 12 hours or more before bedtime. Check out your medications: could any of those be keeping you awake? (Most decongestants contain pseudoephedrine, which is a stimulant.) Is your late-night spicy snack disrupting your slumber? Perhaps you need more time to wind down before bed. A relaxing bath may help.

Get out of bed. If you can't fall asleep after 20 minutes or wake up in the middle of the night and find that you can't get back to sleep, leave the room and read (not a page-turning thriller!) or do something you find boring until you're drowsy enough to get back in bed and nod off.

Relaxation techniques. There aren't many things worse than lying in bed worrying that you can't get to sleep—which then keeps you awake. Self-relaxation techniques are a good way to stop that negative cycle.

Opioid drugs: myth and reality

You've heard that opioids (narcotics) are habit forming. And it's unsettling to know that illegal trafficking of these drugs is rising. But some of your fears about the drugs are likely to be unfounded. Let's shake out the facts from the fears.

Fear: I'll become addicted.
Fact: Addiction is a psychological condition, in which a person craves a drug. Research indicates that only about 1 per cent of pain patients who use opioids become psychologically addicted. However, some people do become *physically* dependent on the drug and if they stop taking it abruptly will have withdrawal symptoms such as restlessness, insomnia, nausea, abdominal cramps and diarrhoea.

Fear: Opioids, if used long term, will damage my body.
Fact: Opioids are very unlikely to damage major organs such as brain, heart, liver or kidneys. The key problem with opioids is psychological—addiction, over-use and misuse.

Fear: When a doctor prescribes narcotics, it means I'm dying.
Fact: A British study found that many cancer patients believe the doctor has written them off once he prescribes morphine. They also fear that they will not be able to function once they take the drug. But the fact is that morphine for pain can improve the quality of the patients' lives, allowing them to function better than they could without it. Its use does not necessarily mean the patient is dying.

'The key problem with opioids is that patients and their doctors rely on the opioid to solve all the pain, but what's required is a holistic approach in which opioids may make a contribution as part of a pain management strategy', says Will Howard, Director, Pain Service, Austin Health, Melbourne. 'And opioids are not appropriate to deal with the psychological distress that is suffered by many patients with chronic pain: that's usually best dealt with by a cognitive behavioural approach.'

Opioids have a range of side effects. So-called minor side effects are common—poor concentration, impaired memory, drowsiness, nausea and constipation. Long-term use can cause diminished production of hormones, especially of the hormones for sexual function. 'Some evidence suggests that opioids can make you more sensitive to pain', says Judith A Turner, PhD, a professor in the department of psychiatry and behaviour sciences at the University of Washington in Seattle. 'And those effects may be long lasting even after you stop taking the drugs.'

Because the drugs can be habit forming, some patients are afraid that they will become hooked on them. 'But only a small subgroup of people ever get addicted', says Fishman. Dr Will Howard agrees, but points out, 'However, many people are overusing these medications. They would achieve a better quality of life by incorporating their opioid medication into a pain management approach to their problem.'

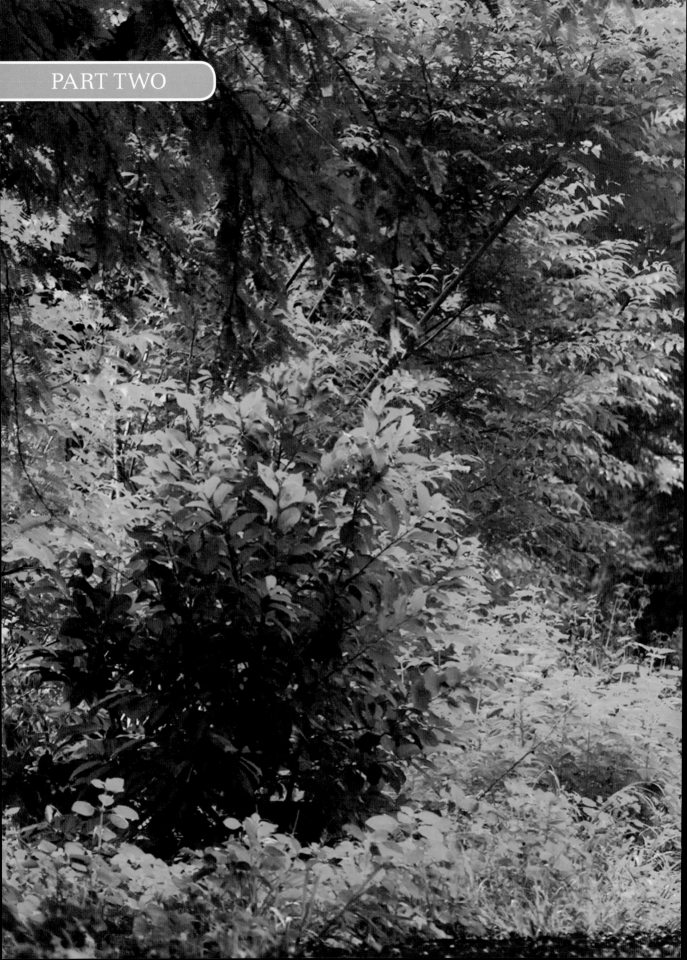

PART TWO

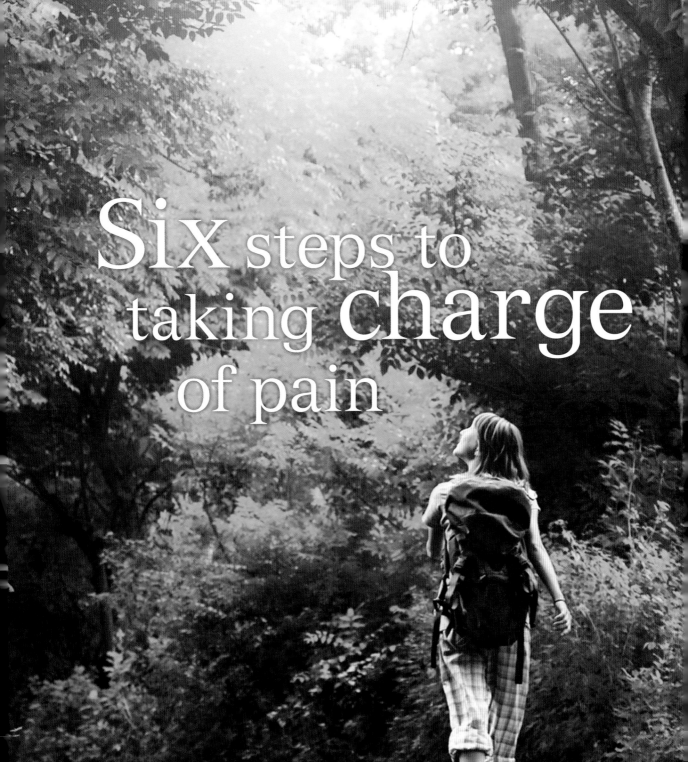

Six steps to taking charge of pain

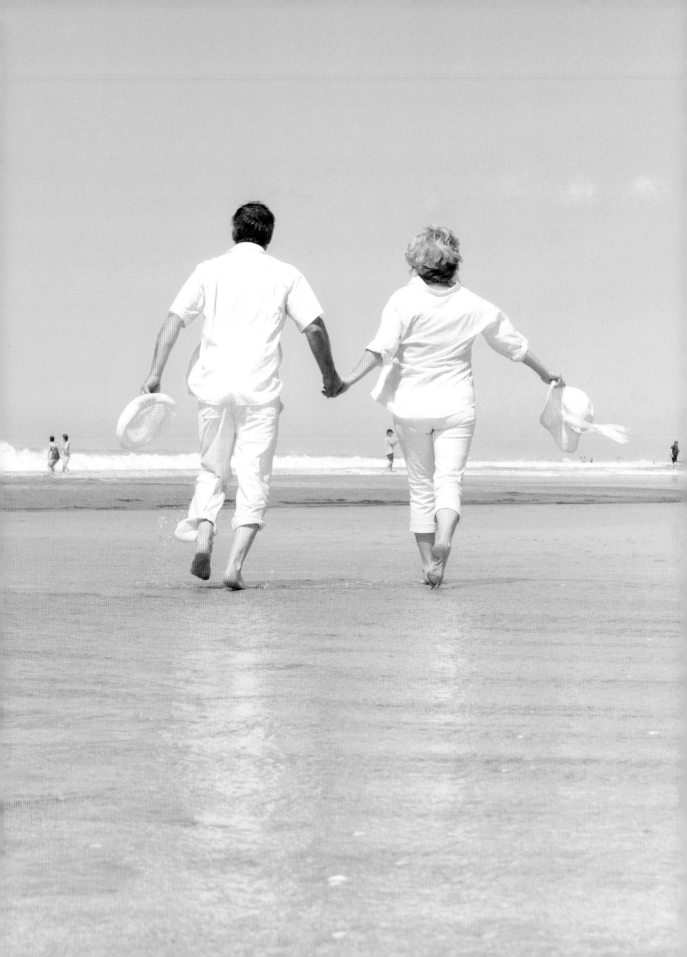

Adopt pain-managing attitudes

As with everything in life, when it comes to managing your pain, your attitude counts a lot. Maintaining a positive, can-do outlook is a surprisingly powerful tool that's always at your disposal. Setting goals, solving problems, rewarding yourself for trying a new strategy, finding support and appreciating your progress are all steps that will help you lead a more fulfilled life.

Acknowledge your pain

Your pain is real, and don't let anyone—including yourself—tell you otherwise. Acknowledging it and being realistic about the ways your condition affects your thoughts, your emotions, your relationships and your day-to-day activities is the first step to managing it. If you're struggling with managing your pain, try these steps.

Talk with friends and family. Explain how your pain affects you. Tell friends and family how they can recognise when you are having a difficult time. For instance, let them know that you may get quiet or grouchy or withdrawn when flare-ups occur. They've probably already noticed, but your acknowledgment will help them understand fully what's going on with you, and they'll be happy that you trust them with your intimate feelings.

Accept help. Letting the people who love you act on your behalf by fixing a meal now and then, doing some household chores or driving with you to a doctor's appointment can help you accept your pain

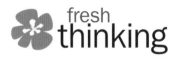

fresh thinking

'Pain severity can be turned up or down by how you think about it. Changing your thoughts to something more helpful can improve your mood and actually lower your pain!'

—Rochelle Cairns, BAppSc (Psych), GradDip (Psych), PhD (Psych), Senior Health and Clinical Psychologist, Pain Service, Austin Health, Melbourne

When flare-ups get you down

Just when you felt that you'd ushered pain out the door, it sneaks in through a window. You're not sure which is worse, the physical pain itself or the emotional hit of its return. Here are some suggestions for raising dashed spirits.

Stay active. Although you may be tempted to withdraw, it's better to continue to think of ways to solve problems, gain information about your condition, see friends if you can and plan light activities, such as a movie night, that keep your anxiety low. Activity is a form of distraction and can often make you feel better.

Be in control. Frustration will only make your pain worse. Try to stay as independent as you can, remembering that managing your pain with the help of others is an act of independence.

Picture better times. Imagine yourself in a place you love, such as the beach, the mountains or the bush. Think about the times ahead when you know you'll feel better.

and feel less isolated by it. The challenge is to maintain a balance between others helping you, and maximising your independence.

Be realistic about what you're feeling. Everyone has a different pain threshold; in fact, researchers now believe that genes affect sensitivity to pain and even how well pain medications work. For instance, redheads are genetically less sensitive to certain kinds of pain medication. The severity of what you feel has nothing to do with how strong or weak you are, no matter what anyone (including you) may think.

Keep a diary. A daily diary can give you a powerful venting tool and also help you recognise pain patterns you may be able to circumvent with lifestyle changes. You'll also realise that while there are times when you experience pain, there are also those really enjoyable experiences and occasions when you can recognise your achievements. It is important to remember these events too.

Vent out loud. If you're having a difficult day, don't try to be stoic and pretend nothing is wrong. Let it out. Cry, yell, express your sadness and frustration to a good friend or a counsellor or to the four walls of your bedroom.

Tell yourself you deserve relief

There's no point in suffering in silence, though many people think they must. If you think yours is a hopeless case, you won't look for the relief that is out there. Here are ways to avoid being pain's victim.

Learn when to say no. Can you forgive yourself if you have to give up cooking for the whole of the football club and lick envelopes instead? Or give up being the first one to make coffee in the morning? Know your limits and stick to them. Be as kind to yourself as you are to others.

Work out what is important. Sometimes we skip doing things for ourselves because we think there are more important things to do. However, sometimes taking time out to practise a breathing exercise, or making time to go for a walk, is the best thing you can do for those around you. By helping yourself, you are helping your family and friends.

Remind yourself that pain is a sensation. This means that working on how you interpret the meaning of pain can have a significant impact on the pain and ultimately the distress you feel.

Develop an attitude of gratitude

You may not be grateful for your condition, but there must be plenty of things in your life for which you do feel thankful. That's good, because focusing on those things is going to make you feel better, both mentally and physically. A number of scientific studies show that people who are able to express gratitude about their lives are happier and healthier. For example, in a study at the University of California, Davis, people were asked to write down five things for which they were grateful once per week for 10 weeks. A control group was asked to think about five problems. At the end of the study, the grateful group felt more optimistic and more satisfied with life, exercised more and had fewer physical symptoms such as headaches. Here are some ways to create an attitude of gratitude.

Give thanks directly. Think about someone who has made a difference in your life. Thank that person through a visit, letter or phone call, describing in detail how he or she changed your life. University of Pennsylvania happiness researchers found that study participants who practised this exercise were immediately happier and less depressed, and that the effects lasted for as long as a month.

Keep a gratitude journal. You don't need to do this every night. In fact, researchers have found writing grateful entries too often can become a chore and lose its effectiveness. But at least once a week, or as often as you feel moved to, write down three to five things that make you glad to be alive. Maybe it's the just-bloomed flower

Scientific studies show that people who are able to express gratitude about their lives are happier and healthier. Think about someone who has made a difference in your life and thank that person through a visit, letter or phone call.

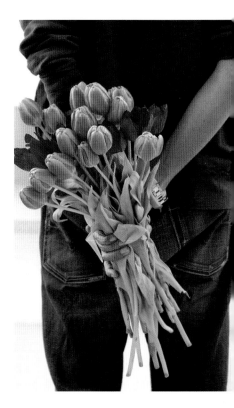

How grateful are you?

Gratitude is a natural painkiller. Are you making it work for you? Take this quiz to find out whether you have a lot or little of the G quotient.

Using this scale as a guide, write a number beside each statement to indicate how much you agree.

1. Strongly disagree
2. Disagree
3. Slightly disagree
4. Neutral
5. Slightly agree
6. Agree
7. Strongly agree

1. I have so much in life to be thankful for.
2. If I had to list everything that I felt grateful for, it would be a very long list.
3. When I look at the world, I don't see much to be grateful for.
4. I am grateful to a wide variety of people.
5. As I get older, I find myself more able to appreciate the people, events and situations that have been part of my life.
6. Long amounts of time can go by before I feel grateful to something or someone.

Scoring instructions

Total your scores for 1, 2, 4, 5.

1. Reverse your scores for items 3 and 6. That is, if you gave 3 a '7' give yourself a '1' instead; if you gave 3 a '6', give yourself a '2', etc.
2. Add the reversed scores for items 3 and 6 to the total from Step 1. This is your total GQ-6 score. This number should be between 6 and 42.

If you scored 35 or below, then you are in the bottom quarter of a survey of 1224 adults in terms of gratitude. If you scored between 36 and 38, you are in the bottom half of people who took the survey. If you scored between 39 and 41, you are in the top quarter (well done!) and if you scored 42, you are in the top eighth (fantastic!). (To increase your G quotient, follow the tips on page 43 in 'Develop an attitude of gratitude'.)

Survey developed by Michael McCullough, PhD, professor of psychology, University of Miami, and Robert Emmons, PhD, professor of psychology, University of California.

Adapted from *Authentic Happiness* by Martin EP Seligman, PhD.

in your garden, or the hot water in your shower or your spouse's smile. Thinking about positive feelings automatically nudges out the negative ones.

Substitute bad for good. Happiness researcher Sonja Lyubomirsky, PhD, suggests that when a spiteful thought comes up ('My neighbour blocked my driveway again. I wish a meteorite would land on her car'), replace it with a grateful one ('I got a call from my daughter today'). Regularly recognising good events diminishes the stress of bad ones.

Focus on something larger than yourself. According to the American Pain Foundation, six in ten Americans have tried prayer to deal with pain and 90 per cent report that it works well; half say it works very well. If you're not religious, try an alternative to prayer, such as a walk in nature. Focusing on a power outside yourself, whether you call it God or the universe or nature, can be psychologically healing, which can translate into fewer physical symptoms.

Use a little mind control

It's not just a hypnotist's trick. You can use your mind to help relieve your pain. Here's how.

Fantasise. A tried-and-true way to make something hurt less is to think about something explosively great. Instead of focusing on an ache, imagine your wedding night or a steamy evening with Mr or Ms Right. Vivid romantic fantasies cut pain sensitivity in half in one study of 40 people by researchers at Johns Hopkins University. Remembering walks on the beach, cuddles under the covers or a special night out not only distracts you from pain, it also reduces anxiety and relaxes you.

Distract yourself. Borrow a PlayStation, Xbox, or Game Boy or grab the controls of the family Wii. Playing a video game lowered pain levels three times more than medications alone in one small study of children. Other research has replicated the finding, and video-game makers report receiving letters from adults who say that gaming is a potent distracter from pain for them, too.

Escape with music. Put on some music. Enjoying your favourite tunes for an hour a day can cut persistent pain by 21 per cent, according to a study of 60 people.

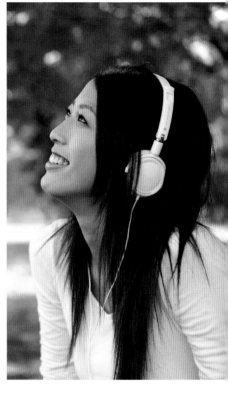

Enjoying your favourite tunes for an hour a day can cut persistent pain by 21 per cent.

Repeat after me

If you hear yourself thinking or speaking unhelpful thoughts or thoughts like these, replace them with more helpful ones:

I can't stand the pain. I am in control of how I respond to my pain.

I can't do anything. I can choose what I do, even if that means doing a little less than I used to.

I hate my life. I love [fill in your favourite pleasures and people].

My situation is hopeless. Some days are better than others.

I feel old and tired. I feel best in the morning.

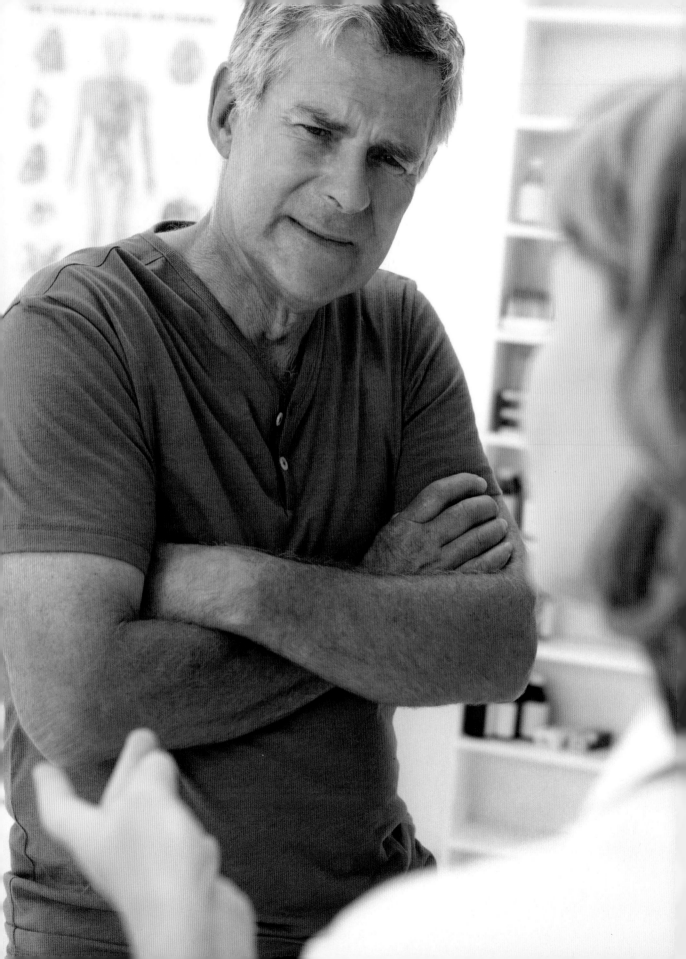

Get the right help

Your family doctor may be wonderful, but the average general practitioner, who has to know about everything from sprained muscles to sore throats, may need some assistance to deal with your situation. If you're still in significant pain—you have more high pain days than low ones—you might need a specialist. In fact, you might need several specialists—a pain management physician along with a physiotherapist, a psychologist and perhaps others. Here's how to get the help you need.

Don't be afraid to ask for another opinion

Addressing your pain is rather like getting your roof fixed: if the first contractor can't mend it, try another. What you don't do is live with a leaky roof. Here's how to know when it's time for you to go elsewhere.

If you still hurt or if your doctor is unfamiliar with your pain. Whether it's your general practitioner or a specialist, you're entitled to ask your doctor about getting another opinion. There should be no embarrassment in this and your doctor should be prepared to offer assistance, if that's what you want, finding another doctor and in sending correspondence summarising your condition to another doctor. (Of course this may take some time and effort so your doctor, or his surgery, may require some reimbursement.)

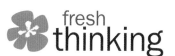
fresh thinking

'Decide that you will manage your pain rather than have your pain manage you.'

—Micke Brown, RN, BSN, director of Advocacy, American Pain Foundation

Educate yourself

To get the right help, you need to know what's missing in the care you've already had. Think through what you need and educate yourself about how to find it.

Learn about your condition. The more you know about the condition that's causing your pain, the clearer it will be who might be able to help you. You can find information about your condition at any number of reputable websites, especially those run by government departments or ministries, medical associations, universities and patient support groups. Learning more about your condition will also make it easier to communicate clearly with your new doctors. Remember that the Internet can be really helpful. However, sometimes the self-help information put there may not be reputable.

Call your local hospital. Hospitals, state health departments and the Australian Health Practitioner Regulation Agency (AHPRA) may be able to refer you to pain specialists. You can also call your health insurance company. No insurance? Call your state health department or a local hospital's social work department. Also ask friends and family for their suggestions and referrals.

Help you can count on

Many organisations exist to assist you in finding the best help.

- Pain Australia
  http://www.painaustralia.org.au/
- Australian Pain Management Association
  http://www.painmanagement.org.au/
- Chronic Pain Australia
  http://www.chronicpainaustralia.org.au/
- Australian Pain Society
  http://www.apsoc.org.au/
- Faculty of Pain Medicine (ANZCA)
  http://www.fpm.anzca.edu.au/
- Australian Physiotherapy Association
  http://www.physiotherapy.asn.au/
- The Pain Society of Singapore
  http://www.pain.org.sg/
- New Zealand Pain Society
  http://www.nzps.org.nz/
- Pain SA (South Africa)
  http://www.painsa.co.za/
- Malaysian Association for the Study of Pain http://www.masp.org.my/

Find Dr Right

You know you want to see a specialist to ease your pain, but your homework's just beginning. Pain specialist, for instance, is an umbrella term for anaesthetists, neurosurgeons, psychiatrists, rehabilitation medicine specialists and others. Some provide only one thing, such as medication, while others offer a multidisciplinary approach. Here's how to sort it all out.

Research your pain centre. If you do opt for a pain centre, educate yourself before you become a patient. Some are pill mills prescribing opiates only; others are needle jockeys offering injections, says David C Miller, MD, medical director of Woodland Pain Center in Michigan City, Indiana. The best bets are pain centres that offer integrated treatments that include cognitive behavioural therapy, physiotherapy and medication management.

Interview your pain specialist. Find out about his expertise. How long has he been practising? Is he certified in pain management? Is he affiliated with a hospital? Does he have experience treating your kind of pain? What are his outcomes? Ask him, 'Can you give me a pain-free life?' Don't expect him to say yes. Do expect him to answer honestly.

Evaluating information on the Internet

The Net is a wealth of information—good and bad. Here are clues to finding reliable websites.

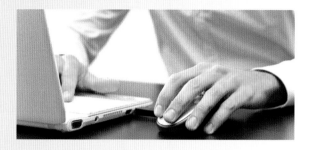

Check medical centres, universities and government sites first. These offer the most accurate information. University sites end in '.edu.au' in Australia and '.ac.nz' in New Zealand; Australian government sites end in '.gov.au' while New Zealand government sites end in '.govt.nz'

Look for the HON logo. The logo from the Health on the Net Foundation is on sites that agree to a standard of credibility, regulated by the HON Code of Conduct.

Try nonprofit research groups. Associations such as the Anti-Cancer Council. Their addresses usually end in '.org.au' in Australia, '.govt.nz' in New Zealand.

Check out the board or reviewers. Make sure that medical advisors review content. A reputable site will have an 'About Us' section on its home page that offers that information.

Look for research studies. See if the information refers to credible studies.

Avoid commercials. If the site makes ads tough to distinguish from information, search elsewhere.

Skip the miracles. Don't bother with sites that offer miracle cures or information that they claim 'your doctor won't tell you'.

Always check more than one site. If you are sceptical about the information you're reading, check another site. Or, if information conflicts, keep searching until you get a sense of the consensus of reputable experts.

Look at the date. It's not helpful to look at information that's 15 years old. Check the review date, usually listed at the bottom of the page, to ensure that the information has been recently reviewed and is still valid.

Check the source of the content. It should be clear where the site got its information. Look for a bibliography listing citations, such as medical journals.

Beware emails and chat rooms. Although you may get interesting information from both, do not consider them factual until you check with your doctor. Beware that some unfortunate people like to dramatise their condition and overstate their pain and disability.

Don't rule out psychological counselling. Considering this option adds to the treatments that address the physical aspects of your pain. But a lot of patients, annoyed by the implication that what's in their head affects their pain, shrug off any suggestion that a psychologist specialising in pain can be helpful. Pain can raise fears about the future, about continuing work, about relationships. A psychologist skilled in pain management can: help identify inappropriate fears and thoughts that can interfere with healthy responses to the challenges of pain; help manage depression and anxiety and help devise realistic goals and plans to deal with chronic pain.

Be a good partner

Once you find a specialist, one key to care is communication. 'Life is all about personal relationships', says Dr Minzter. 'It's no different with your doctor.' Try these tips for getting more out of your next visit.

Do your homework. The more you know about your health problem before you go into a doctor's surgery, the better and more efficient your conversation will be.

Write down your questions, medications and other treatments. Keep a record of your medications and procedures and take a copy with you to every appointment. Your doctor can't remember every detail about every patient, and you may not remember everything about your case, either.

Be an efficient communicator. Keep a pain diary that tracks your levels of pain. Before you see your doctor, whether for a first consultation or for a review, think about, even write down, how you can best describe your pain: its frequency, intensity and location. Your job is to give the doctor a report on your life with pain: the report should balance sufficient detail with an overall view.

Have realistic expectations. If you're leaving one doctor because you're angry that he can't make you 100 per cent pain-free, you may face the same disappointment elsewhere. Most pain won't go away with one visit or treatment, and it's unfair to blame your doctor for that.

State your expectations. Tell the doctor what you want to be able to do again: play with your dog, ride a bike, knit a jumper. Ask him what is a reasonable expectation. A good doctor should be honest, 'You probably will be able to do X and Y but not Z'.

Focus on your main complaint. You may feel as though everything hurts, but reciting a litany of ills will only overwhelm your time-poor doctor. Decide beforehand what you want to be the main focus and outcome of your visit and stick with that.

Follow through on his advice. You can't expect your doctor's advice to help you if you don't act on it.

Learn how to describe your pain

Part of getting the best care is being able to describe your pain, to articulate how pain affects your life. Here are some tips that may help you hone your points.

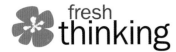

fresh thinking

'Present yourself as a motivated person who wants to work with your physician so that both of you together can improve your pain.'

—Beth Minzter, MD, MS, director of Cancer Pain in the Pain Management Center, Cleveland Clinic, Cleveland

I feel pain in/on . . . At a regular time each day, write down your overall pain, perhaps divided into morning, afternoon, evening and during the night. That way you won't forget.

Record your activities . . . It's important to know what you've been able to achieve.

I feel pain when . . . Describe when you feel pain, for how long, under what circumstances and during what activities.

My pain gets better when . . . Let the doctor know what medications, therapies and situations lessen your pain.

My pain keeps me from . . . Maybe it keeps you from driving, going to church, carrying groceries or playing golf.

Cast a wider net

Pain often requires a combination approach. You may be getting excellent care from a doctor who is prescribing medications, for example, but other treatments, such as physiotherapy or psychological counselling could have a place in your treatment as well. Here's how to safely add other therapies.

Discuss adding other therapists with your doctor. Your doctor may be able to offer referrals to reputable practitioners. Preferably your doctor and other therapists will be used to working with each other and will have well-established lines of communication. Ideally they will work at the same centre.

Red flags

When you choose a doctor, you're keen to find the person whose skills and manner suit you best. It helps to know the red flags that may suggest that a doctor or pain clinic's not the right one. Here are some warning signs to watch for.

The lone ranger. If an alternative practitioner doesn't want to work with your regular doctor or asks you to abandon conventional treatment, he's not the best choice.

The promoter. If your doctor is promoting a particular product or device claiming to cure your ills, walk on by.

The curmudgeon. You don't have to be best friends with your doctor but you should feel you have a good relationship. As Minzter says, 'There are plenty of nice, good doctors'.

The silent type. Your doctor should listen to your observations, encourage you to ask questions and ask you a lot of questions.

Know your rights

You can report poor care. If you feel you've been treated inappropriately you can complain to the hospital (many have a Patient Advocates Office) or to the staff of the Chief Executive Officer or your state may have a Health Services Commissioner.

If you suspect that your doctor or other health-care professional is doing something wrong, you can and should report him to the relevant registration board—in Australia it's the Australian Health Practitioner Regulation Agency AHPRA. AHPRA is responsible for the registration of all health professionals, such as doctors, nurses, physiotherapists and psychologists. Go to http://www.ahpra.gov.au

Consult your pharmacist. Most of us think that the men and women behind the glass partitions simply fill our bottles with the correct medications. But pharmacists have years of training about medications. Pharmacists are a great resource for answering your questions about drugs, their effectiveness and any drug interactions. They can also advise you about nonprescription drugs. Try to use the same pharmacist all the time.

Visit a wellness centre. Wellness centres vary, but you'll probably find a range of services, programs and classes, such as massage therapy, naturopathic medicine, chiropractic, Chinese medicine, acupuncture, fitness programs and nutritional counselling.

Do your research. Just because some studies have shown that acupuncture can be helpful for pain, that doesn't mean it will be helpful for your kind of pain. Before you spend time and money on therapy, research what it is effective for, how to find a reputable therapist and how much time and money you should expect to spend.

Find providers through accrediting agencies. By going to the accrediting agencies' websites, you can find out what credentials you should be looking for when you choose a therapist.

The ABCs of pain specialists

Here is a rundown of various pain specialists and what they do.

Anaesthetists. It used to be that these doctors took care of pain only during surgery. Now, however, they usually meet with and treat patients before, during and after procedures. Anaesthetists have particular expertise in pharmacology and in nerve block techniques such as epidurals. They can manage pain and prescribe drug therapies for patients suffering from acute, chronic and cancer pain.

Neurologists. Neurologists treat diseases and injuries of the nervous system, including the brain and spinal cord, nerves, nerve roots and muscles. You may see a neurologist for your headache, pain after a stroke, pain from damage to nerves as occurs in trigeminal neuralgia, shingles, diabetic peripheral neuropathy, sciatica and other conditions.

Neurosurgeons. Although most people associate neurosurgeons with brain surgery, they are trained to treat the entire nervous system. In fact, they spend about 70 per cent of their time working with spinal problems. Conditions they treat include back pain, sciatica, neck pain, pinched nerves in the neck and carpal tunnel syndrome.

Psychiatrists. It's now widely recognised that pain is affected by your mental health and that chronic pain can cause depression and anxiety. A psychiatrist is a medical doctor who can help assess and manage pain, and act in partnership with your doctor in creating a comprehensive treatment plan that may include medications and psychological therapy to assist treatment of depression and anxiety.

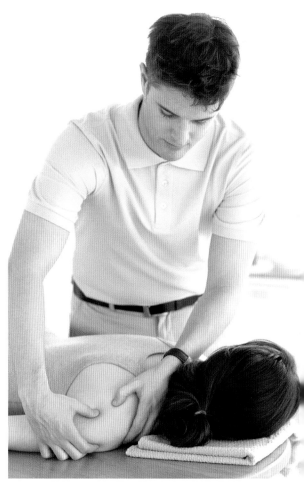

Rehabilitation medicine physicians. These are doctors trained to help people recover function after surgery, injury or illness. They have expertise in developing realistic and comprehensive treatment plans for you, and in coordinating involvement of other doctors and therapists.

Important note. Look for the letters 'FFPM (ANZCA)'. These mean Fellow of the Faculty of Pain Medicine (Australian and New Zealand College of Anaesthetists). A doctor who has this qualification has undertaken two years of study and training at specialist hospital centres, and passed a rigorous written and clinical examination about pain medicine. (This will have been in addition to already having a post-graduate qualification in a medical specialty such as anaesthesia, rehabilitation medicine, psychiatry or other physician's or surgeon's qualification.) You can be confident that a doctor who is a fellow of the FFPM(ANZCA) has an interest in and knowledge of dealing with chronic pain.

Pain often requires a combination approach. Therapies such as physiotherapy, psychology and other counselling, massage and acupuncture could each have a place in your treatment.

Other health professionals

Beyond doctors, a host of other trained health professionals may become part of your pain management plan. Here is a round-up of what they do.

Psychologists. A psychologist is not a medical doctor but has extensive professional training at university and in clinical situations to help people better manage their physical and mental health. They are experts in human behaviour, having studied the brain, memory, learning, human development and the processes determining how people think, feel, behave and react. Psychologists apply their expertise using reliable and scientifically supported methods. Psychologists in Australia don't prescribe medication, rather they are skilled at helping people to recognise and change the thoughts, emotions and behaviours that often go hand in hand with managing chronic pain. This form of psychotherapy is called cognitive behavioural therapy. It can be done in individual sessions or in group programs. (You'll find more information on this at the Australian Psychological Society website http://www.psychology.org.au) Psychologists are excellent sources of training in a variety of strategies to manage situations related to chronic pain; these strategies can supplement medication or reduce the reliance on medication. Examples of these strategies are relaxation and good sleep practices. Psychologists are required to be registered with the Australian Health Practitioner Regulation Agency (AHPRA).

Physiotherapists. A physiotherapist is not a medical doctor, but is a health professional trained to assess and treat physical conditions by helping you to recover strength, flexibility and movement. Physiotherapists work by using stretching and strengthening exercises, ice, heat, manual therapies, hydrotherapy, dry needling (a type of acupuncture) and electrotherapies. Some physiotherapists have special skills in chronic pain management and the prescription of exercise to improve your lifestyle even when pain and/or other physical disability persists. You can expect these specialised physiotherapists to work with you to achieve goals that are important to you. Physiotherapists are required to be registered by the Australian Health Practitioner Regulation Agency (AHPRA) to practise in Australia. The Australian Physiotherapy Association (APA) can help you locate members in your community (see http://www.physiotherapy.asn.au).

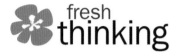

fresh thinking

'Pain is like an alarm clock. It wakes you up so you can attend to a possible problem in your body. But like an alarm clock, you should be able to turn it off.'

—Sheila Sidney Bender, PhD, psychologist and co-author of *The Energy of Belief*

Complementary and alternative medicine (CAM) practitioners

CAM practitioners include massage therapists, osteopaths, chiropractors, acupuncturists, traditional Chinese medicine practitioners and naturopaths. Some of these practitioners deliver services that sit both within and outside of conventional medicine. The scientific evidence to support CAM varies in many areas, pain management included. Some people may want to explore what CAM therapies might offer them. If you wish to consider CAM therapies as a part of your health care, here are some guidelines for doing so safely.

Talk to your doctors about CAM. They may be able to inform you about what scientific evidence exists in favour or against a particular practice and also alert you to any concerns they may have, particularly about practices that may interfere with medications that you are taking. They may be able to refer you to a practitioner.

Do some research on the Internet or at the local library. In 2012 there were over 500 reviews about CAM therapies available for the general public to read in the Cochrane Collaboration database (see http://www.cochrane.org). The Cochrane Collaboration is an international network that helps patients and other health care consumers to assess the potential risks and benefits of treatments and to make well-informed decisions about their own health care. Each review includes a section especially written to make the conclusions understandable by people who are not health professionals.

Gather basic information. Research the CAM practitioners you are considering, looking at things such as education, experience and cost. Interview them in person or by telephone, or they may have a website.

Check their qualifications. Check whether they are registered with a national body such as the Australian Health Professional Regulation Agency (see http://www.ahpra.gov.au).

Look for the words pain specialist or pain management specialist in the description of a health professional you're considering consulting for your condition.

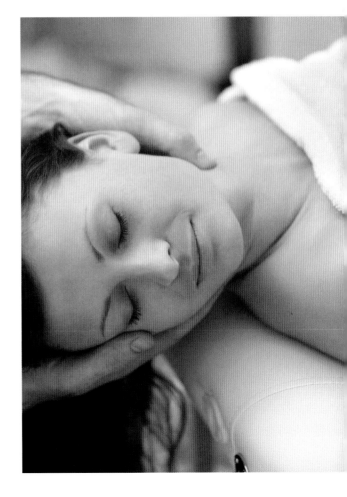

Seeking the right massage

Which massage is for you? For starters, it's best to ask a potential massage therapist if she has worked with your type of pain before. Here are some types of massage to consider.

Relaxation massage. This is the most common kind of gentle massage, designed to relax you and relieve stress. It can include Swedish massage, spa massage, chair massage and others.

Clinical massage. This kind of massage focuses on specific therapeutic goals, such as releasing muscle spasms or working on specific muscles affected by pain or injury. Clinical massage includes deep tissue massage, rehabilitative massage and sports massage, among others.

Evaluate your practitioner after the initial treatment visit. Appraise what you have been told to expect in terms of the outcomes of therapy, time frames and costs.

Inform your medical team. Tell all of your health care providers about any complementary and alternative practices you use, particularly any supplements you have been prescribed. Give them a full picture of what you do to manage your health. This will help ensure coordinated and safe care.

Here are some examples of complementary and alternative medicine practitioners you might be considering.

Acupuncture. Acupuncture is a form of traditional Chinese medicine that has been practised for thousands of years. The therapy involves the placement of tiny needles at specific points in the body to release blocked energy—not an easy concept for some Western practitioners to understand. The National Institutes of Health (USA) says that, in conjunction with standard medical care, acupuncture can be useful for some kinds of pain relief.

Biofeedback therapists. These are often nurses or physiotherapists, trained in biofeedback and physiology, who work with a doctor. A non-invasive treatment, biofeedback can be helpful in treating muscle and stress-related pain. Electrodes that measure temperature, muscle tension and brain-wave functions are attached to the body. Patients are taught how to make changes that help control those functions. Treatment usually involves a series of sessions over several weeks, but, once patients learn the technique, they can do it themselves at home.

Are they right for me?

You have the right to see a doctor or therapist who respects your situation and values your time. Ask yourself these questions to help you figure out if your doctor's the right one for you.

Does she spend at least 15 minutes with you? Does she give you time to discuss new concerns and the effects of any treatments?

Is he routinely late? Your health professional can't always know how much time each patient will take, but he should not keep you waiting half an hour or more without an apology.

Does she investigate new symptoms? If you speak to her about a new ache, does she follow up with appropriate questions and testing?

Is he dismissive of your suggestions? If you bring materials or offer information you've found elsewhere, is he respectful in his response?

Does she discuss options? Does she offer one treatment without discussion or discuss several options, including the pros and cons?

Does your health professional claim to have an exclusive treatment? That's a danger signal. Does he have the statistics and studies to back up assurances about his unique treatment?

It's important to take the time to evaluate whether your doctor is the right one for you.

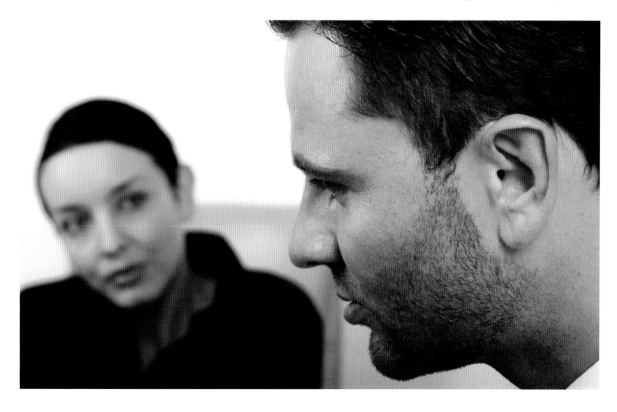

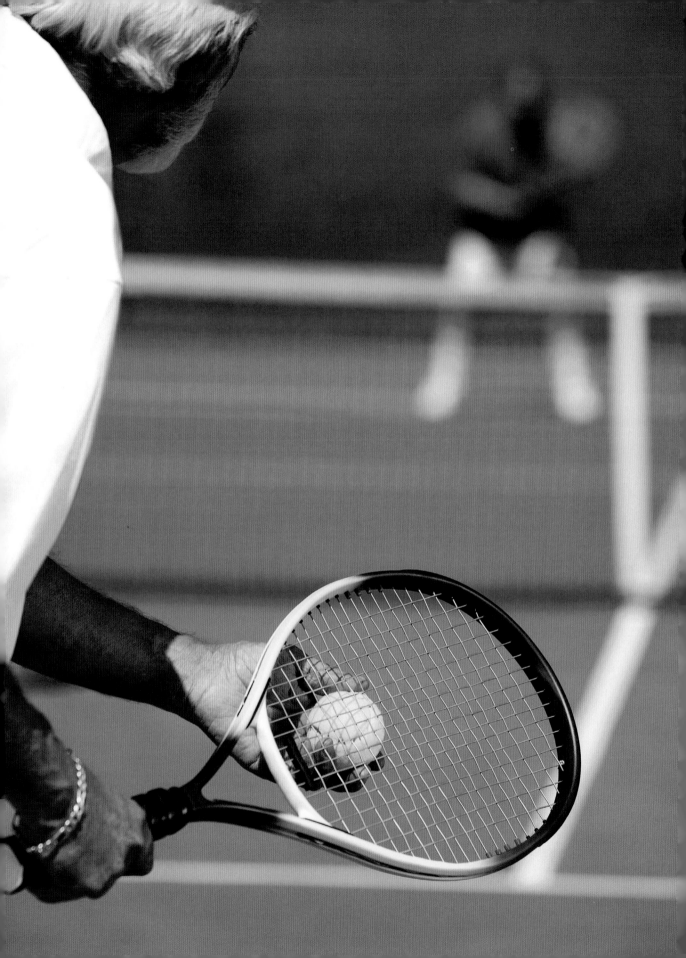

Move more, ache less

Exercise is powerful pain medicine

Getting off the couch is tough when your body hurts; in fact, it's probably the last thing you want to do. But the old advice to climb into bed and rest no longer applies. Why? Researchers now know much more about what exercise does for the body and mind. Does your pain make you grouchy? By exercising for as little as 30 minutes a day, you trigger the flow of feel-good endorphins, the body's natural painkillers that boost mood and lower stress. All that blood and oxygen pumping through your body will begin to make you feel better, happier and more in control.

Does your pain keep you from doing the kinds of things around the house you used to do? By exercising, you have a much better chance of getting back to that go-getting self you miss. You begin to build strength, which, in turn, enables your muscles to take more stress off your bones, and flexibility, which eases movement minus the aches and pains. Each time you take a walk to the supermarket, you'll feel more energy, and, at the same time, you'll fall asleep faster at night and stay asleep, which gives you more energy to resume your life. What's more, you may notice that you're dropping a few kilograms, and weight loss is also a trimmer of aches and pains.

Exercise may sound like a drag, but it's worth the effort. A Harvard study of 135 women with chronic pain found that after a 16-week regimen of walking, strength training and stretching three times per week, starting at about 30 minutes and working up to an hour, their pain was reduced by almost half, enough for

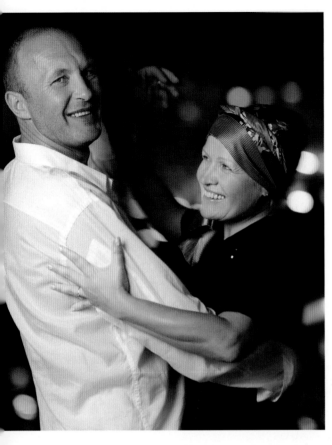

them to get back to many of the activities they missed. People with knee arthritis cut their pain by 43 per cent after 4 months of strength training. Researchers at the University of Tallahassee in Florida found that women with fibromyalgia who entered a strength-training program twice a week for 16 weeks reduced their pain by 39 per cent. And a study at Stanford University of people who did at least an hour a week for 6 weeks of brisk aerobic exercise showed a 25 per cent reduction in the aches and pains of ageing compared with a control group.

You don't have to be an Olympic athlete, buy new exercise clothes or even go to a gym. The important thing is simply moving your body regularly by walking or swimming, gardening or dancing, whatever feels most inviting. Getting the right type of exercise at the right intensity can ease your aches, boost your energy and even prevent future pain.

The important thing is simply moving your body regularly by walking or swimming, gardening or dancing, whatever feels most inviting.

Mapping out a plan

The ideal exercise prescription will vary, depending on your type of pain. 'A good place to start is with something you like to do', says Anne Daly, D Clin Physio, Musculoskeletal Physiotherapist, Pain Service, Austin Health, Melbourne. Here are suggestions she and other pain experts offer for getting started.

Work with your doctor. Before you start any exercise program, ask your doctor to check you and your heart to make sure that you're ready for exercise.

Start slowly. No one expects you to sign up for a marathon. The important thing is to get started, and any activity that gets you moving fits the bill. Walk 10 minutes at lunchtime, get up from your desk every hour and do a few stretches, start lifting your groceries into the car instead of asking someone else to do it. Whenever you have a chance to move, do it. Within a few weeks, you will feel like doing more.

Think time limit, not speed or distance. Initially, it doesn't matter how far or how fast you're moving, but how long. Pretty soon you'll speed up.

Relief you can count on

Still sceptical about how big a bite exercise can take out of your pain? Check out the improvements that researchers have found.

Condition	Potential benefit from exercise	What it takes
Fibromyalgia	45% reduction in pain	Walking, strength training and stretching three times per week
Osteoarthritis	24% improvement in function, 30% improvement in knee pain	Aerobics and strength training three times per week
Migraine	Significant reduction in migraine intensity	30 minutes of aerobic exercise three times per week
Back pain	50% reduction in pain, 60% improvement in back-related function	Yoga, 1 hour and 15 minutes once per week
Breast cancer	11% reduction in fatigue, 5% reduction in pain	3 hours a week of moderate-intensity exercise such as aerobics, strength training and yoga
Plantar fasciitis	75% reduction in pain	Stretching the arch of the foot (pull the toes backwards towards the shins) 10 times, three times per day
Muscle and joint pain	25% reduction in pain	20 to 30 minutes of brisk aerobic exercise three times per week

Be flexible. For instance, if you can't walk at first because your knee hurts, try swimming or a stationary bike instead.

Write exercise on your calendar, just as you would a doctor's appointment. Beware thinking that you'll get to unscheduled exercise at day's end, says Vicki Conn, PhD, RN, FAAN, associate dean of the Sinclair School of Nursing at the University of Missouri in Columbia, who specialises in helping chronically ill people exercise: 'Who has time left over at the end of the day?'

Have a bad-day plan. Some days you may feel your pain makes it impossible to move. But don't take to bed. Instead try to do a little something, even if it's just stretching, suggests Michelle Shufelt, PT, DPT, MS, a physical therapist at the Rehabilitation Institute of Chicago's Center for Pain Studies. 'Most people have a false belief that you have to get rid of pain first before you can get back to activity. But you need to keep moving so that you use your body's natural pump to get toxins out of the painful area.'

Put your fears to bed

You're in pain, and your doctor is telling you to exercise. For a moment, you suspect he may be joking. Of course, you have fears about exercising when you hurt. It can be done, and it will help you. Here are answers to some common worries.

I'm going to hurt more. In fact, the longer you don't use your muscles, the more your pain will increase. It is true that when you start exercising, your muscles may feel a little sore the next day. Strengthening muscles hurts a lot, stop for a while and see what happens. If the extra pain lasts until the next day, try the same exercise for less time or with less vigour, or try a different exercise next time.

I can't walk for 5 minutes. Unless your doctor says you're not ready, you *can* walk for 5 minutes. Tell yourself, 'I'm just going to put one foot in front of the other'. After you've done it once, then you'll know for sure you can do it again.

I won't be able to build up to an hour. That's why you're starting with only 5 to 15 minutes. By adding minutes very gradually (1 minute per week, 3 days per week) your body will become increasingly conditioned, your muscles stronger, your breathing easier. That's how getting fit works.

I don't have time. If you have time to watch television, read a book or take a nap, you have time to exercise.

Exercise will make me tired. Actually, half an hour of moderate exercise usually has the opposite effect. Within several weeks of exercising, you may find you have more energy all the time, perhaps because you're sleeping better and your heart, lungs and muscles have an easier time doing their jobs.

Get your heart pumping

One key to reducing pain is to get your heart rate up. Cardiovascular, or aerobic, exercise increases both your breathing and your heart rate, increasing the flow of oxygen and nutrients to painful areas, which aids in the removal of toxins, speeding healing. Your heart works harder and, like any muscle, grows stronger so that, eventually, you will be able to do the same exercise with less effort.

Exercise boosts energy and lowers stress, which are both common problems for people in pain. It releases tension, loosens tight muscles and makes falling and staying asleep easier, often a difficulty

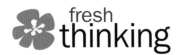

fresh thinking

'We are creatures of habit and influenced by the environment around us. So, to the extent that we set up our environment for exercise, the more successful we will be.'

—Vicki Conn, PhD, RN, FAAN, associate dean of the Sinclair School of Nursing at the University of Missouri in Columbia

for people in pain. It strengthens muscles, which can then carry some of the burden for an aching back or hips. Stronger muscles make day-to-day activities such as shopping and household tasks easier too. You're also apt to lose weight, a boon to sore joints. An 80-kilogram person who stays on the same diet but briskly walks 2 kilometres per day, for example, will lose 6 kilograms in a year.

Giving your heart a work-out also raises your spirits and sharpens your mind. It's a rare soul who returns from even 15 minutes of brisk exercise who doesn't feel a little better about herself, who doesn't have a better perspective on the tasks and problems of the day, who isn't in better spirits. In fact, research shows that your mood will lift after just 10 minutes of exercise and continue improving, reaching its high after about 20 minutes. Other research shows that exercise relieves depression as effectively as antidepressants and psychotherapy. The reason for the lift: exercise releases the mood-boosting brain chemicals serotonin and dopamine, as well as endorphins that act as the body's natural painkillers.

Revved up to give your heart a work-out? Below are experts' top aerobic plans for people in pain.

Your walking work-out

'Walking is a great start for an exercise program', says Anne Daly, Musculoskeletal Physiotherapist, Pain Service, Austin Health, Melbourne. 'It has benefits for your entire body, it's free, requires no equipment and can be done alone or with a friend. Start with 5, 10 or 15 minutes per day and build up the time and effort gradually.'

Oh, my aching muscles

New exercise could make your muscles feel sore the day after. Here's how to make them feel better fast.

Gently massage your muscles. Some studies indicate this can relieve soreness by 30 per cent and also reduce swelling.

Take an Epsom salts bath. Add two cups of Epsom salts to a warm bath and soak for 20 minutes. The magnesium in the salts helps relax muscles and reduces inflammation and swelling.

Apply ice. An ice pack wrapped in a towel placed over the sore spot for 20 minutes reduces swelling. After the pain has peaked, apply a heating pad or warm towel for 20 minutes, which helps by increasing circulation.

Stretch. A few gentle stretches won't necessarily relieve soreness, but they will feel good.

Give it a rest. Go ahead and exercise the next day if you feel like it, but don't try to win any contests.

Continue to build in that way until you are walking at least 30 minutes to an hour per day, 5 days per week. As your fitness improves, you can speed up, walking fast enough to increase your breathing and heart rate but slowly enough so that you can still have a conversation. If you do not feel normal within 10 minutes after you stop, you're pushing too hard. Here are some ways to make walking painless.

- Walk with a friend.
- Listen to music while you walk.
- Wear breathable, loose-fitting clothing, supportive walking shoes and a hat.
- Pick a beautiful or fun spot, such as a path around a lake that has benches, in case you get tired. In bad weather, opt for a shopping complex.
- To protect your joints, walk on soft surfaces, such as a park circuit or sports oval.

Swimming strategies

Swimming can be especially helpful for people with joint pain. Because of the body's buoyancy, you're not thudding down on your bones. The lessened gravity also makes it easier to move with less pain. At the same time, the water provides enough resistance to strengthen muscles. How to get started?

Look for a heated pool. Water between 28°C and 34°C will help relax your muscles and ease your pain.

Start slowly. Swim using any stroke you find comfortable. Swim two or three times a week, working up to 15 to 20 minutes by the end of the first week, 25 to 30 minutes by the end of the second week. Gradually work up to 45 minutes to an hour.

Know when to pause. If you get tired, stop and relax in the water.

Work towards swimming faster. After your second week, begin to swim a little faster. Getting your heart working hard is key to triggering the release of pain-relieving endorphins.

Monitor your pain. If your pain gets worse or you feel new pain, slow down or stop.

Water between 28°C and 34°C will help relax your muscles and ease your pain.

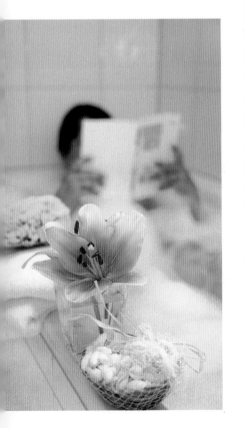

Biking boost

Stationary bikes are perfect for people suffering back, joint and arthritis pain. Cycling builds muscle strength, keeps joints flexible and reduces stiffness. It's also low impact, so it won't cause further pain to your joints. If you have joint or back pain, ask the gym manager whether an upright or recumbent bike would be better for you. Recumbent bikes may be better for people with back pain. If you have knee pain and you're using an upright bike, make sure the seat is high enough that your knee doesn't bend past 90 degrees but not so high that your leg is straight at the bottom of a pedal stroke. If your hips rock when you pedal, lower the seat. To avoid putting undue strain on your knees, push from your heel, not your toe.

Physical medicine and rehabilitation physician Christine Keating often suggests stationary bikes to patients who have trouble walking. As with walking, she suggests the following:

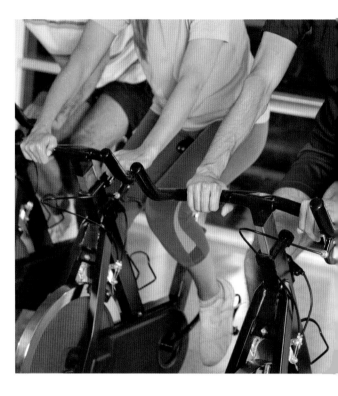

- Start with 5 to 15 minutes 3 days per week.
- Add 1 minute per day each week until you reach 20 minutes.
- Add a fourth day.
- Continue building the same way until you can bike for an hour 5 days per week.

Stronger muscles make everyday tasks such as lifting groceries, climbing out of the car and getting up the stairs much easier. Think of a sturdy bridge versus a wobbly one.

Work your muscles

Your biceps don't have to look like Popeye's, but strengthening your muscles will help relieve pain, and you can do it no matter what your age or current fitness level. Stronger muscles make everyday tasks such as lifting groceries, climbing out of the car and getting up the stairs much easier. Mightier muscles around your joints and back help protect them by lessening strain. Think of a sturdy bridge versus a wobbly one: which would you rather drive your car over? Toning your muscles also helps to keep you trim, since muscle burns more kilojoules than fat, and fewer kilograms lessen the burden on achy joints and back.

Working muscles also stresses bones in a good way, potentially reducing the risk of fracture. The stronger your muscles, the less chance of your falling and injuring yourself.

Hints and tips for pain-free exercise

Warming up for 5 minutes before you exercise, cooling down for 5 afterwards and pacing yourself in between are important ways to fend off pain for almost any condition. In general, it's not a good idea to take anti-inflammatories before exercise because they can mask pain. And when you're dehydrated, which is more likely when you exercise, medication can damage your kidneys, so drink more water during and after exercise. Here are more tips, condition by condition.

Condition	Before exercise	During exercise	After exercise
Back pain	Stretch for 5 minutes.	In the pool, avoid breaststroke and freestyle if they hurt; stick to side stroke.	After any exercise, apply ice for 15 to 20 minutes.
Joint pain	Do range-of-motion exercises for 5 minutes (for instance, rotate your hips in circles one way, then another).	If you hurt, slow down and repeat range-of-motion exercises.	Stretch for 5 minutes; apply ice for 15 to 20 minutes.
Knee pain	Lubricate your knee joints by gently bending and straightening your knee for 3 to 5 minutes.	Use walking poles to help relieve the burden on the joints, and walk on soft surfaces. If you feel pain, slow down and stretch.	Stretch again and apply ice for 15 to 20 minutes.
Cancer pain	Do all-over stretching for 5 minutes. (For example, reach to the ceiling, bend side to side, bend and straighten the knees, etc.)	If you hurt, slow down and repeat stretches.	Do 5 minutes of general stretching as before. Apply ice to painful areas for 15 to 20 minutes.
Plantar fasciitis	Heat about 25 marbles in hot water. Put them in a shoebox and, while sitting, roll your foot over the marbles for 5 minutes. Then place the front of your foot on a fat phone book or stair, and let your heel drop for 20 seconds. Repeat heel drop 5 to 10 times.	When you feel tightness or pain, stop and repeat heel stretch. (A kerb will do.)	Apply ice for 15 to 20 minutes.

Condition	Before exercise	During exercise	After exercise
Achilles tendon pain	Hold on to the kitchen bench and raise heels off the floor, as though you were wearing 7 cm heels. Hold for a one-two count and lower. Repeat 5 to 10 times. Then place the front of your foot on a fat phone book or stair, and let your heel drop for 20 seconds. Repeat 5 to 10 times.	When you feel tightness or pain, stop and repeat stair or kerb stretch.	Apply ice for 15 to 20 minutes.
Leg and foot cramps	Half an hour before exercising, eat half a banana. (Potassium helps prevent cramps.) Drink a cup of water or tonic water. (Dehydration increases cramps.) Do calf and foot stretches for 3 to 5 minutes. (Example: lean against a wall with both hands. Bend one leg and keep the other straight, heel on floor.)	If the cramps resume, repeat stretches and drink a glass of water or sports drink.	Stretch. Include some dairy food in the day's diet. (Calcium helps prevent cramps.)
Headaches	Release neck tension by lying down, head to hip, on a blanket rolled tight (about 15 cm in diameter, 91 cm in length). Spread your arms so you are in a T-shape, let your shoulders drop and your chest open, and relax for 3 to 5 minutes.	To release tension, gently nod your head yes and no.	Do shoulder rolls (raise your shoulders to your ears, move them backwards, down, then up to your ears again in one smooth motion), then lie down on the rolled blanket for another 3 to 5 minutes.
Menstrual pain	Lie on your back with your knees bent, feet on floor. Hug your knees to your chest for a count of five. Rock from your left to right buttock 10 times.	If cramps resume, lie down and do the same thing. Or, standing, rock from foot to foot 10 times.	Repeat floor exercise. Apply ice to your back 15 to 20 minutes if it's sore. If you have stomach cramps, lie on a heating pad for 15 to 20 minutes.

Working at strengthening muscles also increases your endurance and improves the functioning of your heart and lungs. It helps the body use fuel more efficiently, guards you from heart disease and makes you feel better about yourself. The hard part is getting started.

Getting started

Say the words 'strength training', and we picture a body builder heaving gigantic barbells over his head. That image is pretty intimidating, and it's not where we're heading. We're talking about a slow, steady use of your muscles that, over time, will make you stronger. We're talking about an easy, step-by-step program. Ready to get going?

Create a plan. Begin by doing at least one session with a physiotherapist, who can create a comfortable program and show you correct postures that won't add to your pain. Your doctor should be able to refer you to someone.

Work out your exercise baseline. This allows you to be sure that you are starting your exercise program at the level that is right for you. In the 2011 publication *Manage Your Pain* by Dr Michael Nichols, Dr Allan Molloy, Lois Tonkin and Lee Beeston it's recommended that you start with the number of repetitions that you can manage comfortably. Write down this number. Repeat this on the second day of exercise and then average these two numbers. For example, if you did 6 repetitions on day one and 4 on day two, the average will be 5 $(6 + 4 = 10 \div 2 = 5)$. Then work out 80 per cent of this number to get your baseline. In this case, your baseline would be 4 repetitions.

Warm up. Before you begin, walk on the spot for 5 to 10 minutes to warm your muscles.

Leave the weights for later. You can do lots of strengthening by using your body weight alone as resistance. Try slow wall push-ups or climbing stairs.

Work your muscles every alternate day. Leave at least a day between sessions to give your muscles time to repair.

Strength moves

For overall strength: Any aerobics program—walking, swimming, cycling—will begin to condition and strengthen you.

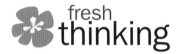
fresh **thinking**

'Forget the old saying "No pain, no gain". If you have persistent pain, the right exercise advice is "Start slow and build up gradually". Using this approach, you *will* get to where you want to go, it just takes time.'

—Anne Daly, D Clin Physio, M Manip Physio, BAppSc (Physio), Musculoskeletal Physiotherapist, Pain Service, Austin Health, Melbourne

For your legs: After you're able to walk 30 minutes, add a small hill to your path. Says Christine Zampach, PT, DPT, MEd, rehabilitation coordinator at the University of California, San Francisco, Pain Center, 'That's the best initial strengthening for your legs and back'. Or you can simply climb stairs, graduating to two stairs at a time, eventually jogging up the stairs. Step up and down on a kitchen stool. Do deep knee bends.

For your arms: Begin with a biceps curl. Pretend you're holding a barbell in each hand, arms by your side, hands in fists. Raise those virtual barbells to your chest, keeping your elbows by your sides. When 10 of those seem easy, start lifting a 500-gram bag of rice or a can of soup, or use hand weights. Gradually build up to 15 then 20 repetitions. When this seems easy, slowly increase the weight. You can also do wall push-ups, which will work your chest, too: stand at arm's length from the wall. Lean forwards and place your hands on the wall, slightly wider than shoulder-width apart.

Posture perfect

Hunching at your desk, slumping into your seat, slouching as you wait in line: these postures strain the neck, shoulder, back and hips, forcing muscles to work harder than they need to, increasing pain.

Good posture isn't a 15-minute exercise. It's 24/7 mindfulness about how you hold your body. But if you haven't been as posture perfect as you should be, you'll feel strange at first as you square your shoulders and sit up straight. Don't worry—that feeling will go away. The good news is that both strengthening and stretching exercises help to improve posture. As the muscles grow stronger and more supple, they'll have an easier time supporting your spine and keeping your body in alignment. Here are some ways to improve posture fast.

Take the mirror test. Standing before a mirror, see if your shoulders are square, not rounded or hunched; your chest is lifted, not sunken; your chin is slightly tucked, not protruding forwards; your

head is directly over your shoulders, not thrust in front of your chest. Pull in your stomach and buttocks and unlock your knees. In this pose, you should look and feel good.

Find a wall. Stand with your back against the wall, with your heels about 15 cm away. Let your head, shoulder blades and buttocks touch the wall. Slip your hand behind your lower back. If there's more than a hand's thickness, tighten your stomach to flatten the curve in your back. If there's too little space, arch your back so that your hand fits. This is your ideal posture.

At your chair. Put both feet on the floor or a foot rest, keeping your knees level with your hips. Tuck your chin slightly so the top of your head points towards the ceiling. Square the small of your back against the back of the chair. For more support, put a rolled towel or cushion behind your lower back.

Breathing into your stretch

It's no coincidence that yoga and breathing techniques are intertwined. Most of us hold our breath when we stretch. But by remembering to breathe slowly in and out, we keep the oxygen flow to our muscles, and we also relax, allowing our muscles to stretch further. Here are three ways to breathe as you do any exercise, including stretching. Combining them will help keep you relaxed and lessen shortness of breath.

Breathe through your nose. This warms and moistens the air, a nice feature in cold, dry air, and also reduces the amount of air pollutants your lungs absorb.

Diaphragmatic breathing. People in pain tend to breathe shallowly. By breathing deeply, you fill your lungs with air, getting more oxygen to the brain and throughout your body. To practise: inhale slowly through your nose as your abdomen—not your chest—expands, breathing in as much as you can. Hold the breath, then exhale as you stretch, fully emptying your lungs. Try to take three breaths with every stretch.

Breathing through pursed lips. Breathe through your nose, expanding your abdomen, following the previous two techniques, and exhale through pursed lips for a longer time than it took to inhale.

Exhale, bend your elbows, and lower your head and chest to the wall, coming close but not touching it. Inhale, then straighten your arms, pushing the weight of your body away from the wall. Start with 10 repetitions, gradually build up to 15 then 20 repetitions.

For your core: Strengthening your core, the area around your trunk and pelvis, helps your posture improve, prevents back pain and makes it easier for you to do things with less pain. Instead of sit-ups—the worst thing for back pain—try this: lie down on your back on a mat, knees bent, feet on the floor. Imagine pulling your navel towards the floor without holding your breath. Bring one knee towards your chest, lower and bring the other towards your chest, doing a slow march. Your legs are your resistance, and keeping your stomach muscles tight protects your back. Keep it flat on the floor; don't let it arch. Work out your baseline and then increase by one or two repetitions each session or each week.

Stretch your limits

Even those of us without chronic pain lose 5 per cent of our flexibility every decade. Pain makes your body tighten, a normal reflex of the muscles to protect from more pain. Even one muscle's tightness can affect us all over: a tight calf, for instance, can cause pain in your knees, shins or feet. When you don't move, tight muscles get tighter, says Zampach. 'You have to reverse that process and teach the body to let go of guarding and return to its normal balance.'

Stretching improves circulation, increasing the blood flow to the areas that hurt you. Stretching also helps your posture, keeping your body in proper alignment so no one part is doing too much work.

Luckily, you don't have to be a rubber band to try stretching. In fact, our range of flexibility is something we're born with. If you couldn't touch your toes at 20, chances are you'll never touch your toes. And that's okay. You want to be somewhere in the middle, where your muscles, ligaments and tendons are taut enough to support you but loose enough that you can move through the full range of motion you had as a young adult. Here are some tips to keep in mind as you stretch.

Reach for tightness, not pain. In other words, stretch until you feel resistance, but don't push so far that you feel pain.

Press, don't bounce. Move slowly into any stretch and hold it for 5 to 10 seconds. Never bounce into a stretch, which can tear muscle fibres.

Stretch everything. Move everything—shoulders, hips, knees, arms, neck—through their full range of motion. It's a good way to get your whole body into balance.

Be symmetrical. Whatever you stretch out on one side of your body, stretch out on the other.

Stretch after exercise. Stretching just after exercise, when your muscles are still warm, is the best way to improve your flexibility.

Stretching improves circulation, increasing the blood flow to the areas that hurt you.

Stretching basics

For an overall stretch: Standing up, reach your arms to the ceiling; hold for 5 to 10 seconds. Bend to one side; hold again. Straighten and bend to the other side.

Neck stretch: Lower your chin to your chest and hold for 5 to 10 seconds.

Shoulder stretch: Reach your right arm across your chest and over your shoulder, placing your hand on your shoulder blade if you can. Hold for 5 to 10 seconds, then switch.

Back stretch: Lie down on your back and bring both knees to your chest. Grasp your hands around your knees and gently pull your legs closer to your chest. Hold for 20 to 30 seconds.

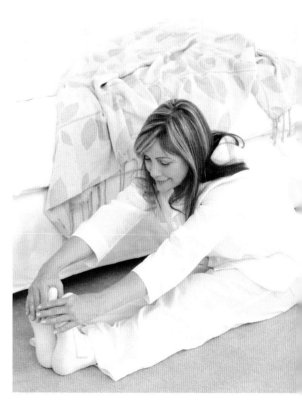

Hamstring stretch: Lie on the floor with your knees bent and your feet flat on the floor. Loop a belt or a large bath towel under one foot, holding the ends. Use it to help you raise your leg towards the ceiling and straighten it as far as you comfortably can, keeping the other leg bent. Hold for 20 seconds, repeat a second time, then switch legs.

Calf stretch: Place your feet about 50 centimetres from a wall. Place your palms on the wall and lean forwards, bending one leg at a time and keeping the other heel on the floor.

Ankle and foot stretch: Sitting, put your right ankle on your left knee. Rotate your foot clockwise 10 times, then anticlockwise 10 times. Switch feet.

Hip stretch: Stand with your feet wider than hip width apart. Shift your weight over your right foot and hold for 20 seconds. Repeat on the other side.

Staying motivated

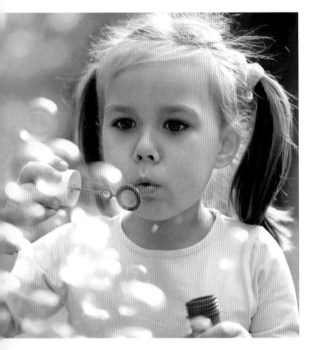

Think of what you used to enjoy doing as a child and find a way to tap into those natural affinities now.

Most doctors, when they recommend exercise, talk about how much it will help our pain or how it will help ward off illnesses such as heart disease and cancer, but it's pretty tough to roll out of a warm bed and get walking for a benefit that may seem intangible. Even though most of us know that moving is the right move for reducing pain, we know what we feel now: we'd so much rather nurse our aching hips in a chair than head outside or to the gym.

People make exercise a habit not by thinking about abstract health improvements but by changing behaviours slowly and consistently, and we have the tips to help you do just that.

Set goals. Write them down. How many times a week do you want to exercise and for how long? What length of time would you like to be exercising in a month? At 6 months? With your doctor or physiotherapist, set realistic goals that you know you can reach.

Keep track. Every time you exercise, mark a calendar on the refrigerator, noting what you did and for how long, suggests Vicki Conn, PhD, RN, FAAN, associate dean of the Sinclair School of Nursing at the University of Missouri in Columbia. 'It's very powerful. Most people forget what they did. But by writing it down, you can look and say, "I really did do this". And you can look at your past behaviour and set new goals.'

quiz
how do *you* like to move it?

You'll have an easier time making exercise a habit if you follow your natural preferences. Ask yourself these questions.

What kind of exercise do you like?

Are you an indoor person or an outdoor person?

Do you like to exercise alone or in groups?

Do you like gym classes or would you prefer video instruction?

At what time of day do you have the most energy?

Do you like to exercise all at once or in 10-minute increments?

Are you someone who likes to get things done?

If walking bores you, you won't do it. If swimming has always drawn you, choose it instead. Think of what you used to enjoy doing as a child—even if it was skipping, kicking a football or roller skating—and find a way to tap into those natural affinities now.

1. If you love to be outside, head to a local park, walk around your neighbourhood, cultivate a garden or put up a ring in the driveway to shoot hoops. In many cities, organisations offer outdoor fitness classes. If you prefer indoors, get a home treadmill or sign up for gym classes.

2. If you prefer exercising alone, pick walking, swimming, cycling. If you like to chat while you sweat, ask a friend to join you or sign up with a trainer or for a class.

3. If you choose a class, make sure the instructor has worked with people who have your condition. If you prefer a video, ask your physiotherapist to recommend one that is safe for you.

4. If you're a morning person, schedule your exercise then. Even if you tell yourself you'll do it later, it's much harder to get out the door when you're tired.

5. If you prefer to exercise in 10-minute bouts, that's fine. Try to fit three of them into your day.

6. Appeal to your practical side. You have to post letters anyway, so why not walk to the nearest postbox? If you want to volunteer your time for charity, why not participate in a charity walk?

Reward yourself. Give yourself weekly rewards (or even daily ones). Finished your first 15-minute walk? Treat yourself to an iced coffee. Reached your weekly exercise goals? Call that faraway friend you miss. Completed 3 weeks of half-hour swims? Get yourself a new swimsuit.

Strike the right balance. It's easy to get overambitious and push yourself too hard. The problem is that your pain may worsen soon after, and you'll feel like giving up. Go slowly, build gradually.

Build in variety. The enemy of exercise is boredom. If you do the same thing, day in, day out, you'll get bored. Change where you walk and who you walk with. Tired of walking? Do some gardening, play backyard badminton or hit the exercise bike.

The where and how of exercise

So, your new prescription is to exercise. Perhaps now you feel overwhelmed by all the choices. Do you try spin classes or yoga, water aerobics or Pilates? How do you know that the instructor can protect you from more pain? Here are some ways to find what you're after.

Consider a rehab program. Many pain and rehabilitation centres offer outpatient programs that will teach you how to move again. Rehab specialists are used to working with people who have all kinds of pain and can help you plan an appropriate exercise program. They can also teach you important skills, such as how to take your pulse, how to determine your target heart rate and how to work with various kinds of equipment, such as resistance bands, exercise balls and dumbbells.

Join the Y or a private gym. YMCAs and gyms offer all kinds of classes, and you can usually try all of them for the price of your membership. If you can't decide between Pilates and aerobics, try each class once or twice to see which one you like and which one made your body feel best. Most gyms have personal trainers who can help you build an exercise program.

Test it with a free offer. Lots of gyms offer guest passes to members or a week's free pass to prospective members. It's a great way to see if you fit with the people who work out there, if the staff is helpful and friendly, and if the location and times suit you.

Be a pain sleuth

If you're not used to exercising, it can be hard to tell the difference between the good pain that can result from exercise and the bad. Here's how.

Good pain. When you begin exercise you're not used to, your muscles get sore because of tiny tears, which cause swelling and pain. Slightly sore muscles are a good thing because, as the muscle repairs, it grows stronger. Unless the soreness is severe or lasts more than a week, don't worry.

Bad pain. Give your pain a number each day before you start exercising. The number should be lower 2 hours after exercise or at least no worse, says physical therapist Michelle Shufelt. If you have new localised pain—in a knee or ankle, for example—that increases while you exercise, stop and have the pain checked by a doctor or physiotherapist.

Is yoga for you?

Once the realm of hard-core devotees, yoga and Pilates have become staples at most gyms. Are they for you? Should you try tai chi? Here is some information to help you decide.

Yoga. Yoga is an ancient practice that involves moving through various postures in conjunction with breathing. Yoga builds strength and flexibility and lowers stress. The postures are done standing, sitting and lying down. There are many different types of yoga to choose from, some gentler than others. Hatha yoga, one of the most popular forms, involves a gentle, slow flow of poses. Iyengar yoga involves longer held poses and uses equipment that allows people with problems such as back pain to modify the poses. Ask the instructor what kind of yoga she teaches and whether it's suitable for your particular health problem. Tell her exactly what ails you, so she can show you how to modify certain postures if necessary.

Pilates. This system of exercises revolves around strengthening and stretching the muscles in your stomach and back that support the spine, called core muscles. The exercises are particularly good at relieving pain in the neck, back and joints. They also help you to be more aware of your body and how you hold it. Some exercises are done on Pilates equipment, others on a mat. If you're a beginner, be sure to take an entry-level class. Find out what credentials the instructor has; Pilates is all about proper form, and using bad form can detract from the benefits and may even cause injury. Comprehensive certifications can take a year or more of study and require many hours spent in the studio as an apprentice teacher. Not all instructors teaching Pilates in gyms are sufficiently trained. To be sure you're getting an expert, go to a studio devoted to Pilates, if possible.

Tai chi. Tai chi, sometimes described as 'meditation in motion', is a Chinese form of standing exercise that involves slow, relaxing movements that improve posture, body alignment and balance. As with yoga, practitioners learn to align their breathing with the movements. It's a particularly good choice for back and joint pain. Most tai chi classes are gentle enough to be appropriate for just about anyone.

Cue up your exercise

It takes several weeks to create a new habit. Until exercise becomes as ingrained as brushing your teeth, and even after, use these cues to keep you glued to your exercise schedule.

- Put your walking shoes by the bedroom door so you see them first thing in the morning.
- Put a Post-it note on your refrigerator reminding you to exercise.
- Ask a friend to call to remind you.
- Schedule your exercise as you would a dental appointment—in your calendar.
- Set an alarm clock for when it's time to exercise.

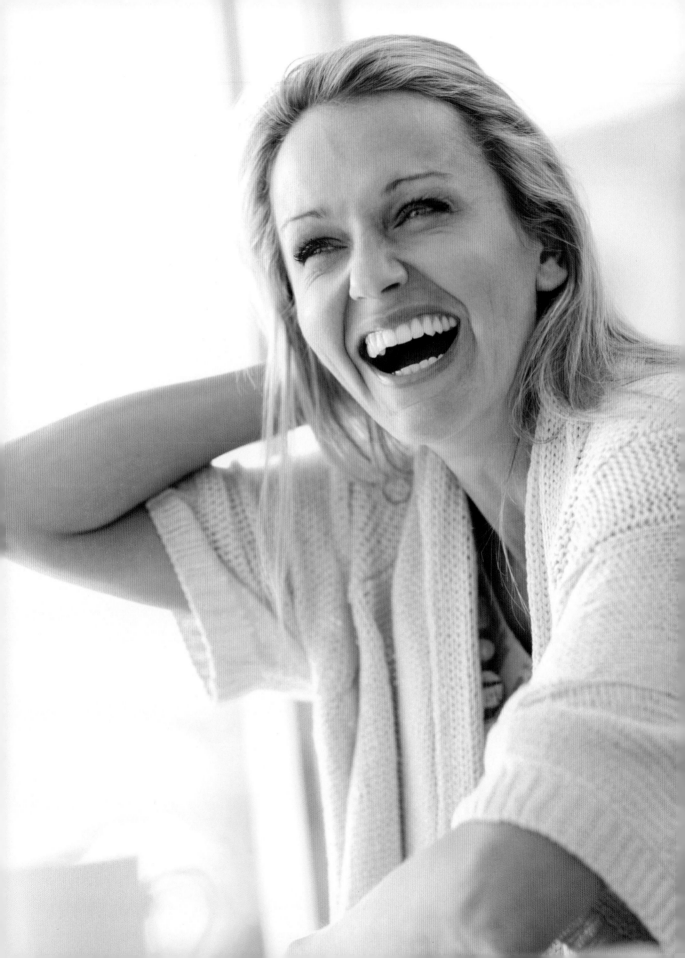

Laugh it away... and other mind–body solutions

Your pain is most certainly not all in your head. That said, your mind can profoundly influence how your body feels. Doctors know that pain is a physical, emotional and cognitive experience influenced by how a person interprets his pain signals. 'Pain is so tied to emotions that, a lot of times, if you release those emotions, you release the pain', says Larry Altshuler, MD, founder and medical director of the Balanced Healing Medical Center in Oklahoma City.

The sensation of pain comes from nerve impulses that travel from the painful spot to the brain, which registers the site and nature of the pain. Brain images taken of people in pain show that pain stimulates activity in areas that control sensations and in those that regulate emotions and thought processes. This helps explain why there is a two-way relationship between pain sensation and emotion. 'Two people can have the very same condition and give it two different numbers on a 0-to-10 pain scale. And two people can give the same number for wildly different sorts of pain. Someone can give an eight for a stubbed toe and another eight for cancer pain', says Steven D Hickman, PsyD, a clinical psychologist and director of the University of California, San Diego, Center for Mindfulness. That begins to explain why your relationship to pain matters. Let's say that you have a pain you rate as an eight, but four of those points come from distress. 'Even if you can't do anything medical for the pain, you can do something about the distress', says Hickman. 'The degree to which you come to terms with your pain can relieve a lot of suffering.' So simple techniques, from laughter to relaxation, from meditation to distraction, can help you establish a new relationship with your pain. After his experiences in Hickman's class on mindfulness, one of Hickman's patients, a former football player who had once played through his pain, said, 'I fought with my pain for years, and what I learned to do in this class was to dance with it'. You can, too.

Find the funny

You may know the story: many years ago, journalist and author Norman Cousins suffered from a painful spinal disease. He discovered by chance that when he watched funny movies and laughed for at least 10 minutes, his pain receded for several hours, allowing him to get some sleep. He eventually regained his health and attributed much of that to laughter. Groucho Marx had the same idea when he said, 'A clown is like an aspirin, only he works twice as fast'.

Regular laughs aren't miracle cures, but they do have a real effect on the body. Have a good laugh, and the pituitary gland releases chemicals, including endorphins, which act as the body's natural painkillers. Immune cells and illness-fighting antibodies increase, stress hormones drop by as much as 70 per cent and the flow of blood and oxygen improves. So does pain tolerance. A recent study at the University of California, Los Angeles, found that when children were watching funny videos, they were much more able to tolerate the pain of submersing their hands in ice-cold water, and their stress hormone levels fell to boot. Those who laughed the most remembered their pain least.

Of course, not all of us are keen to laugh, especially when we're in pain. Some of us grow up in difficult families and have had more than our share of burdens, both physical and emotional. That need not matter, says social worker Katherine Puckett, PhD, national director of Mind–Body Medicine at the Cancer Treatment Centers of America in Zion, Illinois. We can fake it until it's real. 'Laughter is something that is innate. But in people in pain who haven't felt like laughing in a long time, laughter may be dormant. So we start with simulated laughter, and even if a person doesn't feel like laughing, the simulation soon grows into authentic laughter.'

Puckett offers patients a laughter club based on a kind of laughter yoga, combining breathing and laughing, developed in India. The club doesn't spend its time watching funny movies; its members start by simply practising laughter sounds: heehee, hoho, haha. 'If

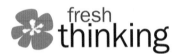

fresh thinking

'The struggle or suffering is not so much in the things we face, but in our relationship to them. If you go waist-deep into the ocean determined to face the next wave, more than likely it will knock you on your butt. But if you ride with that wave, you have a better chance of still standing after the wave.'

—Steven D Hickman, PsyD, clinical psychologist and director of the University of California, San Diego, Center for Mindfulness

The incredible painkilling power of endorphins

Larry Altshuler, MD, tells the story of a lung cancer patient who came to his centre in intractable pain. She was dying but wasn't ready to go. An acupuncturist guided her through a mind-body technique called interactive imagery. He knew she was religious and explained that after he had led her through several relaxation exercises, he would guide her down an imagined road where she could talk to whatever image represented her God. The acupuncturist went to do his work but quickly came back out of the sick woman's room. 'She's no longer in pain', he said to Altshuler. She had turned off her morphine pump and remained pain-free until dying peacefully a week later. In writing, she told her family what had happened in that imagined visit. She had told the image that she wanted to live. The figure responded: 'What are you doing down on Earth? I have a place by my side for you. Let go, and come join me.'

Stress and pain had caused her body to steadily pump out cortisol, noradrenaline and adrenaline, all chemicals that over time damage the body. Relax the body and mind, and the production of the harmful chemicals slows. 'When she realised that her death was the way it was supposed to be and thought, "I'm going to heaven", she probably began to produce endorphins', says Altshuler. It doesn't take a deeply religious experience to produce these chemicals. Everything from exercising hard to having a good laugh can trigger their release, too.

one person starts really laughing, then another does and it becomes contagious and just spreads.' Puckett might suggest that two people pretend they are meeting for the first time, reaching towards each other to shake hands. But instead of saying the expected 'How do you do?' they say in the same cadence, 'Heeheeheehee'. It's so absurd that the laughter soon becomes real.

Laughing can make you feel better even if you have to force it. 'I see people dealing with serious problems of life and death who come in, and when they start laughing it's fake', says Puckett. 'But in almost all cases people leave feeling better, more relaxed, with less pain and not thinking about cancer.'

Your laughter prescription

Laughter works. It will lessen your pain and allow your problems to fade for a while. As Puckett says, 'In the actual moment of laughing, that's all the brain can be doing. You can't be mad or sad. It's a great distraction'. On the next page are some exercises to get you mirthful. Make it your goal to laugh at least 10 times per day. (Children laugh an average of 300 times per day.) The more you do it, the more you'll want to.

Talk to your pain

How you think about your pain can affect whether it spends the night or packs up to go elsewhere. Here are a few examples of how to turn unhelpful thoughts into still-realistic better ones.

Not helpful: Oh, here's my pain again. The day's only going to get worse from here.
Helpful: Let's see how I'm feeling. How about if I get out of bed and give things a try?

Not helpful: This shower feels great, but when I get out, my pain will start all over again.
Helpful: This shower feels great. Maybe I'll feel well enough afterwards to go shopping.

Not helpful: My pain has ruined my life. I can't do anything.
Helpful: My pain has changed my life. But, because of it, I now take better care of myself. And I can still [fill in the blank].

Not helpful: My family doesn't believe I'm in pain, and they're angry that I don't do the things I used to. I'm really letting them down.
Helpful: I'm doing the best I can. It's up to me to help my family better understand how my condition affects me.

Try a pencil smile. Okay, this isn't laughing, but it's guaranteed to make you want to. Hold a pencil in your teeth and smile for 30 seconds. You won't be able to let go of the smile, and if you do it while driving, guaranteed it will make you and other snarly drivers laugh. You'll fool your brain into replacing those stress chemicals with feel-good ones.

Hang out with the king of comedy. If you have funny relatives or friends, now's the time to spend time with them. Studies have shown that laughter is 30 times more frequent in social settings than when a person is alone.

Join a laughter club. Yes, 6000 laughter clubs laugh on in 60 countries, born of the Indian laughter yoga practice. To find one near you, go to http://www.laughteryoga.org. The site also offers laughter yoga books, DVDs and videos.

Learn to relax

The school calls: your child is sick. Your boss emails and wants you in his office, immediately. Your car has a flat tyre. Do you feel a headache coming on? Of course. Stress, well, stresses us out. You know the signs: your shoulders tense, your breath speeds up, your heart races, you clench your teeth, all of which can make chronic pain worse. That can create a cycle: your stress worsens your pain, and your pain stresses you out.

Under normal circumstances, some stress is a good thing—it can stimulate us into action and get us going. But if you're stressed all the time, learning how to let go is key. Start by learning to relax. It's a skill like any other. Relaxation techniques such as deep breathing, visualisation, progressive muscle relaxation and meditation all work by reversing the tension stress causes. Stress hormones fall, your heart and breathing rate slow and your muscles relax, lessening pain. In fact, relaxation decreases signals to your brain's pain centre. Relaxation doesn't just undo the bad effects of stress; it also adds to the balance sheet, increasing your energy and focus, boosting your immune system and even letting you home in on solutions instead of problems. Ever wonder why you come out of a hot shower or back from a walk knowing the solution to a tricky problem? That's the power of relaxation working.

Take a mental getaway

Relaxation techniques aren't hard, but, as with exercise, to get the most benefit you need to do them every day. They work by relaxing your body and also your mind, offering a way for you to step aside mentally, draw a breath and regain perspective. Here are just a few of your options.

Guided imagery. With this technique, close your eyes and imagine yourself in a place that makes you feel happy and relaxed, such as a beach or mountaintop. Try making your own 20-minute tape,

Why aren't you laughing now?

Before you can start laughing, it may be helpful to check out why you don't laugh enough now. Yes, you're in pain. What else might be holding you back?

Too much stress. Before you try to start laughing, take some deep breaths and exhale some of that stress away. Imagine that you're breathing out your stress and pain.

Seriousness in overdrive. Maybe you take yourself or your day-to-day events too seriously. If you catch yourself in what seems a dire moment, picture yourself—or the person who is annoying you—as a cartoon character, such as Elmer Fudd or Daisy Duck.

Too much gloom in the room. No one wants to trivialise her pain or problems. But a flying superhero hanging on a living room plant or a framed grinning monkey in your bathroom, for example, can remind you that moments can be funny even during dark times.

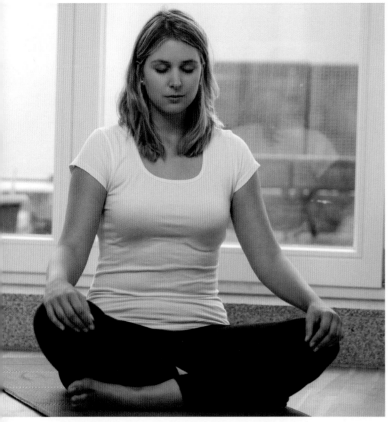

Mindfulness meditation: sit quietly, focusing on your breathing, and allow your thoughts to flow through you without reacting to them.

asking yourself to travel to the places you love, describing the scene, the sensations it evokes.

Interactive imagery. This technique takes 20 to 30 minutes. It resembles guided imagery, but instead of summoning a specific image, you allow images to come spontaneously, accessing the unconscious by talking about the images and what they mean to you. Here's how to do it.

• Begin with progressive relaxation, starting from your toes, clenching, then relaxing each muscle group or body part until you reach your head.
• Breathe in, imagining you are inhaling healthy nutrients and wholesome air. Hold for 6 to 8 seconds. Breathe out, imagining all the toxins leaving your body.
• Count backwards slowly from 10.
• Visualise a stream. Use all your senses to see, feel, smell and taste the surroundings.
• Walk down a path and, at the end, see an image that may represent your pain, your anger. Talk to the image about what you're thinking and feeling. Don't worry if you don't understand the images that come to mind.

Mindfulness meditation. This meditation technique involves what psychologist Steven D Hickman, PsyD, calls moment-to-moment nonjudgmental awareness. First, you sit quietly, focusing on your breathing, and allow your thoughts to flow through you without reacting to them. This is not focusing on your pain but letting go of the struggle over its presence. One variation is a walking meditation: find a 3-to-6-metre path you can walk on. First, stand, allowing yourself to tune in to your body, its tensions. Then begin to walk, and as you do, repeat the words *lifting, shifting, planting*. Focus on the shift of your body as you move through each step. 'The point is to let go of expectation', says Hickman. 'It's about noticing whatever happens, to attend to the process of walking. You allow what happens to pass through you instead of being buffeted by it.'

Instant stress busters and mood lifters

You can't always eliminate the cause of your stress, but you can still get stress relief instantly. Try a few of these stress busters.

Breathe. Take a deep breath through your nose, hold for 4 to 6 seconds, then purse your lips and let the air escape through your mouth. Continue for 5 minutes, and you'll be so relaxed no one will know you.

Avoidance. Hate the highway traffic jam? Take the back way home. Too much on your plate? Say *no* to the next request. Worried about world events? Turn off the news.

Run early. Stressed by time pressures? Leave for events 15 minutes earlier than usual. When you arrive a bit early, take the opportunity to breathe and relax.

Don't do it all. Once you take a breath, you'll realise that maybe not everything has to be done, or done yesterday. The leaves *can* wait until next week. The big project *can* be broken into small steps. Pizza *can* replace a home-cooked meal. Perfection is a pain.

Dealing with depression

You might say that depression and pain are sisters. Both affect how we feel, our mood, our behaviour, our ability to enjoy life. And, in fact, the pair is joined: someone with chronic pain is three times more likely to suffer from depression than someone without pain. The reverse is also true: people who are depressed are three times as likely to have chronic pain, especially back, stomach or joint pain, or headaches. Both intensify the other. Both, if they go on too long, can alter the way the nervous system works, extending one or both conditions indefinitely. In fact, some scientists believe that depressed people may be more sensitive to pain than other people. Fibromyalgia may be a good example: it involves chronic muscle pain with no signs of damage, lower thresholds for pain and a higher rate of depression than any other pain disorder.

Unfortunately, many people who have pain don't realise the link between pain and depression. Fifty per cent of depressed people who see a family doctor mention only their physical complaints. Some people are embarrassed to talk about depression. That's a shame, because many of the treatment approaches for one can affect the other, from antidepressants to exercise to relaxation techniques. If you think you suffer from depression, here are some ways to help you cope that may also help you manage your pain.

Speak up. If you know you are vulnerable to depression, share that information with your doctor as soon as any pain treatment begins. Your doctor may be able to help your pain from becoming chronic

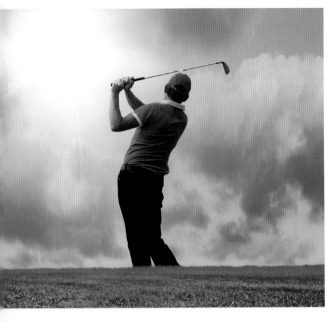

by addressing depression simultaneously. This knowledge may affect the doctor's choice of treatments: some antidepressants are more effective than others for treating pain as well as depression.

Exercise. You've already heard the advice to exercise. Exercise not only helps relieve pain but is a powerful mood lifter. As little as 10 to 15 minutes at a time can sweeten your spirits. That's because exercise boosts mood-altering neurotransmitters in your brain just as antidepressants do, and it stimulates the release of endorphins, the body's natural painkillers. While depression often chases off sleep, exercise improves it. And that 10-minute jog lowers stress hormones and increases body temperature, which can calm you.

Exercise not only helps relieve pain but is a powerful mood lifter. As little as 10 to 15 minutes at a time can sweeten your spirits.

Stay involved. Both pain and depression are isolating. Walking with a friend, joining a club or support group or volunteering to help someone else can boost your spirits.

Stressed, angry or depressed?

Sometimes it's hard to tell stress, anger and depression apart. Try answering the questions below to find out which may play the biggest role in your life. Circle the five statements that most apply to you.

1. I feel sad and hopeless most of the time.
2. I spend most of my time alone.
3. I have trouble sleeping most nights.
4. I have a hard time making decisions.
5. I often have trouble concentrating.
6. I often dislike my bosses.
7. I have trouble meeting deadlines.
8. I let small things get under my skin.
9. I'm more of an observer than a participant.
10. I have a sarcastic sense of humour.
11. I drink and smoke more than I like.
12. I often feel tired.
13. I have a sensitive stomach.
14. I often feel anxious and insecure.
15. I tend to see the glass half empty.

If most of your answers fall in 1 to 5, you may be depressed. If most of your answers fall in 6 to 10, chances are that anger is contributing to your pain. And if most of your answers fall within 11 to 15, stress is your address.

Treating pain *and* depression

Pain centres, medical centres that focus on pain, often treat pain and depression simultaneously. Here are some approaches that help address both problems.

Antidepressants. Of the tricyclic antidepressants, amitriptyline (Endep) affects both pain and depression, in part because it acts as a sedative and increases the neurotransmitters noradrenaline and serotonin, as does a newer drug, venlafaxine (Effexor).

Psychotherapy. Talk therapy can help people make connections among their pain, depression and other difficulties such as problems in relationships or at work, and help them find ways to feel better.

Cognitive behavioural therapy. This type of psychotherapy helps people learn how to change unhelpful thought patterns that may heighten pain and increase depression. (See 'Learning to cope', below.)

Sleep. One sign of depression is sleeping too much or too little. Sleeping well doesn't banish pain or depression, but it can help. Skip tempting daytime naps, and cut back on caffeine, alcohol and smoking. Regularise your sleep routine, getting up at the same time every day. Your goal: 8 hours of refreshing sleep per night.

1-minute zone out

When you feel ready to explode from stress, try one of these instant timeouts:

• Stare for 1 minute into a fire (or a fish tank, the clouds, the ocean), a form of meditation.
• Close your eyes for 60 seconds, breathe deeply, and repeat a soothing word such as *calm, relax* or *peace*.
• Breathe slowly as you imagine yourself descending a stairway.

Learning to cope

When Kate Muller, PsyD, director of the Cognitive Behavior Therapy Program at Albert Einstein College of Medicine in New York City, began seeing a woman in her late forties, the woman complained of terrible joint and muscle pain, the result of treatments for hepatitis C. She woke up stiff and, tired by lunchtime, was unable to work because of pain. Often she would feel so lousy when she woke that she went back to bed, thinking, 'What's the point of getting up?' Even when something helped, such as a warm shower, she responded by remembering that the soothing effects would quickly fade. She was haunted by guilt about letting her family down and, at the same time, angry that pain was eroding her relationships. When she did feel an energy boost, she raced around doing errands until she dropped.

Muller responded by asking the woman to monitor her pain, noting both its intensity and whatever thoughts sprang into her head when she experienced it. The next session they worked together on coming up with more balanced statements that didn't involve judgments. For example, instead of thinking upon waking, 'I hate this pain. The day is only going to go downhill from here', she might say, 'Let me do a body scan and see how I'm feeling now. Let's see if I can get out of bed'. In three to four hour-long sessions, the woman's rating of her pain had decreased by 30 to 40 per cent.

What Muller's patient experienced is the essence of *cognitive behavioural therapy*, a therapy based on the belief that the thoughts and emotions people have about pain affect the pain itself and also influence the behaviours they use to address pain. Says Muller, 'Change a thought, and you will affect behaviour, emotion and physiology. What research has shown is that after cognitive behavioural therapy people report less distress and impairment from pain. And they are better able to go back to daily activities.'

Numerous studies have proven cognitive behavioural therapy to be effective in addressing back pain, arthritis pain and cancer-related pain, and in easing the sleeplessness that often accompanies pain.

Practise distraction

Although tuning in to pain and developing a relationship with it instead of fighting or ignoring it are helpful ways of managing it, distraction has its place as well. Here are some ways to take your mind off pain.

Take an inner vacation. Dale Weinert, a physical therapist, cancer survivor and founder of Inner Vacations Tool Kits, suggests stepping into the shower and imagining that the warm water is massaging away the tension and pain in your muscles, washing them down the drain.

Play a video game. Carl G Arinoldo, a psychologist in Stony Brook, New York, has found computer games to be one of the most effective distractions from pain. Pick the action-packed ones, which require more concentration.

Listen to music. In a study done at the Cleveland Clinic Foundation, patients who endured years of chronic pain cut their pain levels by up to 21 per cent and their depression by 25 per cent by listening to music for up to an hour per day. Other studies have shown that before bed, listening to music can also improve sleep. Researchers suspect that listening to music lessens the focus on pain.

The therapist won't ask you to become a Pollyanna. No one loves pain. But if you can manage to say, 'I don't like it, but I am going about my day', that's better than pulling the covers over your head and sulking, and may even lessen your pain.

Pain-managing techniques

If cognitive behavioural therapy sounds good to you, why wait for your appointment to get started? You can use these techniques in the comfort of your home.

Cognitive restructuring. That's a way of saying that you're going to reframe your thoughts. Whenever you feel pain, write down its intensity (give it a number from 0 to 10, for example) and the thoughts that go through your mind. Then rewrite the thought without the negative adjectives. Drop 'horrible' and say something like this instead: 'I hurt today, but let's see what I can try.'

Body scan. Sit in a quiet space for 20 to 30 minutes. With your eyes closed, imagine that you are scanning your body from head to toe. Imagine that a light is moving very slowly, looking for sensations, tension, pain. Spend about 2 minutes on each body part, moving from your head to your neck and shoulders, your torso, your arms and hands, your abdomen, thighs, knees, feet. When you observe tension or pain, describe it to yourself without judgment: 'it feels like a tingling' or 'my left shoulder feels tight'. Once you get to your feet, recall what you felt, returning to the places where you felt pain. The point of this exercise is to sharpen your observations of your body, says Muller. 'Over time, because you notice where the tension is, you get better at looking for triggers, like lying in bed a certain way. Even your observations about pain can help you tolerate it better.'

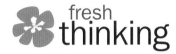

fresh
thinking

'The things you tell yourself about pain can actually make the pain worse or make it more tolerable.'

—Kate Muller, PsyD, director of the Cognitive Behavior Therapy Program at Albert Einstein College of Medicine, New York City

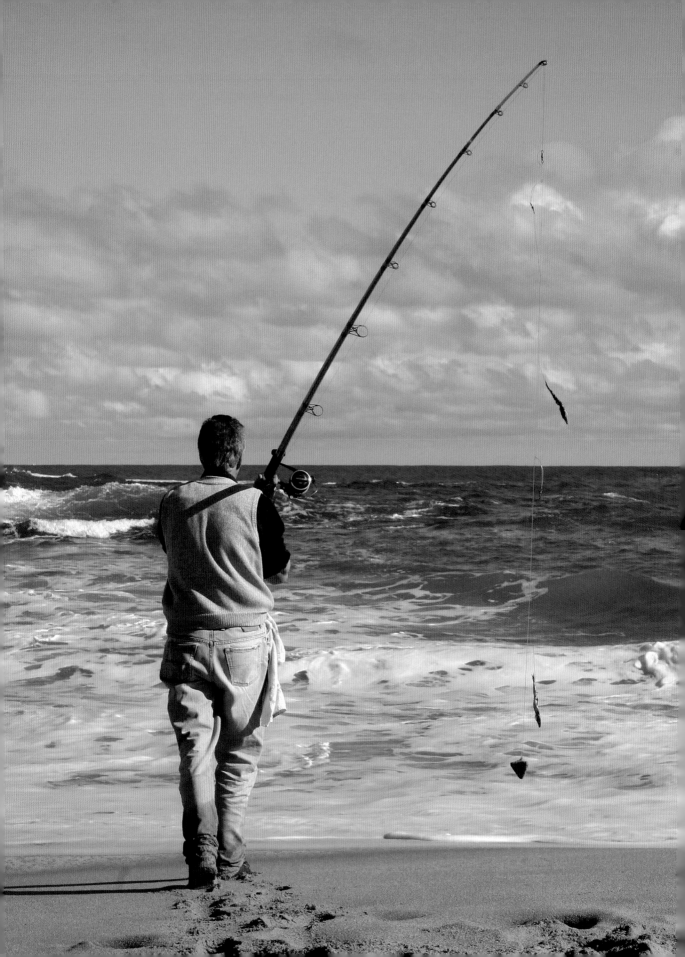

Sidestep your pain triggers

Learning to know and manage your own personal pain triggers can give you more control over your condition. Although you have no sway over the weather or your hormones, you can avoid overexertion, eating too much of the wrong things, smoking, sitting the wrong way or getting overly stressed.

Some triggers may be obvious: as children, most of us had stomach-aches only on school days. That wasn't a coincidence. And people with arthritis learn that on wet, cold days, chances are that sore muscles will seize up and joints will ache a bit more. It's less obvious that your response to a critical boss or an overbearing friend may also stoke your pain. Even anticipating pain can be a trigger. You know you're going on a long car trip, and even as you head to the car, you feel your back muscles tighten, remembering the discomfort of your last long car journey. In fact, in a study at Emory University in Atlanta, pain control centres of the brain lit up in the MRI scans of people anticipating an electric shock. The more people dreaded the shock, the more alert the brain's pain centres were. In anticipating our pain, we can become our own worst trigger.

Sometimes, triggers sneak up on you. A simple twist or turn can activate back pain; a sip of cold water, tooth pain. The timing of triggers can make them tricky to identify as well. Sometimes, for example, it may take 24 to 36 hours before a physical action can take effect.

But triggers can become your best friends. By knowing that perfumed stores activate your migraines, you can skip them. By recognising that sleeping on the same side each night stirs up neck and shoulder pain, you can practise sleeping on your back or buy yourself a neck pillow that lessens the strain on your neck and shoulder muscles. Determining your triggers can be tricky, and you won't learn them all overnight. If you work with your doctor to become your own trigger sleuth, the results will be less pain and frustration.

Take a trigger inventory

A huge part of dealing with pain, as with any relationship, is learning what works best, what soothes it, what leads to conflict and what makes it mellow. You are in training to be your own best pain detective. Ask yourself the following questions and see if your answers can help you learn what makes your pain lion roar.

How's your sleep lately?

• Do you have a mattress that's more than 10 years old? Consider replacing it.
• Bright lights? Dim them.
• New noises or neighbours? Try turning on a fan, even in winter, to block the sounds.
• Are you exercising or eating within 3 hours of bedtime? Doing either shortly before bed will make falling asleep tough.
• Do you have a brightly lit clock by your head? Its glow could be disturbing. Turn its face away from you.
• How do you spend the hour before bed? Instead of doing your taxes, try reading or listening to music that relaxes you.

Why anger augments pain

Stuck in traffic, you find yourself in a fury at the waste of time. When you get home to a sink of dirty dishes, you imagine walking away and yelling. And when the third solicitor calls on the phone, you feel your back or neck muscles go into spasm. Your pain response is probably no coincidence. For years, studies have linked anger, both suppressed and expressed, to chronic pain such as headaches and back pain. Anger's no sleeping pill either. It rouses your fight-or-flight response, increasing your adrenaline, raising your blood pressure and speeding your heartbeat.

A recent study at Vanderbilt University in Nashville sheds a new light on the connection.

It found that people who vented their anger explosively or who got angry easily had more intense pain and produced fewer naturally occurring opioids than people who had healthier ways of managing their anger.

If you're someone who is often angry, especially if you suppress anger, you may benefit from cognitive behavioural therapy. The therapist will focus on teaching you ways to express your anger constructively and on changing the attitudes and thoughts that make you angry. Try this, for example: when you feel yourself getting angry, take several slow, deep breaths.

• How many hours of sleep do you get per night? You need 7 to 8. One clue: if you have trouble getting up because you're tired, you're not getting enough.

• How many hours do you spend in bed? If you spend many more hours than you actually sleep, trying using your bed for sleep and sex only. Associating your bed with wakeful activities won't help your shut-eye.

• Do you get up at the same time each day? Keeping a regular routine will help your body prepare for sleep.

What are your eating habits?

• Do you eat only one or two large meals each day? A heavy meal can aggravate conditions such as heartburn and IBS. Try cutting down the size of your meal and eating less, more often.

• Do you eat a lot of foods with additives such as nitrates (hot dogs, cured meats)? Try switching to unprocessed meats and eating proportionately more fresh fruit, vegetables and cereal grains.

• How many alcoholic drinks do you have per week? Alcohol can exacerbate many conditions, such as gout and heartburn, and interferes with sleep, which increases pain. Try cutting back or switching to water.

• What kind of fats do you eat? The saturated and trans fats in fatty meats and many commercial biscuits and cakes may increase inflammation. Switch to low-fat dairy products, use plant oils such as olive oil and cut back on red meats in favour of fish.

• Do you eat a lot of highly spiced food such as chilli and salsa? Hot spices can aggravate some conditions such as heartburn and IBS. Try replacing them with more soothing spices, such as ginger or fennel.

• How much coffee do you drink? Caffeine is no stomach soother and can stir up pain for those with heartburn or gastrointestinal disorders. Remember that many soft drinks contain caffeine, as does chocolate. Too much caffeine can also interfere with sleep.

• How much water do you drink per day? For some conditions such as migraines, dehydration may play a part. Drink at least eight glasses of liquid per day, mostly water.

• Do you chew gum? Sounds harmless, but, in some people, it can activate headaches.

• Do you eat a lot of diet foods and drinks? Some people react to the flavouring and sweetening additives in these products.

What new activities have you taken on?

• Are you taking a new exercise class? Have you been scrubbing the bathroom or weeding the garden? Carrying more groceries than usual?

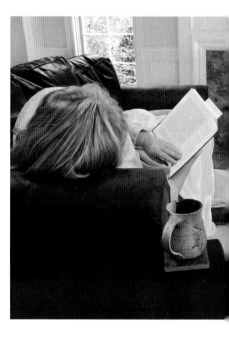

How do you spend the hour before bed?

Has your home or work environment changed recently?

• Changed your desk chair or desk height? Even small shifts like that can affect your posture and the amount of strain on already painful muscles. Try to adjust new furniture so that you're sitting with your feet on the floor, your knees slightly higher than your hips and with some support for the small of your back.

• Bought new furniture, carpeting or office equipment? They could be emitting fumes that could trigger a headache. Try letting new furniture air out in fresh air or in an open garage for several weeks. If you can, keep your windows at least partly open so that you get some fresh air.

• Changed your lighting? Glare and flickers from overhead lights can trigger headaches. Try minimising their use and using individual lamps and dimmer switches instead.

• Carrying a laptop every day? Whether it's an oversized bag, a laptop or a baby, if you're carrying a big load around the house or to and from work, you're putting pressure and strains on your muscles, increasing your pain. Get someone else to carry heavy loads for you, make several trips yourself instead of trying to carry several things at once or buy a holder with wheels and roll it.

Find your food triggers

As anyone who's ever had indigestion or heartburn knows, food can switch on pain. Certain foods are common triggers for people with conditions such as irritable bowel syndrome, gout and migraines. Eating a plate of beef with a big glass of wine, for instance, is a bad idea for anyone with gout. Other food triggers are less obvious. These tips can help you pin them down.

Find out about your condition. Talk to your doctor and look up reputable websites for information about foods that tend to exacerbate the pain of your condition. There's no reason to reinvent the wheel. If certain foods are common triggers, it's logical to start by finding out what they are.

Keep a pain/food diary. Write down when you feel pain, the severity of the pain on a 0-to-10 scale and the foods you have eaten within the last 24 hours. Also, take note of other factors such as stress, sleep and menstruation that may have contributed to pain.

Eliminate individual foods. After you've kept a food diary for a week, try eliminating the food or foods that seem to be the common

Common pain triggers

Ailment	Common triggers
Arthritis	Stress, overdoing it, junk foods, fatty meats, sugar and fast foods may increase inflammation
Back, shoulder, neck pain	Straining muscles with excessive exercise or poor posture (waking or sleeping), stress and carrying or lifting heavy objects
Chronic fatigue syndrome	Poor sleep, stress and overexertion
Dental pain	Hot or cold foods, hard foods, chewing gum and tension (TMD)
Fibromyalgia	Stress and fatigue
Gastrointestinal pain	Spicy and fatty foods, lactose, coffee, tea and alcohol; cigarettes; late-night meals and stress
Gout	Alcohol, excess meat and seafood, fatty foods and excess weight
Haemorrhoids	Sitting too long, straining on the toilet, excess weight, low-fibre diet, dehydration and delaying trips to the toilet
Headaches	Stress, strong odours, fatigue, bright lights, loud noises, menstruation, excess weight, alcohol and smoking
Leg and foot pain	Lying down, walking, smoking, over- or sudden exercising, shoes that lack adequate support and being overweight
Lupus	Sun exposure, smoking, stress, fatigue
Psoriasis	Stress, smoking, cold weather; infections and conditions that weaken the immune system such as alcoholism, HIV and arthritis; some medicines such as those for high blood pressure and malaria
Trigeminal neuralgia	Drinking hot beverages, getting too little sleep, walking in frigid weather, chewing, touching your face and brushing your teeth

factor whenever your pain increases. You can start by eliminating one food at a time and if, after 3 months, your condition remains the same, return the food to your diet and eliminate another. Consult a dietitian if you're worried about more than a few different foods, or if a whole food group (such as dairy foods, or all wheat products) is suspected. The process may take a while.

Skip junk and fatty foods. Certain groups of foods are much more apt to stir up inflammation than others, including fast foods, fatty

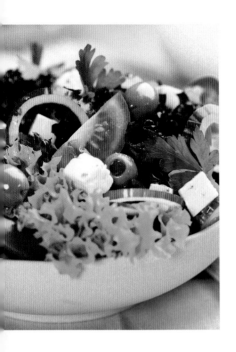

meats, sugary foods and fatty snacks. Some food additives, such as nitrates in hot dogs and bacon, can trigger headaches.

Suspect the spices. Spices such as chilli, garlic, pepper and cinnamon are a concentrated source of flavour and beneficial natural substances such as anti-oxidants, but also substances that cause intolerance reactions in some people. Try avoiding spiced foods and see whether this helps.

Check the size of your portions. Sometimes, it's not individual foods that cause pain but simply eating too much food. Carrying extra kilos can add to the pain of any joint condition, such as osteoarthritis or rheumatoid arthritis. If you are overweight, try eating more fruit, vegetables and whole grains in place of fatty or sugary foods. Aim to exercise at least 30 minutes most days of the week.

Try switching to foods free of chemical additives, such as fresh fruit, vegetables and grains.

Recognise when stress is to blame

Stress is the biggest of all pain triggers, worsening almost every kind of pain. When you're stressed, your body responds by revving its motor, releasing a flood of stress hormones, including adrenaline and cortisol. As a result, your heart beats faster, your blood pressure rises, you breathe faster, your muscles tighten and your arthritis pain, migraine pain, stomach pain or fibromyalgia gets worse.

The key to controlling this pain trigger is to learn to recognise your own personal stress signals, so that you can take active steps to relax. You may feel frazzled or depressed. You may be grouchy and moody, picking fights with friends. You may respond to stress by driving faster, smoking or drinking more or reaching for the potato chips in front of an endless parade of TV programs. You may be distracted, forgetful, jumpy. Or you may simply feel unable to act, paralysed, and without energy.

Once you recognise how stressed you are, you can take the following measures to decrease your stress.

Ask yourself what role stress plays in your life. If you're always stressed, what purpose does it serve, and is that purpose still necessary? For example, maybe you pile on stressful activities so that you don't have to think about the future, a sour relationship, a loss. It would be easier on your system to focus on resolving those issues, perhaps with the help of a counsellor.

Build in relaxation. Make a list of the things you do for fun, such as seeing friends or reading a book, and carve out more time for them.

Set up fun as an appointment on your daily calendar, so the allotted time won't get filled up with obligations. See friends who relax you or make you laugh, and dump the ones who criticise or pressure you.

Exercise. Few people ever return from a long walk saying how stressed they feel. Getting outside to walk or ride a bike for at least 30 minutes every day is relaxing and stimulates chemicals that can boost your mood.

Consider therapy. With the help of a biofeedback therapist, for example, you can learn to monitor and control your physical response to stress. For instance, once you can see that your muscles contract when you are getting a headache, you can learn how to relax those muscles, helping your body avoid pain. Another therapy is hypnosis. A trained therapist can help you learn how to move into an extremely relaxed state, releasing tension and stress. The hypnotist may make suggestions to help you deal with setting limits on work or to help you give up stress-inducing habits, such as smoking.

Try these feel-good moves

Reducing stress by recognising what triggers it is essential to managing your pain; so is recognising what makes your body feel good. For some people, a massage is torture. For others, it's a pathway to bliss. Most of us are aware of at least some feel-good triggers that help us forget our pain, or at least send it away for a while. Here are some other possibilities to explore.

Exercise. Just try asking a postrace runner to wipe that smile off his face. You don't have to run to get the feeling: swimming, tennis or a 30-minute stint on a stationary bike can all trigger great feelings and stir the production of endorphins, the body's natural painkillers.

Make love. There's no more pleasurable way to release a flood of endorphins.

Pat a pet. Even a few minutes spent patting a dog or cat can trigger the release of serotonin, prolactin and oxytocin, all hormones that make us feel good. And the purring or tail wagging you get in return is sure to put a smile on your face.

Savour some dark chocolate. There may be a reason that we love chocolate. Like exercise and sex, chocolate releases endorphins that kill pain. Don't overdo it; a square or two will do the trick.

Get some sun. Ever notice how much better you feel on a sunny day? Wear sunscreen, of course.

Turn to suspense. Watch a few scary movies or ride a roller coaster. In the aftermath of fear comes a burst of endorphins that will leave you feeling a rush.

Talk to your funniest friend. People who are happy and optimistic tend to relax us and make us laugh.

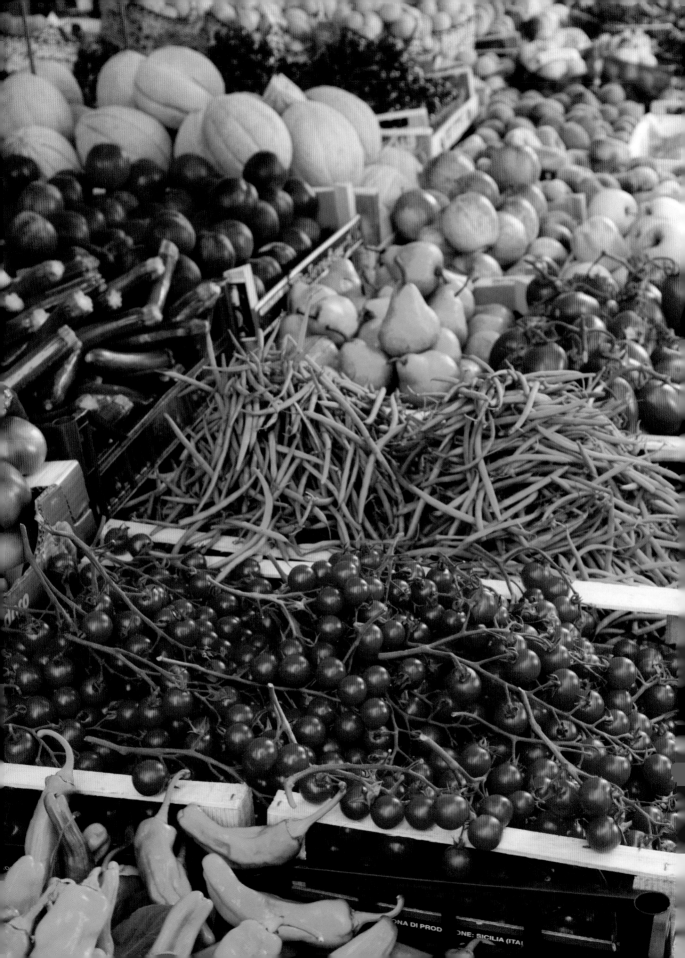

Pain-proof your diet

Your diet can make it easier or harder for you to deal with your pain. People in pain tend to self-medicate with comfort foods, including refined carbohydrates such as mashed potatoes, sugary treats and piles of pasta, as well as fatty, salty convenience foods loaded with 'bad' fats. The trouble is, these foods can make pain worse in several ways. Foods containing trans fat and saturated fat can trigger inflammation in the body that can exacerbate everything from arthritis to bursitis, carpal tunnel syndrome, diverticulosis, fibromyalgia, irritable bowel syndrome and premenstrual syndrome. Refined carbohydrates can promote inflammation and send you on a blood glucose roller coaster that ultimately saps your energy, so it's even harder to cope with your pain. Fatty, starchy high-energy foods can also lead to weight gain, which worsens pain either directly, or indirectly by making you feel less inclined to get up and move around.

Food doesn't have to be the enemy, however. Some foods, such as fatty fish, actually soothe inflammation. Switching to whole grains can help boost your energy. Read on to discover how the right diet can take a big bite out of your pain.

Your pain-fighting shopping list

Instead of focusing right away on foods to cut from your diet, start by adding delicious foods that nourish your body, protect against cell damage and ease inflammation, especially when they begin to crowd out fatty foods and junk food.

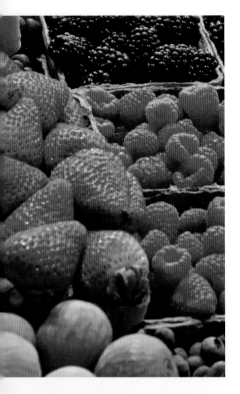

Raspberries and strawberries contain strong inflammation fighters. Why not pop at least half a cup a day of these low-kilojoule, no-fat fruits?

Apples. These contain an anti-oxidant plant chemical called quercetin, which fights inflammation. Most brightly coloured fruit and vegetables have chemicals that tamp down inflammation.

Broccoli. This vegetable contains glutathione, which is a power anti-oxidant that may guard against arthritis. Other foods rich in the anti-oxidant include asparagus, cabbage, cauliflower, potatoes, tomatoes, avocados, grapefruit, oranges, peaches and watermelons.

Brown rice. Brown rice and other whole grains can fight the constipation of irritable bowel syndrome. According to a Harvard University study, women who eat brown rice are less likely to be overweight than those who don't. (In painful conditions such as arthritis and joint pain, less weight means less pain.) Whole grains, such as brown rice, are a good source of magnesium, which appears to cut the frequency of migraines by helping to relax nerves, blood vessels and muscles.

Cherries and berries. Cherries contain chemicals called anthocyanins that fight inflammation in somewhat the same way that aspirin does. Raspberries and strawberries also contain this inflammation fighter. Berries are not only a good source of fibre but they are low in kilojoules as well.

Chocolate. Now we're talking. Dark chocolate contains chemicals that help fight inflammation. According to a large Italian study, people who ate about 30 grams of dark chocolate every 3 days had significantly lower measures of a protein associated with inflammation than those who ate no chocolate.

Cranberry juice. This juice is known for quelling painful bladder infections. Researchers at Harvard University found that women who drank 300 millilitres of the juice a day had bladder infections only 42 per cent as often as those who did not drink it. The scientists believe that an ingredient in the juice may inhibit bacteria from invading the bladder wall.

Fish. Oily fish such as salmon, trout and anchovies, along with walnuts, linseeds and pumpkin seeds and olive and canola oils, contain omega-3 fatty acids that act as powerful anti-inflammatories. A University of Pittsburgh study found that people with back and neck pain who took omega-3 fatty acids in supplement form for 3 months had less pain. Eat fatty fish at least twice a week, and consider taking a daily omega-3 fatty acid supplement of 3 grams of fish or linseed oil (also known as flaxseed oil).

Grapes. Down some grapes, or wine, or mulberries, and you're getting a dose of resveratrol, which inhibits inflammatory enzymes in much the same way aspirin does but without the stomach irritation.

Green or black tea. Tea, along with colourful fruit and vegetables, contains flavonoids that may protect against cell damage that can worsen conditions such as arthritis. It also contains a chemical that fights inflammation.

Olive oil. Researchers at the University of Pennsylvania have found that a chemical in olive oil, oleocanthal, inhibits inflammatory enzymes in the same way that ibuprofen does.

Onions and garlic. This family of bulb vegetables are high in anti-inflammatory substances, as well as sulfur compounds that help stimulate the immune system.

Orange juice. British researchers who analysed the diets of 25,000 people found that those who ate foods with a chemical common in oranges and other orange fruits such as apricots and nectarines were less likely to have painful inflammatory joint conditions. Just one or two serves of fruit per day made a difference.

Peanuts and other nuts and seeds. Foods high in an amino acid (tryptophan) may lower pain sensitivity 1 hour after you ingest them. Other foods with tryptophan are hazelnuts, sesame seeds, sunflower seeds, turkey, dairy products, soy, seafood, whole grains, rice, beans and lentils.

Pineapple. Bromelain, a protein-digesting enzyme derived from pineapple reduces inflammation. Studies show that eating pine-apple may reduce pain in those with knee osteoarthritis and rheumatoid arthritis, and reduces swelling in those with carpal tunnel syndrome.

Spinach. Green leafy vegetables, including kale, chard, bok choy and silverbeet, are full of anti-inflammatory carotenoids, plant pigments that give green and orange fruit and vegetables their vibrant colour.

Soy protein. Researchers at Oklahoma State University found that people with osteoarthritis, especially men, who ate 40 grams of soy protein per day for 3 months had less pain and moved more easily than those who didn't. It's tough to eat that much pure soy protein (soya beans, for instance, are only 35 per cent protein) a day unless you add soy protein powder to a shake or smoothie, but it is still worth adding soya beans, tofu and soy milk to your daily intake.

Creating a soothing spice rack

Although some spices can cause reactions in some individuals, most people can benefit from their power to block inflammation and pain. Below is a list of pain busting spices and the reasons that they help.

Spice	What it does	How to use it
Chilli	Encourages the draining of mucus, helpful for sinusitis.	Use fresh chillis or powder to spice up soups, casseroles, salads and breads.
Curry powder and pastes	This combination of spices, including turmeric, garlic, cumin and cinnamon, contains anti-oxidants that also help relieve inflammation and pain.	Use in meat, rice, pasta dishes, soups and stews.
Garlic	Garlic acts as an anti-inflammatory and also helps boost the activity of the immune system.	Add garlic to pretty much everything, from meat dishes to pasta to vegetables.
Ginger	Ginger inhibits enzymes that help produce inflammatory chemicals.	Add to stir-fries, salsas, tea or soups.
Mint	Mint contains menthol, which, applied to the skin, acts as an anti-inflammatory that soothes joint pain and can also relieve itching. Scientists at the University of Edinburgh found that the chemicals in mint activate a nerve receptor that inhibits pain messages. Peppermint helps soothe stomach upset by relaxing the muscles of the intestinal wall and so may be effective for IBS or cramps.	Make a mint tea, adding 30 g of mint leaves to 475 ml of boiling water. You can also buy mint-infused ointments and massage oils.
Thyme	Several studies have shown that thyme helps inhibit pain responses, especially gastrointestinal pain.	Use to season chicken, meats, fish, vegetables and soups.
Turmeric	Some studies suggest that curcumin, a chemical in turmeric, fights inflammation and pain, particularly of rheumatoid arthritis.	Use as you would curry in meat, rice and pasta dishes, soups and stews. Or add a sprinkle to vegetables.

Weight loss for pain relief

Carrying extra weight can make pain worse, and excess fat stores can be a source of inflammation in their own right. People who are obese suffer six times as many migraines as those of normal weight.

According to one study, the risk of knee osteoarthritis increases by 36 per cent with every 5-kilogram weight gain. In another study, when obese patients lost an average of 39 kilograms through bariatric surgery, their back pain decreased by 44 per cent.

Of course, losing weight can be a tough battle, and dealing with chronic pain doesn't make changing old habits any easier. But there are ways to lose weight without starving yourself, shutting yourself in a steam room or putting a padlock on your refrigerator. Here are tips to get you started.

Think of losing weight as a prescription. Chances are your doctor has given you several prescriptions to combat your pain that you wouldn't dream of leaving unfilled. Think of weight loss as another one.

Reset your table. Brian Wansink, PhD, a professor of nutritional science at Cornell University and author of *Mindless Eating,* has found that people can make big strides towards eating less simply by making small changes. For instance, by serving food on smaller plates, you will automatically give yourself smaller helpings. By preparing plates in the kitchen and eating in the dining room, you make seconds much less likely.

Use sensory cues. If you're someone whose downfall is TV snacking, try this, suggests Wansink: put a loose rubber band on each of your wrists. Every time you reach into the snack bowl, snap the rubber band on that wrist. That small change will make you more aware of how much you're eating.

Right size your portions

Changing the kinds of foods you eat—more fruit, vegetables, whole grains and lean meats and less sugary, fatty food—is key to losing weight. Those changes won't do you much good if you continue to overeat even the healthy stuff. That's where portion control comes in. You not only have to eat more healthily to lose weight, you also have to eat 1000 fewer kilojoules per day to lose a kilogram per week. Here are some tips for keeping portions the right size for weight loss.

Read the serving size on the package. What you thought was a single-serving package might contain two or three servings. Note the serving size and the kilojoules per serving.

Get out your measuring cup. You're retraining your eyes to recognise a reasonable serving. So, for a week or two, confirm the

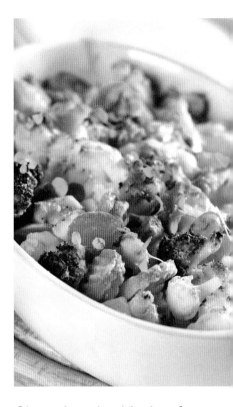

Changing the kinds of foods you eat—more fruit, vegetables, whole grains and lean meats and less sugary, fatty food—is the key to losing weight.

suggested serving size in a measuring cup. Three-quarters of a cup is an average serving size for cereal, for instance.

Consider portion control measures. If you find it too easy to go back to oversized servings, you can buy kitchen gadgets to help you. There are plates designed to help you visualise the proper portions of meat, rice, and so on. You can also buy a sectioned dish that offers the right-size portions for protein, carbs and vegies.

Divide and conquer. When you're dining out, share a main dish with someone else or ask the waiter to put half the meal in a doggie bag before he serves it.

Eat as though you have time. It takes about 20 minutes for your brain to get the message that you've had enough to eat. If you eat slowly, you're likely to feel full even before you've finished what's on your plate.

Crunch and munch. Keep crunchy 'free' foods such as carrots and celery sticks on the table and munch a few between more fattening bites. Put your fork down after each bite to slow yourself down.

Skip the all-you-can-eat buffets. Don't make this hard. All of us want to get the most for our money. But piling your plate at a buffet or supersizing your serving because it only costs just a little bit more does you and your pain no favours.

Practise mindful eating

Becoming more aware of what and how much you eat makes you much less apt to down a handful of M&Ms as you pass through the kitchen or open a bag of chips and eat the whole thing while perched in front of the television. Here are a few tips to help you become a more conscious diner.

Learn to savour food. Try this simple exercise: put a nut in your mouth, close your eyes and let the nut roll around in your mouth. Think about what the salt tastes like, feel the curve of the nut. Bite down and focus on how the nut cracking feels to your teeth. Chew very slowly, noticing the flavour of the nut filling your mouth. This is mindful eating, and once you try it, you'll realise how often you eat food without really paying attention to it.

Eat at the table. When you're having a meal or snack, give your full attention to that moment. If you can, sit at a table with a plate, enjoying nothing but your food. Eating while you work, read,

Studies show that if you can stick to your healthy plate for 3 weeks, your cravings for sugary, fatty foods will all but vanish.

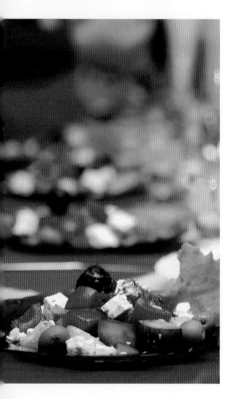

Sweetening your pain: can sugar lower pain perception?

Most of us aren't in pain when we're eating lollies. Researchers have found that table sugar actually lowers the perception of pain, at least in infants, perhaps by triggering the release of the body's natural pain-relieving chemicals. When infants drank sugar water before immunisations, their pain scores dropped by an average of 78 per cent. Of course, sugar adds weight and no nutrition, so try this remedy sparingly. When pain's got the better of you, for example, try adding a teaspoon of sugar to a cup of green tea. At least you'll feel soothed.

drive or watch television is the fast route to eating more than you realise without tasting a bit of it.

Love what you eat. Make healthy meals even more enjoyable by choosing enticing new recipes, cooking your family's favourite vegetables and setting a beautiful table, adding flowers and turning on a little music.

Cut your cravings

Biscuits, lollies, desserts: we can't resist. Or can we? Studies show that if you can stick to your healthy plate for 3 weeks, your cravings for sugary, fatty foods will all but vanish. A Belgian study found that when people refuse tempting foods, they have stronger willpower the next time. Still, temptation will strike. Fight back with these strategies.

Create a diversion. You can hear the corn chips calling to you from the cupboard, and nothing will do until you feel their salty, fatty crunch between your teeth. Such cravings usually pass, especially if you divert your attention. Try getting up and doing a household task for a few minutes or playing a CD. Chances are by the time the first song is over, your craving will be, too.

Don't get too hungry between meals. One reason you start dreaming of chocolate cake may be that you're actually too hungry. No diet will last if you starve yourself and are hungry all the time. So keep your appetite calm. If you get hungry between meals, have a healthy snack, such as a crunchy sweet apple and a handful of raisins and nuts. Sit down and drink a cup of hot tea, then settle in and enjoy the snack. Let yourself feel pampered and well fed.

Put the fatty snacks at the back. The easiest way to fend off temptation is to clear your cupboards of sugary, fatty snacks. If that causes a family revolt, at least put the foods that tempt you where you can't see or easily reach them. Buy them in tiny amounts. Buying the economy pack makes it easy to feel as though you've eaten less than you have.

Taste the temptation. Every once in a while, give in a little. If a life without chocolate depresses you, have a small piece now and then. That's not what hurts us. It's the piece that turns into the whole bar, or the bite that turns into the whole cake.

Sneak in more vegetables

You consider meatballs and pasta a well-rounded meal. Your idea of heaven is steak and a baked potato. Green vegetables, even fruit, are not on your radar. They remind you of your mother's canned peas and mushy asparagus. As you've read, vegetables and fruit hold many of the anti-inflammatory plant chemicals that can help lessen your pain, as well as anti-oxidants, vitamins and minerals that improve health. They also offer bulk and crunch for few kilojoules. In short, it's worth establishing a rapport with plants.

Get intimate with stir-fries. Quick-frying broccoli, onions, snow peas—well, just about any vegetable—in a little peanut oil and soy sauce transforms vegetables into savoury bites that actually make you want to overeat. Serve them over half a cup of brown rice, and you have a tasty meal that will in no way resemble wimpy, boiled, grey greens.

Make them easy to reach. Buy ready-to-eat cut-up fruit and vegetables (or cut them yourself) and put them at the front of your top refrigerator shelf. That way, when you're snooping for a snack, a crunchy fresh one will be right in front of you.

Change the recipe. Whenever you make a soup, a stew or a casserole, halve the meat and double the vegetables.

Sneak them in. If you're having a sandwich, add a layer of onions and tomatoes, a slice of avocado, some curls of carrots. They will add crunch, flavour and bulk to your meal. The same goes for hamburger or pizza. Vegetables make great toppings.

Add to salads. Maybe you're used to tossing lettuce and tomatoes together and calling it a salad. Add some variety and extra vegies by adding some shredded cabbage, carrots or zucchini.

Get out the barbecue. Like stir-frying, barbecuing vegetables transforms them. Brush onions, asparagus, yellow squash, mushrooms and eggplant with olive oil and throw them on the barbecue. Barbecuing, like roasting, brings out vegetables' inherent sweetness. Guaranteed: you'll never find vegetables boring again.

Water's winning ways

Water can be a great boon for diet success. A glass or two before meals helps you feel full. Water is essential for good health: it helps regulate body temperature, remove waste and carry healing nutrients and oxygen throughout your body. In fact, some of the signs of dehydration are chronic pain in your joints and muscles, headaches and constipation. Getting enough water is key to less pain, but, let's face it, water doesn't taste like a milkshake, and lots of people simply don't like drinking it. Like eating more healthily, drinking water is a new habit to establish. Here's how to work more water into your day.

Keep a jug of cold water in the fridge. Refrigerator-cold water tastes better than cool water from the tap. By keeping a jug in the fridge, you can easily see how much you have or haven't drunk.

Spice it up. Make water more appetising by adding orange or lemon slices to each glass or jug (as long as you change them daily). Or, if water's too dull, drink caffeine-free herbal teas.

Carry it with you. Get in the habit of keeping a bottle of water by your side at home, at work or in the car. The bottle will remind you to drink, and with easy access, you'll take more sips during the day.

Ritualise it. Use daily habits as cues to drink. For instance, have a glass when you wake up, after you brush your teeth and before meals. If you always drink a glass of juice in the morning, make half of it water. It's easier to start a new habit when you fold it into old ones.

Know the signs of dehydration. Along with more pain and thirst, the signs that tell you to get sipping are a dry mouth, fatigue, less urinating, weakness and dizziness. Your urine should be a pale straw colour if you are well hydrated.

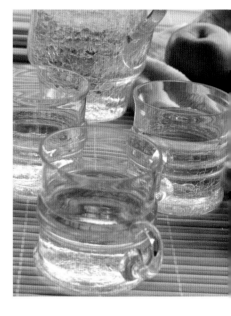

Like eating more healthily, drinking water is a new habit to establish.

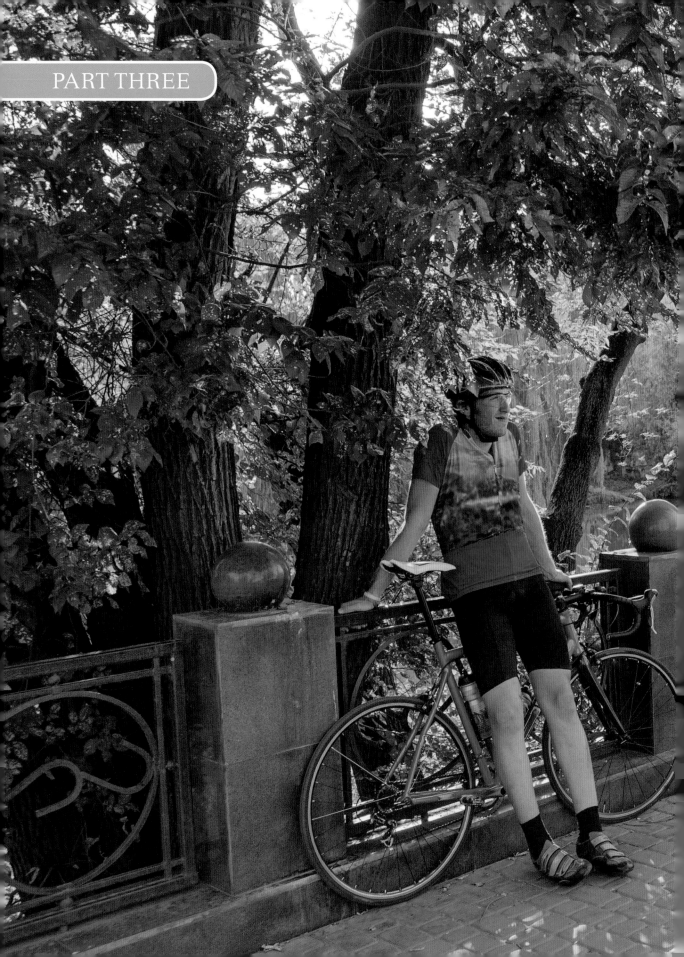

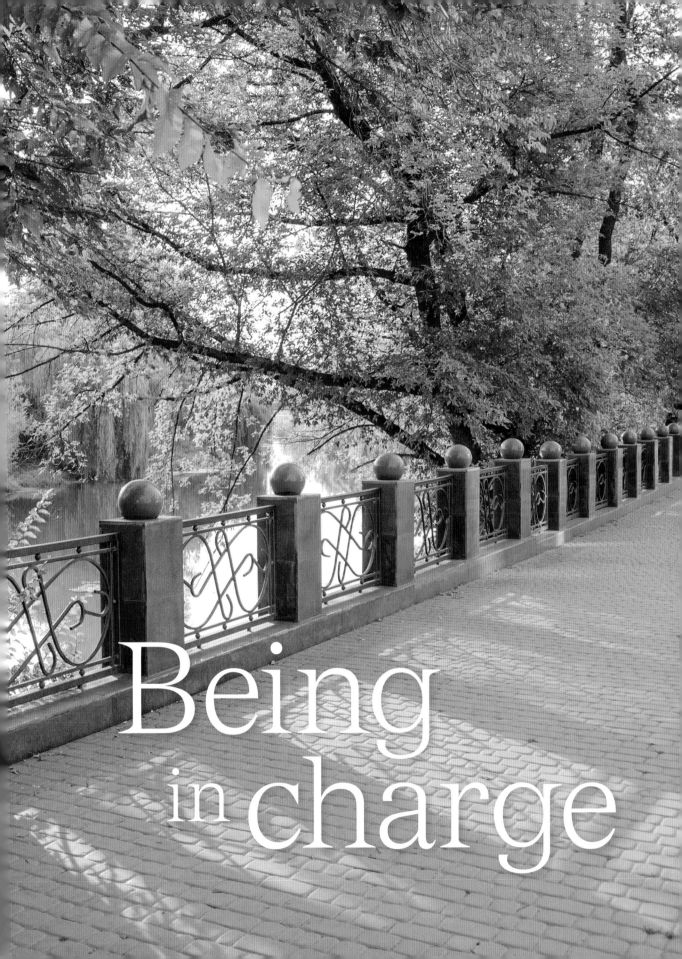

PART THREE

Being
in charge

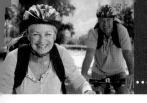

Back pain

Back pain is second only to headaches as a source of pain. Back pain can be a dull ache or an agonising stab. It's usually in the lower back but can occur higher, too. Lower back pain can be associated with pain into the legs. Most back pain settles within a few weeks but it can linger longer than an unwelcome guest. Back pain can often recur, but there's a lot we can do to keep our backs healthy.

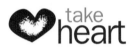
take heart

Ninety per cent of people with lower back pain get better **within 2 months,** even if they don't do a thing about it.

Common origins of back pain are from the discs (the 'cushions' that sit between each vertebral level), the facet joints (that sit at the back of each vertebral junction and guide the movement of the spine) and the muscles and ligaments that attach to the spine.

Fortunately, back pain can be managed. You have a wide range of options for getting your back pain to back off.

✔ Best first steps

You spend Sunday pulling weeds and Monday morning can barely get out of bed. Or you finally carry that heavy chair onto the porch, and when you try to stand up, well, you can't. What can you do?

1. Cease and desist.
Don't take to bed for a week. A number of studies have shown that bed rest doesn't help and may even make matters worse. If you can, keep up your normal activities. A little aggravation of your pain should be tolerable but avoid things that make your pain a lot worse.

2. Take a nonprescription painkiller.
Take paracetamol or an anti-inflammatory such as ibuprofen or naproxen. There is no clear evidence to show that one of these agents is superior to any other. Follow the directions on the package. The sooner you take it, the better it will work and the less you may need in the end, so don't wait until you're doubled over or laid

flat. These drugs work best when taken regularly through the day. You can expect these nonprescription painkillers to reduce severe pain to a moderate level or moderate pain to mild pain.

3. Haul out an ice pack.

If you've just hurt yourself, an ice pack applied to your back will make you feel better.

4. Call your doctor.

You should see your doctor if the pain is: worsening; worse at night; associated with bladder difficulties or leg weakness; or fails to improve significantly within 6 weeks.

Doctor's bag

If straightforward, at-home measures such as ice, gentle stretching and nonprescription anti-inflammatories don't do the trick and you're in real pain, your doctor can offer several medications that can attack the pain and give you relief until nature takes over. Here are a few low-risk options.

Muscle relaxants. If you're in severe pain and can barely move, a muscle relaxant can work wonders. Medications such as diazepam (Valium) are effective either alone or taken with nonprescription anti-inflammatories. They are best taken at bedtime, because they may cause drowsiness. They can also be habit forming and generally their use should be restricted to 1 week or so.

Opioids. An episode of severe pain may require the use of an opioid such as Panadeine or OxyNorm to help keep you moving. Long-term use of opioids is controversial. Experts recommend that if long-term use of opioids is considered, non-drug management should be fully utilised (see 'Your pain toolbox', page 110). Also the opioid should be a slow-release formulation such as Kapanol, OxyContin or Jurnista, or a patch such as Durogesic or Norspan that releases the drug slowly via the skin.

Antidepressants. These are used because they have properties that modify pain signalling in some situations. Medications that are sometimes useful for subacute and chronic back pain are amitriptyline (Endep) and duloxetine (Cymbalta).

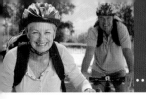

🍴 Your pain toolbox

Most back pain will settle within a couple of weeks. It usually doesn't need powerful painkillers or special tests, so usually you don't need to see your doctor. Listed below are several interventions that have some evidence to support their use for back pain that has lasted more than 6 weeks and where a significant underlying pathology (such as infection or cancer) has been excluded by your doctor. In terms of outcome, there is little to choose between the different interventions. Because back pain often recurs, the cheapest option for you is usually to work with your physiotherapist to set up a personalised program of exercise, including stretches, core stabilising, postural correction and general activity, which you can self-manage after a few appointments.

Exercise. Keeping moving within a day or two of the onset of your back pain will help to settle your immediate pain and to prevent many unhappy returns of your back pain. Walking is a good start, as is riding a stationary bike. If you're buying a bike, choose a style that is comfortable for you. If you have osteoarthritis or spinal stenosis, you may prefer an upright bike, which lets you lean forwards; if you have degenerative disc disease you may be more comfortable with the back support and reclining position of a recumbent bike. Swimming is another good choice—the sidestroke or backstroke may hurt your back less than freestyle or breaststroke. Working with a physiotherapist to set up a routine will also protect you from overdoing it.

'Back School'. Learning ways to move and position yourself that don't stress your back can help. In fact, a recent review of 24 studies found that patients with lower back pain who learnt, through discussion with a health care provider, a class, a pamphlet or a video, how to address back pain and protect their back returned to work earlier than those who received no education. It's worth asking your doctor for back-care materials and a training session with a physiotherapist.

Yoga. Yoga is a reasonable treatment for back pain to try in addition to medications and self-care. Researchers in Seattle found that back patients who took 12 weekly yoga sessions not only had less pain than those who did therapeutic exercises and education, but their relief lasted 14 weeks longer.

Acupuncture. Current guidelines suggest that for back pain of less than 1 year's duration, a trial of up to 10 sessions of acupuncture over 12 weeks may be helpful in alleviating pain.

Massage therapy. So-called soft tissue manipulation helps relax muscles and ease tension, and it may temporarily override pain signals. Make sure your massage therapist is certified and accustomed to working with people who have back pain.

Spinal manipulation. This therapy, performed by a chiropractor, osteopath, physiotherapist or other trained medical professional, is recommended for both acute and chronic back pain. The therapist uses his hands or a device to move a joint of the spine beyond its normal range of motion. Studies show that it can provide mild to moderate relief as effectively as other medical treatments. Guidelines from expert panels recommend a maximum of nine sessions delivered over a 12-week period.

Instant relief

Sick of gnarly back pain at the end of a long day? Here are some 5-minute pain stoppers:

Heat. Take a hot shower or bath. Or microwave a towel or gel pack, or plug in a heating pad, then apply to your back. The heat increases blood flow to the back, diminishes pain signals and helps the spinal muscles relax and stretch.

Squats. Replace all that bending you do with squatting. Bending overstretches your back muscles and weakens your back. Squats strengthen the back, as well as the supporting muscles of your butt and thighs. Bonus: a better booty.

Back stretch. Lie facedown on the floor and, keeping your hips on the floor, gently rise on your elbows. This move feels good and helps counter back spasm.

Chair stretch. Slouching isn't good for your back, but neither is ramrod stiffness. Several times per day, lean back in your chair with your feet on the ground, making sure there's a slight curve in your back. That posture distributes your weight more evenly, taking some pressure off your spine.

A stroll. The best thing you can do is change position every half an hour or so by getting up from your chair, taking a 5-minute walk or even making a phone call standing up.

A tennis ball. Lie down on the ball, allowing the ball to press into your sore spot, then let your body relax. The pressure will create a small stretch and release of your muscles.

A rest. Just lying down for a few minutes—not a few days—will help relieve the pain.

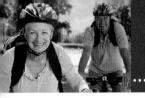

Cognitive behavioural therapy. Your pain is real but so is how your mind deals with it. Cognitive behavioural therapy is an effective intervention that counters subconscious mental and physical habits that can aggravate pain and worsen the disability that you may experience. It involves learning, analysis and activity sessions.

Serious help

Back surgery is a serious matter, one to consider only when all nonsurgical treatments have failed. Before your doctor recommends any of the following options, he will likely perform several diagnostic tests, such as X-rays, CT scans or MRI scans. That information, along with a physical examination and your account of your symptoms, will help you and the doctor decide what's best for you.

Discectomy. This surgery is considered when a nerve is squeezed and irritated by a prolapsed disc causing pain or weakness in the leg or loss of bladder control. The surgeon removes the bulging, gel-like centre of the disc, relieving pressure on the nerve.

Spinal fusion. This surgery is indicated when there are many months of severe back pain associated with inability to perform usual daily activities. There are a variety of surgical techniques to achieve the fusion, usually involving plates and screws to the spine combined with bone grafts. Consideration of fusion should include discussion of the long-term effects on your spine.

Artificial discs. Until recently, the only choice if a disc had a significant tear, which is a common cause of back pain, was fusing the two vertebrae, thus sandwiching the disc. Now surgeons can replace the damaged disc with a polyethylene or metal core that slides between the damaged plates. This procedure is not widely available. It should be considered only if there has been an inadequate response to an intensive physiotherapy program combined with an intensive cognitive behavioural program.

Minimally invasive back surgery. Techniques are being evolved to lessen the extent of tissue trauma that is caused by conventional surgery. The intent is to speed up the rehabilitation process for you and to improve long-term results from surgery.

Neurostimulation therapy. This technique involves the implanting of a device into the space between the spinal cord and spinal column—the epidural space—to help relieve pain in patients with nerve-related back pain. The device sends electrical signals that block the pain signals headed for the brain. You control the signals with a remote control, customising your pain therapy. A multicentre study of the therapy found that among patients with herniated, or ruptured, discs whose back surgeries did not relieve pain, 48 per cent had a 50 per cent improvement in leg pain, as well as significant improvement in back pain and function after 6 months.

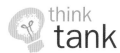

think
tank

'Because back pain sometimes
lingers and often recurs,
your goal should be to set
up an approach that you can
do yourself without endless
attendances with doctors
and therapists.'

—Dr Will Howard, FFPM (ANZCA), Director,
Pain Service, Austin Health, Melbourne

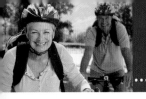

Neck pain

When a deadline looms, the relatives are coming for dinner or the kids scream, our neck muscles soak up tension like those superabsorbent paper towels, and the next thing we know we're in pain. It doesn't help that we also strain those neck muscles by hunching over our desks, computers and laptops all day. The result: up to 50 per cent of us suffer from neck pain every year. Tension and poor posture aren't the only causes, of course: some neck pain is the result of whiplash, worn joints or wear in the discs between the neck vertebrae.

The good news is that the most common neck pain, that caused by stress and bad posture, usually gets better in several days. As for other kinds of neck pain, new treatments can help.

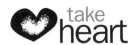

In a Flemish study, 79 per cent of patients with neck pain recovered by using **anti-inflammatories** or **muscle relaxants, heat** and **exercise**.

✅ Best first steps

You've been working long hours at your sewing machine, your desk, your workbench. Now your neck burns or refuses to budge when you try to turn your head. Here's what to try.

1. Nonprescription pain relievers.
Take paracetamol or an anti-inflammatory such as ibuprofen or naproxen. These drugs work best when taken regularly through the day according to the directions on the package. You can expect these nonprescription painkillers to reduce severe pain to a moderate level, or moderate pain to mild.

2. Apply ice and heat.
An ice pack in a towel, resting against your neck for 20 minutes several times a day, will numb the pain and reduce inflammation. You can also alternate the cold pack with a heat pack.

3. When to see the doctor.
Symptoms such as numbness or pain running down your shoulder, arms or legs are your signal to get to your doctor or an emergency

department straightaway. Your spinal cord may be at risk. You should also seek medical care if, at the same time as developing your neck pain, you have any change in your bladder or bowel habits, which may indicate that the neck pain is linked to a neurological problem. Neck pain with neurological problems is uncommon; most neck pain does not need a visit to the doctor.

Doctor's bag

Neck pain may be, well, a pain in the neck, but it's remarkably easy to treat. A 7-year international study on neck pain has found that your best options can be the simplest ones, like exercise. Here are the latest in recommended therapies.

Neck and shoulder exercises. A 10-week Danish study found that patients with neck pain who did specific strength-training exercises for neck and shoulder muscles three times per week had significantly less pain than patients who did general fitness training only. See a physiotherapist to be prescribed specific, individualised exercises to suit your neck condition.

Transcutaneous electrical nerve stimulation (TENS). This therapy involves placing electrodes on the affected areas. A stimulator sends mild electrical pulses through the skin: the stimulation of the underlying nerves may result in decreased pain signalling at the relay points in the spinal cord.

Injections. Injections may be used to treat muscles in spasm: the injection may use various agents including saline, local anaesthetic or Botox or even no drug at all—this is called dry needling. Other injections may be aimed at relieving pain from the facet joints of the cervical spine: this requires precise targeting, so a form of medical imaging is involved—a fluoroscope, or CT-scanner or ultrasound.

Spinal manual therapy. This therapy is performed by a chiropractor, osteopath or physiotherapist. It may provide immediate or short-term relief of neck pain. Up to 12 sessions may be required but usually only a few are needed. This involves the therapist using her hands or a device to move a spinal joint rhythmically and repetitively (mobilisation) or rapidly, often accompanied by a cracking or popping noise (manipulation). While these techniques are generally considered to be safe and well tolerated when delivered by a

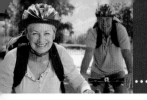

well-trained health professional, there are reports of severe adverse events such as stroke or neurological trauma occurring after manipulation and some mobilisation techniques. Feel free to mention any concerns you have and to discuss alternative treatments with your health professional.

Acupuncture. There is some limited evidence that acupuncture can help to relieve chronic neck pain. In one study, patients found acupuncture more effective than spinal injections. Several studies have shown acupuncture to be more effective than massage.

Your pain toolbox

No one wants to be a prisoner to pain or passive in the efforts to squelch it. However, you can do a lot on your own to drive away neck pain.

Posture. Slumping in your chair with your head forwards can strain your neck muscles. Every so often, check your position. Straighten up, push your chest forwards and make your shoulders square and your head in line with your shoulders. Better still, get up and walk around at regular intervals, adopting a good posture when you sit down again.

Instant relief

Neck pain is like a shrill note that doesn't end. Luckily, you can make moves to cut the pain in minutes. Here are a few suggestions.

Hot rice. Pour some uncooked rice into a small pillowcase, knot the top and warm it in the microwave for a perfect, pliable heating pad that can custom fit to your neck.

Hairdryer. For instant relief, blow a hairdryer on your neck (be careful not to burn yourself).

Neck stretches. Lower your chin towards your chest and allow the back of your neck to stretch briefly, also try tilting your ear towards your shoulder allowing the other side of your neck to stretch. Repeat on the other side.

Rest breaks. Lie down for a few minutes several times during the day to give your neck a break from holding up your head.

Creams. Creams or gels containing menthol, camphor or salicylate (an ingredient similar to aspirin) rubbed on your neck can temporarily relieve pain, and the light massage feels good, too.

Weightlessness. The sunscreen, the chequebook, the coloured markers for the kids: does it all really have to be in your handbag? The more you leave behind on the kitchen table, the more weight you'll take off your neck and shoulder muscles.

Ergonomics. Raise your computer screen so that your eyes are aimed at the top of the screen. You won't have to bend your neck to read the bottom.

Neck pillows. A contour pillow, curved to support your head and neck allows you to keep your head parallel to the bed. There are a number of contour pillows on the market. You can also fashion your own using an everyday pillow and a small towel. Roll the towel up so that you have a 5-centimetre-wide roll running across the width of your pillowcase, place this inside the pillowcase and adjust the position of the roll to fit the contour between your shoulder and ears.

On the phone. Don't cradle your phone between your ear and your shoulder. It hurts! Use headphones, especially if you are keyboarding at the same time.

Omega-3 fatty acids. Patients with neck pain who took 1200 milligrams of omega-3 fatty acids (the anti-inflammatory nutrients in oily fish) daily for an average of 75 days had a 60 per cent improvement in pain, according to one University of Pittsburgh study. Check with your doctor if taking more than 1000 milligrams per day as it can interact with other medications.

Serious help

Surgery is rarely needed for neck pain. However, it is sometimes done to address a compressed nerve root or compressed portion of the spinal cord. Currently we don't have the diagnostic processes or surgical answers to treat most conditions where pain, rather than neurologic function, is the indication for surgery. Here are some situations where cervical spinal procedures are indicated.

Facet joint denervation. Australian studies have demonstrated that in some situations after whiplash injuries, turning off the nerve supply to the facet joints at the back of the spine provides long-lasting pain relief. The nerves are turned off by placing a special needle close to the facet joint, using imaging by fluoroscopy to ensure accurate positioning, and heating or freezing the nerves.

Cervical spinal fusion. In patients whose spines are unstable to the extent that the spinal cord is at risk, fusion is performed using metal work and sometimes bone to stabilise the neck.

Spinal decompression. If abnormal bone formation, disc herniation or scar tissue is causing pressure on the spinal cord or a nerve root to the extent that neural function is threatened, the doctor may suggest removing part of a bone or disc in the neck to reduce the pressure.

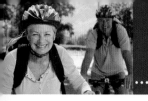

Shoulder pain

The shoulders of models, athletes and others with good posture can seem so regal, unburdened by the body's bulk. The complex shoulder joint forms the junction of the arm bone with the shoulder blade. Add the rotator cuff and four muscles surrounding the arm bone and now the cricketer can bowl a fast ball, the driver reach into the back seat, the ballerina circle her arms. However, all that wonderful movement is what can leave you feeling locked up as tight as a vice. Most shoulder pain stems from these culprits: tendinopathy, bursitis, injury, instability and arthritis.

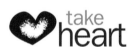

Ninety per cent of shoulder pain resolves with **rest, exercise** and **medication**.

Tendinopathy results from overuse of your shoulder tendons, the cords that connect muscle to bone. The tendons lodge their complaint, first with inflammation and pain, then by fraying like a used rope. Bursitis, often the sidekick of tendinopathy, is the inflammation of the bursae, small fluid-filled sacs around your joints that normally cushion your shoulder from the friction that all those reaching, swinging, circling movements cause.

Injuries, of course, are wild cards that can cause a bone in the shoulder joint to move, dislocating a joint. Although joints can be put back into place, dislocations can recur. Osteoarthritis, too, sneaks up on our shoulders, the result of wear and tear on the joint surface, or cartilage, that leads to joint inflammation, swelling, pain and stiffness.

Fortunately, the pain is rarely intractable. With rest, medication, exercise or, in some cases, surgery, you can throw the pain out.

✅ Best first steps

You reach for the jar of pickles on the top shelf and pain shoots through your shoulder like an arrow. Here are a few relieving moves.

1. Skip that movement.
Whatever move you were making when the pain struck, leave off for now. Skip any heavy lifting and tomorrow's game of tennis. Generally speaking, keeping your hand at shoulder level or below will help you sidestep pain.

2. Take an anti-inflammatory.

Take an anti-inflammatory such as ibuprofen or naproxen; there is no clear evidence to show that one of these agents is superior to any other. Follow the directions on the package—these drugs work best when taken regularly through the day. These painkillers can reduce severe pain to a moderate level, or moderate pain to mild.

3. Add ice.

Place an ice pack wrapped in a cloth on the aching spot for 15 minutes, then take it off for 15 minutes. Repeat several times. Ice tamps down swelling and numbs pain. For chronic conditions, moist heat may be a better choice.

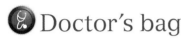 Doctor's bag

If pain and limitation of movement are not settling, your doctor may suggest investigations to clarify the source of the problem. An ultrasound may detect wear or calcium in the tendons; an X-ray may detect wear in the joint itself. She may also suggest an injection.

Tendon injections. Tendon pain is often treated with steroids. In recent times there have been studies looking at injections of your own blood that contains factors that promote healing pain.

Bursa and joint injections. Steroids have an accepted role when the bursa or joint is inflamed. Sodium hyaluronate injections also appear useful for adhesive capsulitis and osteoarthritis. Sodium hyaluronate is one of the natural components of joints. In Australia the Therapeutic Goods Administration has approved it for use in osteoarthritis in knees, so its use for shoulder conditions is what's called 'off label' for now.

Your pain toolbox

Soothing shoulder pain doesn't have to be complicated. In fact, you already possess the most important tools for recovery.

Exercise. After the initial pain has subsided, it's time to get moving (carefully) again; avoiding movement when your shoulders hurt sometimes just makes matters worse, reducing your range of motion and weakening your shoulder muscles. In fact, a Danish study found that therapeutic exercise was as effective as surgery for rotator cuff injuries.

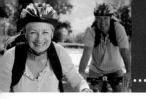

Relaxation. Throughout the day, remind yourself to release your shoulder muscles. Sit quietly for 10 minutes and relax your shoulders and neck, sitting with your arms comfortably supported. Every few hours, roll your shoulders forwards and back. In an Italian study, office workers who tried these tricks for 8 months saw their shoulder pain drop by 43 per cent.

Serious help

Shoulder pain that stems from repeated dislocation involving a torn ligament, rotator cuff tears or arthritis can require surgery. Here are several options.

Arthroscopic repair. Your shoulder's unstable, or your rotator cuff's torn. The doctor can insert an arthroscope, a tiny telescope about the size of a pencil, into your joint cavity through a 1.25 centimetre incision, repairing a tear with tiny instruments.

Shoulder replacement. If you have severe arthritis in your shoulder, your doctor may recommend shoulder replacement. Smaller incisions and longer-lasting materials make this procedure far more appealing than before. Your arthritic joint surfaces are replaced with a plastic socket and a metal ball attached to a porous stem that fits into your arm bone. The aim of the surgery is to reduce your pain; the trade-off is likely to be a reduced range of movement.

Instant relief

Your shoulder pain has been bothering you all day and you've had it. Try these moves for quick relief.

Deep breathing. Tension loves to lodge in shoulders. Lie on your back, your knees bent. Breathe in deeply, letting your stomach rise; exhale, noticing the release of tension in your shoulders (and elsewhere). Repeat for 3 minutes.

Soup can do the trick. While standing, hold a small soup can in the hand on the side with the painful shoulder. Bend over at the waist, letting your arms hang. Keeping your shoulder relaxed (let the arm just dangle), slowly trace a figure eight with the soup can. Repeat 10 to 20 times. Stop if you feel numbness, pain or tingling.

Pendulum swing. With one hand on a table for support, slowly swing the arm with the painful shoulder back and forth and around in a circle. It will release the shoulder muscles and keep them from stiffening.

Pillow padding. Lie on your good side, then use a pillow to support the arm with shoulder pain in front of your body. Lying on your back, place a pillow under the arm of the achy shoulder.

Chronic fatigue syndrome

For years, many people with medically unexplained chronic fatigue and pain were told by doctors, friends and family that their distressing complaints were imaginary (or 'all in their mind'). We now have good scientific research that rejects this stigmatising proposition. For example, scientists at the University of London have identified 88 genes that are expressed differently in people with chronic fatigue syndrome (CFS), formerly known as myalgic encephalomyelitis (ME).

A study by the US Centers for Disease Control and Prevention found that women with CFS have abnormally low morning levels of the stress hormone cortisol. People with CFS also have higher levels of a cytokine molecule (involved in cell-to-cell communication) called tumour necrosis factor alpha. This molecule has been linked to fatigue.

It seems that CFS sufferers may have suffered from an infection that has left their immune system chronically activated. A number of genes that are active in the immune response seem to be involved, particularly those involved in fighting infection.

Scientists suggest that one of the main problems in CFS sufferers resides in the hypothalamus, an almond-sized part of the brain that controls sleep. The hypothalamus also controls hormonal function, as well as autonomic function (the system that regulates many bodily systems such as blood pressure, sweating and bowel function).

In short, CFS is a complex condition (or conditions) that appears to be associated with genetics, stress hormones and the disordered operation of the immune system.

Although the challenges of your condition may leave you blue, recent follow-up studies suggest that some people improve with time. However, many remain with impaired physical and mental

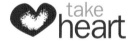

Moderate exercise **lessens fatigue** and **improves functioning** in 75 per cent of people with CFS.

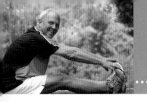

function for several years. Only when there is a clear understanding of the mechanisms of CFS will curative treatment become possible.

Best first steps

You are not lazy or trying to get attention. Rather, you have an illness that needs to be treated. Remember that, and take these first steps down the road to feeling better.

1. Get a diagnosis.

An obvious suggestion, of course, but you shouldn't assume that you have CFS. Chronic fatigue can be a symptom of other illnesses such as thyroid deficiency, anaemia, cancer, infection and autoimmune diseases, so it's important to rule out other health problems (be patient, as this may take a while). Forty per cent of people who report chronic fatigue turn out to have a treatable cause of this symptom. If your doctor isn't very familiar with treating chronic fatigue syndrome, or doesn't believe in it, look for someone else to investigate and treat you. You might like to check with the Australian Medical Association or the New Zealand Medical Association when conducting your search for a more knowledgeable physician.

2. Become educated.

Find out as much as you can about CFS and how it's likely to affect you. In addition to the information you get from your doctor, you can go to several websites, including these following ones.

Diagnosing CFS

There are no specific tests that definitively diagnose CFS. Most sufferers are young adults and, in addition to extreme fatigue, often experience sleep disturbance, difficulties with memory and concentration, headache, sore throat, tender lymph glands, aching muscles and joints and slow recovery from the effects of exercise. The presence of four or more of these symptoms for 6 months puts you in this category, provided other causes of fatigue have been ruled out. People with CFS are more likely than others in the community to recall episodes of traumatic childhood events (sexual, physical, emotional abuse; emotional and physical neglect).

Adding insult to injury, there are some doctors who will intimate that you are not really sick. This could be your signal to find another doctor.

- Bridges & Pathways Institute Incorporated, http://www.fibromyalgiaaustralia.com.au/
- ME/CFS Australia (Victoria), http://www.mecfs-vic.org.au/fibromyalgia
- Associated New Zealand ME Society (ANZMES), http://www.anzmes.org.nz/

These groups can steer you to the latest research, information on complementary therapies and support groups in your area.

3. Remind yourself to be patient.

Though you want relief *now*, impatience will only add to your stress and frustration. Working with your doctor to manage symptoms such as pain and sleeplessness may initially be a game of trial and error, as you figure out what medication and activity levels work best for you. Slowly, you will be able to put together a plan that tackles CFS from several directions, lessening your pain and increasing your energy.

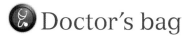 Doctor's bag

No one medication or therapy is the entire answer to CFS. Together, you and your doctor can put together a multipronged plan to address your particular symptoms. Here are some helpful treatments.

Drugs for disordered sleep patterns. Your doctor may recommend sedative medications, but only for short-term use, or the drugs gabapentin (Neurontin) or pregabalin (Lyrica). Neither of the latter medications is currently available on the Pharmaceutical Benefits Scheme in Australia or PHARMAC in New Zealand for CFS.

Drugs for pain. CFS can be associated with widespread pain and it then overlaps clinically with Fibromyalgia Syndrome, although they do appear to be different conditions. Your pain typically does not respond to nonsteroidal anti-inflammatory drugs, such as ibuprofen, but may be helped by drugs such as the opioid-like tramadol (Tramal), or by the pain-modifying drugs gabapentin (Neurontin), pregabalin (Lyrica) or by antidepressants such as duloxetine (Cymbalta).

Antidepressants. Drugs such as fluoxetine (Prozac) or sertraline (Zoloft) may elevate the mood of some CFS sufferers. Others such as duloxetine (Cymbalta) and milnaciprin (Savella) may relieve pain,

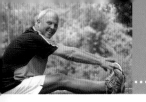

as well as improve mood. They can do this by boosting your brain levels of neurotransmitters serotonin, nordrenaline and dopamine, which tend to be low in this condition. The pain-relieving effects tend to occur at lower doses than those given for major depression.

Cognitive behavioural therapy (CBT). This therapy works by helping people change how they think about their circumstances and alter their behaviour. If you have CFS, it can be helpful to shift how you think about your fatigue—from the more hopeless 'I'll always be this way', for example, to the more optimistic but realistic 'I'm tired, but I'm working with my doctor on getting more energy'. A cognitive therapist can also help you learn to deal with stress and set appropriate limits on your activities. Patients usually meet with a therapist for hour-long sessions and do exercises, such as keeping a diary or trying out different behaviour between sessions.

Stimulant medications. Although sometimes prescribed for the purpose of improving ability to concentrate and remember, stimulant medications such as methylphenidate (Ritalin) have no place in CFS treatment.

Complementary and alternative medicine (CAM). Although they are popular, a recent systematic review concluded that there is extremely limited evidence for the effectiveness of CAM in relieving symptoms of CFS. However, the available studies were of low quality and showed quite a high risk of bias that precluded any firm conclusions being reached regarding their effectiveness. You might prefer to save your money until more rigorous trials have been conducted.

Your pain toolbox

Your doctor can't cure CFS, but there's plenty you can do on your own at home to feel better.

Good sleep habits. People with CFS often have disturbed sleep. The key to good *zzz*s is to create the best possible conditions for falling and staying asleep for 6 or so hours. Go to sleep and get up at the same time every day. Make sure your mattress is comfortable and that your bedroom is cool, dark and used only for sleeping and sex. Taking a warm bath or playing a relaxation tape or soothing music before bed can be great sleepy time rituals.

Moderate exercise. Working up a sweat is not the way to go when you first start exercising. At least five recent studies have found that a gradual increase in the amount of regular exercise will slowly lower levels of fatigue, reduce joint and muscle pain and build up your general physical condition. Commence with just 3 to 5 minutes of daily exercise, increasing by a few minutes a day until you can exercise for an hour and build up fitness. If you feel exhausted the day after a longer walk, rest for a day, then resume your program, but decrease your walking distance and time by a few minutes. Your doctor and/or physiotherapist can advise on other types of exercise that may suit you. Make sure you drink plenty of water (whether you're exercising or not), since many people with CFS tend to have low blood pressure.

An energy diary. Keep a record of when you feel most and least fatigued and what activities or people tend to tire you out. This can help you bump up the activities that boost your energy and weed out those that drain it.

Foods that supply sustained energy. No studies suggest that a healthy, low-fat diet helps CFS, but eating plenty of fruit, vegetables and whole grains while cutting back on sugary foods and drinks (as well as processed carbs such as white bread and baked goods) will keep you healthier and help you make the most of your energy. In some people, CFS is worsened by food intolerances, and if you suspect that your fatigue is linked to what you eat, it is worth investigating. A dietitian specialising in food allergy and intolerance can help you to identify the triggers.

Help from family and friends. Living with CFS can be tough emotionally and also logistically. You may not always have the energy to do all the things that need doing, so plan to enlist help. Begin by sharing information with loved ones about the condition and talking about the kinds of things you may need help with, from feeding the dog to shopping for groceries. If you can afford it, pay someone to help with household chores or looking after your children. Friendly neighbourhood teenagers might be a source of help at a modest cost.

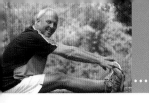

Fibromyalgia

Your muscles ache, you droop through the day, you have more stress than a taut rubber band and you've lost your keys again. Like most fibromyalgia sufferers, you find this syndrome both puzzling and painful. The pain can range from a persistent muscle ache to sharp shooting pain to tingling or burning, all at their worst in the morning.

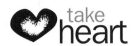

Exercise may sound like a drag, but according to researchers at the University of Tallahassee in Florida, women with fibromyalgia who participated in a **strength-training program** twice a week for 16 weeks **reduced their pain** by 39 per cent.

Fibromyalgia is pain in the muscles and fibrous tissues. The pain is widespread (felt on both sides of the body and both below and above the waist). It is not a form of arthritis because its pain centres deep within the muscles and the joints do not swell. As if the aching and soreness weren't enough, fibromyalgia is often accompanied by fatigue, headaches, sleep disturbances, mood change and a type of forgetfulness sometimes referred to as 'fibrofog'.

Although no one is certain what causes fibromyalgia, scientists are beginning to piece together the clues. There is no shortage of theories out there. However, we now recognise that the constellation of symptoms resemble those seen in sick or injured animals and are known as the stress or sickness response. There are many possible triggers of the response, and these include bodily trauma, infection and psychologically traumatic experiences. Usually stress responses turn themselves off when they are no longer needed, but it appears that in patients with fibromyalgia, they are no longer able to do so. We know that when they are prolonged, stress responses both consume a lot of energy and can be damaging to the body.

Researchers are now thinking along the lines that, because fibromyalgia is a general bodily system disturbance, singly prescribed modalities of treatment (for example, medications, acupuncture) result in little benefit. However, when combined with graded exercise, these modalities do tend to perform somewhat better.

✔ Best first steps

Having pain that never lets up is enough to wear anyone down. Here are some steps to consider taking in your search for pain relief.

1. Get a diagnosis.

Fibromyalgia can be a tough condition to diagnose. A series of tests will be ordered, but they will more than likely come back 'normal'. The sooner you see someone who knows its symptoms, the better. Don't settle for a doctor who tells you it's all in your mind, or doesn't have experience with fibromyalgia. If you're not satisfied, ask for a referral to a rheumatologist, a specialist who deals with musculoskeletal problems.

2. Dealing with flare-ups of pain.

Flare-ups are part of the usual pattern of chronic pain conditions. They will settle so don't let them overwhelm you. Nonprescription analgesic medications such as paracetamol or one of the nonsteroidal anti-inflammatory drugs (such as ibuprofen or naproxen) may be of little help. You might end up trying these medications in combination. High doses of either of them can land you in more trouble, with serious damage to your stomach or liver. Taking hot showers, applying hot packs and using an electric blanket are some readily available non-drug options.

3. Educate yourself.

Learn all you can about the condition and its treatment. Ask your doctor about the whole range of available drug and non-drug treatment options. Follow-up questions you might ask concern obtaining up-to-date information about the known benefits and risks of each form of treatment. The more you know about treatment possibilities, the better you will be able to manage this condition. You can go to several websites, including:

- Arthritis Australia Fibromyalgia: http://www.arthritisaustralia. com. au/images/stories/documents/info_sheets/2012/ Fibromyalgia.pdf
- Arthritis Foundation of South Africa: http://www.arthritis. org.za/
- Arthritis New Zealand: http://www.arthritis.org.nz/

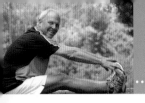

Doctor's bag

Since blood tests and X-rays are little help for diagnosing fibromyalgia, for years many doctors believed that it was a psychological condition. Thanks to advanced neuro-imaging techniques, many researchers are now convinced that the syndrome reflects a malfunction of the central nervous system. The information has led to new drugs and therapies.

Neuropathic analgesics. Pregabalin (Lyrica) was the first drug approved specifically to treat fibromyalgia pain. According to an 8-week trial at the University of Kentucky, almost half of the 529 patients studied had a 30 per cent reduction in pain, and 29 per cent had a 50 per cent reduction. What's more, many improved in the first week of treatment, sleeping better and feeling more energetic, a sure route to better spirits. Originally developed as an anti-epileptic drug, pregabalin appears to work by curbing the excitability of some of the nerve fibres in the central nervous system that are involved in generating pain.

Serotonin-noradrenaline reuptake inhibitors (SNRIs). Duloxetine (Cymbalta), part of a class of antidepressants known as SNRIs, was the second drug approved in the USA for fibromyalgia patients. In a study at the University of Cincinnati, duloxetine significantly reduced pain and improved function in more than half of the women treated,

Instant relief

Even when you're following doctor's orders, fibromyalgia pain doesn't necessarily behave. For those moments, here are suggestions for quick soothers.

A warm bath. Not only will a warm bath help soothe frazzled nerves, but it will relax tense muscles, always a good way to feel better.

Stretching. After your bath, light stretching exercises such as head circling and shoulder shrugs can help you feel good.

5 minutes of breathing deeply. Feeling stressed worsens your pain. 'To relax, stand up and take a deep breath through your nose', says Karen Moore

Schaefer, PhD, who conducts research into fibromyalgia at Temple University, Philadelphia USA. 'Then open your mouth as if you are going to kiss someone and gently blow out. Repeat several times.'

Sports creams. Sports creams or creams containing capsaicin, which is the stuff that makes chillies hot, rubbed on sore spots can temporarily relieve pain by a mechanism known as counter-irritation.

whether or not they suffered from depression. Duloxetine works by increasing levels of serotonin and noradrenaline, two neurotransmitters involved in the brain's ability to down-regulate the pain experience.

Opioid (opium-like) drugs. Strong opioids, such as codeine, oxycodone, morphine and hydromorphone are not helpful in fibromyalgia and can even worsen widespread pain. This phenomenon is called opioid-induced hyperalgesia. However, tramadol (Tramal) taken in combination with paracetamol has been found helpful in one study of 3 months' duration. Tramadol acts on a number of circuits within the brain that are involved in dampening down pain as well as reducing depression and anxiety.

Anti-Parkinson's disease drugs. Although classified as a drug for Parkinson's disease, a central nervous system disorder, pramipexole (Sifrol) helps relieve pain by affecting dopamine receptors. However, in Australia and New Zealand, pramipexole is not approved for indications other than Parkinson's disease.

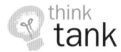

think
tank

'You should make regular exercise your most important therapeutic strategy.'

—John Quintner, FFPM (ANZCA), Consultant Physician in Rheumatology and Pain Medicine, Pain Medicine Unit, Fremantle Hospital, WA

Your pain toolbox

When it comes to a condition such as fibromyalgia, anything you can do to gain a sense of control will help. There are several approaches you can take on your own.

Exercise. This is the most important step you can take to lessen pain. Vigorous exercise boosts levels of the feel-good brain chemical serotonin, which reduces pain, boosts your mood, increases your energy and helps you sleep better. Swimming or water aerobics classes in a heated pool are good choices. The warm water relaxes muscles and eases pain. Walking and cycling are other easy, low-impact options. Begin with just 5 minutes of exercise per day and work up to at least an hour a day.

A coping plan. Planning for days when you feel your worst can save you a lot of disappointment. For instance, write down the tasks that have to be done each day, underlining the ones you feel can't be postponed. Then schedule when you'll do those, and plan to rest in between them. Write down names and phone numbers of people you can call on for help. Pace your activities on the days you feel well: be mindful of the temptation to overdo things or you'll hit a slump the next day.

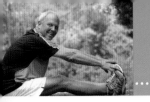

Chilling out. Take a warm bath or listen to your favourite music when you feel overcome by pain or fatigue. Dispense with too many deadlines, visits from relatives and screaming kids. You can tell the kids to tone it down, work with your employer to set more realistic deadlines and have your partner explain your situation to the relatives.

Yoga. Insert a few relaxing yoga moves into your day. A small Brazilian study showed that eight 50-minute weekly sessions of hatha yoga, a gentle style of yoga that includes deep breathing and stretching, lowered pain in people with fibromyalgia by as much as 30 per cent.

Cognitive behavioural therapy (CBT). A review of studies found that CBT, which helps patients shift their thought patterns and behaviours, worked well with other treatments to reduce fibromyalgia pain and improve coping and function. Stress management, relaxation, mindfulness and hypnosis come under this heading.

Acupuncture. A recent study at the Mayo Clinic found that acupuncture significantly reduced pain, fatigue and anxiety in fibromyalgia patients.

The sleepy side of fibromyalgia

Some scientists believe sleeplessness itself may be the main trigger that causes fibromyalgia. When you sleep deeply you release a hormone called somatomedin-C, essential for nerve and muscle health. However, fibromyalgia patients, robbed of deep sleep, release much lower levels of the hormone. Another hormone released during deep sleep is insulin growth factor (IGF). People with fibromyalgia produce much less of this hormone, too. The possibility that poor sleep may cause or worsen fibromyalgia suggests that more attention needs to be paid to help you rectify any sleep disturbance. So how can you go about this?

Establish and stick to a regular sleep schedule. Try to go to bed and arise at the same times each day. Tempting as it may be to sleep during the day when you feel exhausted, do not nap; it may diminish your chances of sleeping at night.

Perfect your bedroom. Plump the pillows, buy a fan, invest in a more comfortable mattress (if yours is more than 10 years old, it's time) and move the computer, the TV and the bonging grandfather clock elsewhere. Make your bedroom a shrine to sleep, not to extra office work or gruesome crime shows.

No caffeine after 11.00 am. Caffeine can be a powerful stimulant that keeps you awake, and its effects may not wear off for up to 10 hours.

Lupus

Lupus can be a baffling disease affecting any part of the body—skin, joints or major organs. It is a disturbance of the immune system: instead of going about its usual function of clearing up debris from day-to-day cell turnover, it becomes super efficient and attacks the cells of various parts of the body as if they were foreign invaders.

Lupus can mimic other diseases. One person may have fatigue and fever, another joint pain and symptoms involving the heart, kidney or central nervous system. Some may complain of widespread pain. Other symptoms include a telltale butterfly-shaped rash on the face, a variety of skin rashes worsened by sun exposure, mouth ulcers, hair loss, cold and blue fingers and toes, chest pain (pleurisy), dry eyes, easy bruising, mood changes such as anxiety or depression and memory loss. Symptoms can often come and go for no good reason. This pattern can happen over a number of years.

There are four varieties of lupus. One, discoid lupus erythematosus (DLE), affects only the skin. Another, drug-induced lupus, is caused by any of approximately 38 drugs, most commonly procainamide, a heart medication; hydralazine, a blood pressure medication or quinidine, also for the heart. This variety usually disappears once the medication is stopped. A third, lupus in newborns, usually disappears within 6 months. The most common variety, systemic lupus erythematosus (SLE), is also the most serious. Effective drug treatment for SLE is available and, together with lifestyle changes, a good quality of life is achievable for most sufferers.

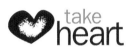

CellCept has been an **important advance** in the treatment of lupus-related kidney disease.

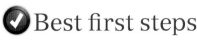 Best first steps

Even if you're not certain you have lupus, you know for sure that you're in pain. Here are some initial steps you can take to feel better.

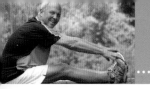

1. Pain relief with nonprescription medications.
Anti-inflammatories such as ibuprofen or naproxen can both ease pain and reduce inflammation. Be sure to follow the dosage information that appears on the package. Paracetamol can ease pain but does not reduce inflammation.

2. Get a diagnosis.
It's tough to do much until you know what you're dealing with. If you have a rash, fever, sore joints and feel tired all the time, make an appointment with your doctor for a thorough check-up.

Doctor's bag

Because of the variability and unpredictability of its symptoms, SLE may be difficult to diagnose. Before your doctor (GP or specialist physician) offers treatment, she'll get your medical history, your family history and the drugs you may be taking for other conditions. You would expect to undergo a thorough physical examination and to be sent for diagnostic screening tests. Other tests might need to be undertaken to detect any damage to your kidneys, liver, lungs or heart. Skin and liver biopsies might be necessary in individual cases. When the diagnosis is made, you will in all likelihood be offered one or more of the following treatment options.

Prescription NSAIDs. If nonprescription painkillers such as ibuprofen aren't relieving your pain, your doctor may offer stronger prescription versions. However, NSAIDs can cause stomach problems, as well as increase your risk of heart attacks and strokes. They can also affect the kidneys and increase blood pressure readings.

Corticosteroids. People with SLE commonly take a corticosteroid called prednisolone, taken by mouth. This drug acts quickly to lessen pain as well as joint stiffness and swelling. Once you respond, your doctor will likely lower the dose slowly until you can stop taking it. When taken over the long term, corticosteroids can have a number of side effects, such as weight gain, easy bruising and osteoporosis (bone thinning). Corticosteroid creams can be helpful for skin rashes and injectable preparations are injected into joints to reduce inflammation.

Antimalarial drugs. Hydroxychloroquine (Plaquenil) is an anti-malarial drug that has been found useful in treating both the arthritis and skin rashes of SLE. It may also prevent attacks of pleurisy (inflamed membranes around the lungs) that are not infre-quent occurrences associated with general flare-ups of the disease.

Chemotherapy drugs. Some of these drugs are in the category of disease-modifying antirheumatic drugs (DMARDs), which means that they can slow the progression of SLE, as well as reduce the dose of corticosteroids that would otherwise be necessary to control the disease process. These drugs include methotrexate (Methoblastin, Ledertrexate) and azathioprine (Imuran). A newer drug is called mycophenolate mofetil (CellCept), which was originally used to pre-vent rejection of transplanted organs. An immune-system suppressor, CellCept appears particularly helpful in the treatment of kidney com-plications, but it can also be used to reduce overall disease activity and your daily dose of corticosteroids.

Your pain toolbox

Lupus has the power to put you in a really bad mood. One way to take care of it is to take care of yourself by eating well, exercising and getting plenty of sleep. These tips will also help.

Sunscreen. Sunlight can trigger a flare-up and skin rashes. When-ever you are exposed to the sun make sure that you wear a sunscreen with a 30 SPF or higher to protect you from UVB rays. To protect you from UVA rays, something such as Parsol 1789 is a necessary ingredient. Cover yourself up by wearing a hat, long pants and a long-sleeved shirt whenever you're in the sun.

Instant relief

Lupus means *wolf* in Latin. You may have, right at home, an arsenal to keep the beast from your door.

Rest. When the fatigue that so often accompanies lupus hits you, you may be tempted to fight through it, but don't. Rest up for short periods during the day; your body will thank you. There's no virtue in struggling through exhaustion. Don't nap, as this will risk spoiling your night-time sleep.

Lavender baths. Draw a warm bath, especially before bedtime, and sprinkle in several drops of lavender essential oil. Lavender has a relaxing and sedative effect.

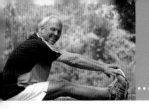

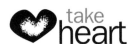
take **heart**

Combining **lifestyle changes** with **self-education** about lupus will pay off for you.

Good sleep habits. Whether your sleepless nights are caused by pain or not, you can boost the chances of uninterrupted slumber by going to bed and getting up at the same time each day. Don't make your bed a business or entertainment centre if you expect to get any sleep there.

Exercise. The more you can exercise, the greater will be the benefit to you. These benefits might include: improved sleep pattern; improved mood; a lessened risk of a flare-up and stronger bones. The last one is particularly important to combat the bone-thinning effects of corticosteroid therapy. Consider including a physiotherapist on your team to help you devise a regimen that you can routinely follow. This will combine muscle stretching, weight training and general aerobic exercise such as walking.

A smoke-free life. If you smoke tobacco, quit. Smoking adds to your risk of developing cardiovascular disease and lung cancer.

Good fat. Numerous animal studies have found a decrease in lupus symptoms when the animals were fed a low-energy, low-fat diet. However, good fats, such as those in fish, seem to reduce symptoms. Scale back the steak dinners and put fish on the menu, along with vegetables and whole grains. Fatty fish such as salmon contain omega-3 fatty acids that help decrease inflammation.

Water. Hydration is important in lupus, but avoid drinks containing caffeine or sugar, both of which are suspected to worsen symptoms.

Oranges. According to a Japanese study over 4 years, vitamin C supplementation lessened the risk of activation of SLE. Other studies suggest that fibre is beneficial too. Add more vitamin-C rich foods, such as citrus fruits and berries to your diet. Unlike juice, the whole fruit provides the benefits of fibre as well as vitamin C.

Me time. One of the most important things you can do is have time each day that is for you. Set aside half an hour to read, listen to music or meditate. It will help you manage stress, keep your perspective and remember that there is much in life for you to enjoy.

Recognising when a flare-up is coming. Being alert to flare-ups can help you take steps early to manage them. Signs to watch for include feeling really tired, dizziness, increased pain, a rash or fever or a headache. Such indications should signal you to get more rest, avoid the sun and stay calm.

Cancer pain

Many people with cancer are worried that they will get severe pain. Pain can be due to the cancer itself or from pressure on organs or bones. It can also be the result of treatment, including surgery, chemotherapy and radiotherapy. However, while half of all cancer patients and 70 per cent of people with advanced cancer will experience some pain during the course of their disease, this pain can be well controlled.

Fortunately, there are now many different ways that cancer pain can be treated. It is important that you tell your GP or oncologist if you have any pain. Cancer pain is unlikely to go away with time so you must talk to your doctor sooner rather than later. Your doctor may need to do an examination or investigations to determine the cause of the pain. The treatment plan will be specific to the type of pain, taking into consideration your medications and any other medical problems. You need to take the medications as prescribed. Let your doctor know if the medicine is not working or is causing side effects. You should not put up with pain—constant pain can make you miserable and less able to deal with your cancer treatment.

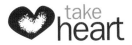

According to the World Health Organization, cancer pain can be **satisfactorily controlled** in up to 90 per cent of cases.

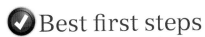 Best first steps

1. Tell your doctor you have pain.
You can work with your doctor to control the pain and maintain your quality of life. Before your appointment, write some notes about the pain—where it is, what words describe it (dull, throbbing, sharp, aching), what makes it worse and what makes it better. You may be asked to rate your pain on a scale from 0 (no pain) to 10 (worst pain you can imagine).

2. Take the prescribed medicines.
Once your doctor has decided on the best type of medicine, then it's essential that you take it as prescribed. Don't be alarmed if your

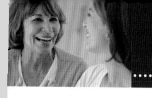

doctor suggests morphine or similar drugs (see 'Morphine myths' page 137). Morphine and other opioids are very useful drugs that are usually well tolerated when used properly. If you are nervous about morphine, discuss it with your doctor at the time that it is suggested.

3. Treat 'breakthrough' pain.

Breakthrough pain is a burst of pain that can occur at any time, although it is often related to specific activities, such as showering. Often the regular medicine that you have been prescribed isn't enough to control this pain. You will also have been given a fast-acting medicine. You can take this extra 'top-up' or 'breakthrough' medicine whenever you are uncomfortable. If you persistently get pain during certain tasks, then it is a good idea to take the breakthrough medication before this activity.

4. Avoid constipation.

Strong pain-relieving medicine (such as morphine) usually causes constipation. Most people need to start taking laxatives when they start taking the morphine. Talk with your pharmacist or doctor about which are the best medicines to take. It is good to have a lot of water and fibre in your diet, but in most cases this will not be enough to prevent constipation. Exercise can help, too.

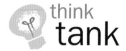

think tank

'Never skip a dose or wait for the pain to get worse before taking your medicine. The longer you wait, the harder it is to get the pain back under control.'

—Dr Juli Moran, MBBS, FRACP, PGDipPallMed, Director of Palliative Care Services, Austin Health, Melbourne

Doctor's bag

Depending on the cause of your pain, more than one pain-relieving medicine may be needed. With the medicines that your doctor has asked you to take regularly it is important that you take them when you are meant to, even if your pain is better at the time. Here are some medicines that may be prescribed.

Paracetamol. Even when you are taking stronger pain relief, it is important to continue the paracetamol. Do not take more tablets than your pharmacist or doctor recommend.

Opioids. Opioid (narcotic) medicines have been used to treat cancer pain for many years. In Australia, they include morphine (MS Contin, Kapanol), oxycodone (Oxycontin), fentanyl (Durogesic), hydromorphone (Jurnista) and methadone (Physeptone). They come in the form of tablets, patches or injections. Most regular opioids are available in a slow-release form so they need to be taken only once or twice a day. You'll usually also be prescribed a smaller dose of fast-acting opioid that is used to 'top up' your regular opioid when you have breakthrough pain.

Anti-inflammatories. Drugs such as ibuprofen and naproxen work particularly well for bone and muscle pain and are often used before or with opioids.

Steroids. Including prednisolone and dexamethasone, these drugs are often used for cancer pain, but they are also effective for reduced energy or appetite. They are often used in combination with other pain-relieving medications.

Adjuvant medications. These are medications that were developed for other conditions. The two most commonly used are antidepressants and anticonvulsants. These drugs act differently from paracetamol, opioids and anti-inflammatories and can be a good addition to these medications if pain proves hard to control.

Morphine myths

Many people are reluctant to take morphine due to a variety of fears. Some of these are based on the way that morphine was used many years ago; others are simply not true. The most common fear is that patients will get addicted to morphine. This is not possible. When morphine is used to relieve cancer pain it is not addictive. If you need to increase your dose of morphine then it is usually because the pain has become worse. Another common belief is that morphine is used only 'at the end' and a suggestion that you need morphine means that you are close to death. While this may have been true in the past, morphine is now used for a wide variety of reasons because it is such a good pain reliever. It is given to people with broken bones and after operations, to children and to women having babies. Another fear from the past is that morphine hastens death. These days, we use much smaller doses of morphine and increase the doses slowly and safely so it is very unlikely to make people die more quickly; in fact, the converse may be true—if pain relief is poor, your body may not cope as well with cancer. Some people won't use morphine as they want to 'save it for later', in case the pain gets worse and the morphine won't work anymore. This is unnecessary as morphine is started at very low doses and can be increased to high levels, meaning that there will always be relief for your pain. The same applies to the other opioids, such as oxycodone, fentanyl, methadone and hydromorphone, which are used for cancer pain.

In particular, they are used for pain due to damage to nerves (neuropathic pain). Antidepressants include amitriptyline (Endep) and nortriptyline (Allegron), while anticonvulsants include gabapentin, pregabalin (Lyrica), carbamazepine (Tegretol) and clonazepam (Rivotril, Paxamation). These drugs can cause a range of side effects, so are often started at low doses and increased slowly. Side effects such as drowsiness will often improve after a few days.

Your pain toolbox

Once you and your doctor have worked out a plan for managing your pain, try some of these self-care measures.

A pain diary. If your pain is not well controlled a pain diary will help you record information to discuss with your doctor. This includes when you got the pain, how severe it was (rate it from 0 to 10), how long it lasted, what made it worse and what made it better. In particular, if you take a dose of breakthrough medication, it is important to note how long it took to work and how well it relieved your pain.

Wellness and supportive care. There are many non-drug therapies that have been found to help with pain. Allied health interventions

Instant relief

You'll have days when the pain medication just won't work quickly enough, when you simply want the pain to vanish *now*. Here are some tips for chasing pain out the door fast.

Heat. Some people find that heat packs can give pain relief. Make sure that the packs are not too hot. Don't use them on areas where you have recently had radiotherapy. Avoid areas where sensation or circulation are abnormal. Never apply heat over an opioid patch: it can cause a dangerous rise in blood level of the opioid.

Cold. Others find that cold packs (wrapped in a cloth to avoid ice-burns) can reduce inflammation and pain, including nerve pain. Use for 10 to 20 minutes at a time. Again, you should avoid areas of abnormal sensation or circulation.

Progressive muscle relaxation. Lie down and go through your body, clenching and then relaxing each group of muscles, eventually focusing on those that are causing you pain. This can help relax tight muscles and may reduce pain.

Distraction. Take your thoughts off pain by listening to a favourite CD, watching a movie or talking to an entertaining friend.

Visualisation. Imagine locking your pain in a closet, making it walk the plank or dousing its fire with cool, refreshing water. Images such as these can diminish pain.

such as physiotherapy and music therapy have clearly been shown to improve pain in certain situations. Complementary approaches such as massage, acupuncture and relaxation therapy have also been shown to help with specific types of pain. Talk to your doctor or your oncologist; many new cancer centres have palliative care or supportive care and wellness programs that offer a range of treatments that have been shown by research to be effective.

Exercise. Exercise has many benefits even when you have cancer, including for pain and mood. However, if you are constantly tired, then it is more important to find ways to save your energy, such as asking others to help, or doing jobs in small stages.

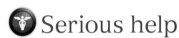 Serious help

In some cases, when drugs can't control the pain, the doctors will treat your cancer itself to help improve the pain. Your doctor may try one of the following measures.

Surgery. Surgery can reduce the size of the tumour, or move it, to relieve pressure on the nerves and other body parts.

Chemotherapy. Chemotherapy can work by reducing the tumour size, which relieves pain from the tumour itself, or by reducing pressure on adjacent structures if that is causing the pain.

Radiotherapy. This can significantly reduce tumour growth and pain in selected areas. It is particularly useful for cancer in the bones.

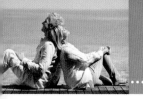

Burning mouth syndrome

You wake up, and without warning your tongue, lips or huge sections of your mouth are burning, as though you'd just taken a gulp of scalding coffee. The pain starts slowly, building through the day, reaching its peak in the evening. Sometimes the pain subsides at night, but other times it can be so severe it keeps you awake. For some people, the pain can be constant. For others, it can blink on and off like a light in fog. Burning mouth syndrome can persist for months, even years.

Burning mouth syndrome (BMS) is as odd a condition as it sounds. Its symptoms include burning, tingling, dryness, a taste of metal or bitterness in your mouth and depression. No one knows what causes this syndrome, which affects up to 15 per cent of people worldwide. Because it appears most frequently in postmenopausal women and in seven times as many women as men, shifting hormones may play a part. It may be linked to other conditions: anxiety and depression; other chronic pain conditions such as headaches; high blood glucose levels and deficiency in B vitamins, iron and zinc. Dry mouth or other oral conditions such as thrush, a yeast infection or geographic tongue (in which patches of the normal bumps, or papillae, on the tongue are missing, giving the tongue a maplike look) may also play a part. Some studies suggest BMS may be caused when certain nerves affecting taste are out of whack.

Because the syndrome has many possible causes and symptoms, treatment has to be customised. In general, it's treated as other nerve pain conditions are, with low doses of drugs used for anxiety, depression and convulsions because these medications also decrease pain signalling.

✔ Best first steps

Besides pain, your first reaction to burning mouth syndrome will probably be bewilderment. However, as with any painful condition, there are steps you can take straightaway to help.

1. See your doctor or dentist for a diagnosis and treatment.
Don't delay. If you have persistent pain or burning in your tongue, lips, gums and any areas in your mouth, take a trip to your doctor or dentist. He or she should rule out other conditions, such as diabetes, Sjögren's syndrome (an autoimmune disease affecting the body's moisture-producing glands), or a thyroid problem, that could be causing your symptoms. Treating those conditions may clear up BMS.

2. Read the fine print on drug inserts.
Some medications, including blood pressure drugs, can cause a burning or dry mouth. Your doctor may be able to switch you to a different drug.

🩺 Doctor's bag

When it comes to BMS, your doctor's bag is brimming with effective treatments. The most important step is figuring out what triggered your symptoms. Your doctor (or dentist) will begin by examining your mouth, taking your medical history and asking about your oral routine. She may also give you blood and allergy tests. Depending on what she finds, she may then refer you to a specialist (an oral medicine or pain specialist) who can help relieve your symptoms. Below are some of the treatments that may help you.

🕐 Instant relief

On days when that burning sensation inside your mouth becomes too much, or your burning tongue is burning you up, try these steps for an on-the-spot reprieve.

Ice. Chewing on ice chips may help dull the pain.

Sugarless gum. Chewing it increases saliva production, which helps wash away food and neutralises acid.

Drink more fluids. Drinking water won't affect your pain, but it will help ease the feeling of a dry mouth.

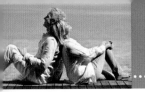

Anti-anxicty drugs. If your doctor or dental specialist suspects a nerve-related cause he may prescribe benzodiazepines, such as clonazepam (Rivotril).

Tricyclic antidepressants. In low doses, tricyclic antidepressants such as amitriptyline (Endep) appear to lower pain.

Anticonvulsants. Although there is mixed evidence about the usefulness of gabapentin or pregabalin (Lyrica), these anticonvulsant medications reduce pain in some patients.

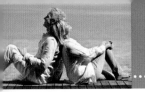 Your pain toolbox

A few nonmedical strategies may help you get relief.

Vitamin supplements. You may lack certain nutrients such as B_1, B_2, B_6, zinc and iron, something a blood test can confirm. Ask your doctor whether you need supplements or changes in your diet and a multivitamin.

Mouth TLC. Skip the astringent mouthwash and potentially irritating toothpaste (including cinnamon and mint flavours), and brush with a milder toothpaste or bicarbonate of soda instead. If you smoke, quit. Lay off acidic drinks, such as orange juice and coffee, as well as alcohol. Skip the spicy food, too.

Denture adjustments. If you have loose or irritating dentures, now's the time to get them adjusted.

Dental pain

We've all seen the cartoons: the kid with an ice bag clamped to his cheek, trapped in purgatory by an aching tooth, the father getting ready to dive in with pliers. Dental pain can be a relentless yowl that we want to stop now, or a mild but steady pain that dogs us all day long. The first step in stamping out dental pain is finding its cause.

Toothache has many possible causes, but the most common are trauma, a cracked tooth, cavities or erosion, hypersensitivity or pain that shows up in your teeth but starts elsewhere, such as in infected ears or sinuses, known as referred pain. A toothache can also be a sign of a heart problem, such as angina (chest pain caused by restricted blood flow) or a heart attack. It can also be caused by gum disease, which damages the gums and bones that support the teeth.

'Many people avoid the dentist in the hope that the pain will go away', says Mina Borromeo BDSc, PhD, University of Melbourne. 'But if tackled at the very start of symptoms, people can avoid a lot of pain and trouble. People don't realise that dental pain can trigger significant health issues if left untreated. An abscess can cause swellings that are potentially life threatening.'

Unfortunately, most of us associate trips to the dentist with more pain: the drilling, the poking, the injections. For lasting relief, however, a trip to our dentist is the smartest strategy (and may be less painful than you think). You can also take soothing steps at home to address dental pain and prevent a reprise.

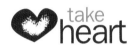 take heart

Eliminating sports drinks, lemonade and **soft drinks** from your diet can provide a significant reduction in the erosion of your dental enamel.

✅ Best first steps

The longer you wait to treat tooth pain, the larger the problem becomes. So, it's important to act fast.

1. Call the dentist and tell the receptionist you're in pain.
Most people would rather give a speech than go to a dentist, but only a dentist can diagnose and treat your pain. You want the receptionist

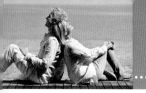

to know you have a toothache so she gives you an appointment as soon as possible. If they cannot give you an urgent appointment when you are in pain then find another dentist who can.

2. 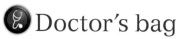Take an anti-inflammatory.

If you can't reach your dentist immediately, take ibuprofen or paracetamol. Take regularly but do not exceed the maximum recommended dosage. Just remember that dousing pain won't keep your dental problem from getting worse—you should still make that dental appointment. If you have any swelling in your mouth or face you should see a dentist immediately. The swelling can have dangerous consequences if left untreated.

Doctor's bag

Put the pliers away. Your dentist will diagnose the cause of your pain and likely offer one of the following treatments.

Cavity filling. These holes in your teeth, caused by decay, can pack a wallop of pain. Your doctor will remove the decayed part of the tooth, replacing it with a filling or, if the decay is more extensive, a crown. (Prevention is key here: brush and floss regularly so that the sweet dessert or biscuit you love isn't turned into an acidic etching solution by the bacteria in your mouth.)

Periodontal cleaning. You'll know that you have the beginning of gum disease (gingivitis) if your gums bleed when you brush. It does not mean you should stop brushing your teeth, but rather that you should get your gums checked by the dentist. Let gingivitis go and it becomes periodontitis, a condition in which gums pull away from the teeth, allowing in bacteria that can eventually erode the

Instant relief

When it hurts a lot and you're waiting for your dentist appointment, try these tricks.

Room-temperature food and drinks. Sweet, hot or cold food and drinks can get your dental nerves jangling.

Salt water. Give yourself a warm saltwater rinse to decrease swelling.

Aloe vera. Fresh aloe vera gel, squeezed from a cut leaf and then applied around the tooth, can temporarily ease pain.

supporting bone. Although you may have no pain with gingivitis, your gums may be swollen and tender. Periodontitis will inflame your gums, and you may feel pain as a tooth loosens or from a resulting abscess, a localised infection. Gum disease is the result of poor dental hygiene, that is, not brushing often or thoroughly enough and thinking that using a toothpick to prise popcorn out of your teeth every once in a while is a substitute for daily flossing. Your first step is a professional periodontal cleaning, attacking the pockets of bacteria, plaque and tartar, which is the hardened build-up of food, salt, minerals and other debris on your teeth at the gum line. In severe cases, the dentist will cut away unhealthy tissue. You may also have to take a course of antibiotics.

Damage repair. Sometimes pain originates from a tooth that you have cracked, chipped or broken. The damage extends into the centre of the tooth, alerting the nerve. Ouch. The pain may come and go or be constant as a wailing siren. Or it may hurt only when you bite down. Depending on the extent of the damage, your dentist will fill, file or crown your tooth. Or she may have to do a root canal or extraction.

Toothpaste for sensitive teeth. Sometimes dentine, the middle part of your tooth, is exposed, usually because of receding gums or gum disease, although overenthusiastic brushing, abrasive toothpaste, an acidic diet or bulimia can cause it, too. Your dentist may switch you to desensitising toothpaste with fluoride that will help prevent decay. Most contain a potassium salt that helps soothe the excited nerves in sensitive teeth.

Your pain toolbox

Although your dentist is your best bet for stopping dental pain, you can help prevent it in the first place. Below are a few suggestions for staying pain-free.

A good brushing. The best way to prevent dental pain from gum disease, cavities or hypersensitivity is to brush at least twice per day with a soft toothbrush and floss your teeth and gums at least once per day.

Tooth-protecting foods. Cheese, meats and nuts help protect teeth enamel by neutralising acids. Stock up on fruit, vegetables and whole

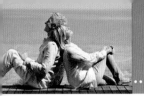

grains as well. Crunchy foods such as carrots, celery and apples can help dislodge food debris that contributes to tooth decay, gum disease and bad breath. Avoid sugary drinks and foods, including dried fruit, and acidic ones, such as pickles and lemons; all partner with bacteria to create acid in your mouth, the fast route to more cavities, gum disease and sensitivity.

Sugarless gum. This helps root out food stuck between your teeth and increases your saliva, which helps neutralise decay-causing acids.

Serious help

Sometimes damage to the tooth and gums is severe enough to require more complicated repair. Below are several options.

Root canal. If the decay has damaged the nerve or pulp, your dentist may perform a root canal, removing the nerve in the centre of the tooth. The root is sealed and the tooth capped. And your pain is gone. You may also need a root canal if a tooth break damages the nerve. Despite what you've heard, a root canal procedure is not the worst thing you can experience, especially if you put yourself in the hands of a good specialist, called an endodontist.

Surgery for broken teeth. If your tooth has split vertically, you may need minor surgery to remove the root or to have the tooth removed. Cracks that begin at the tooth's root may also require extraction. If a fracture happens below the gum line, you may need surgery to remove enough bone so that the crown can fit over the root.

Gum disease surgery. If your gum disease has caused deep pockets between your teeth and gums, your dentist may recommend surgery to reduce their size. Or you may need surgery to remove diseased tissue, reshape the bone or create new gum and bone tissue to replace what you have lost. Again, you should put yourself in the hands of a good gum specialist, called a periodontist.

Sinusitis

Your head and eyes ache, and your nose is stuffed more tightly than an olive. Even your teeth hurt. In other words, you have sinusitis—inflammation of the mucous membranes in your sinus cavities, which are the passages around your nose and throat. It usually begins after a cold or allergy attack. Fluid builds, blocking your sinus cavity, and pretty soon the whole nasal drainage system is clogged. If the build-up of fluids lasts longer than a week or so, it may lead to bacterial infection.

Other conditions can predispose you to sinusitis: a nasal blockage from an injury can impede the normal drainage of mucus; or complications from other diseases such as cystic fibrosis or HIV.

A British study found that antibiotics or steroid nasal sprays were no better at speeding recovery of mild sinusitis than no medicine at all. Such findings press home this point: the power to banish the pain lies in your hands. Taking a dose of paracetamol or ibuprofen, inhaling steam or flushing out your sinuses with salt water—all simple to do at home—may provide all the relief you need.

✅ Best first steps

A mild sinus infection may run its course in about 2 weeks. Use these strategies below to move it along. But if you have sinusitis accompanied by a fever of more than 38.5°C or severe pain, see your doctor. In very rare cases, untreated sinusitis, especially in children, can cause meningitis and vision problems. You should also see your doctor if the sinusitis fails to clear up within 2 weeks or is recurrent.

1. Steam your sinuses.
Steam from a humidifier will help the mucus flow, clearing out your sinuses. Or fill a bowl with steaming water, add a few drops of eucalyptus oil, throw a towel over your head and the bowl and breathe deeply.

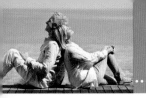

2. Take a decongestant.

Nonprescription decongestants can help relieve pressure and dry up excess mucus. Some combine decongestants and pain relievers. Don't use a decongestant nasal spray for more than 3 days: the blood vessels become accustomed to the presence of the decongestant. When you stop the spray, rebound swelling and blockage occurs and can persist.

Doctor's bag

To assess the cause of your sinusitis, your doctor may look into the nostrils. She may also order an MRI or a CT scan, tests that can identify inflammation and obstructions. Or she may ask for allergy tests or cultures of throat and sinus to determine if bacteria's behind the infection. Treatments include:

Ipratropium (Atrovent) spray. This spray reduces nasal mucus production without causing the tendency to rebound congestion.

Antibiotics. If your infection is caused by bacteria, your doctor will prescribe a prolonged course of antibiotics until you are without symptoms for at least a week.

Corticosteroids. To relieve the painful swelling of chronic sinusitis, your doctor may prescribe steroid sprays. These ease inflammation, lowering mucus production and shrinking swollen nasal passages and sinuses so they can drain. Sometimes, if there are nasal polyps or severe swelling in the nostrils, the steroids need to be taken as tablets.

Allergy medications or injections. If the sinusitis is caused by allergies, your doctor may prescribe allergy medications or injections that stimulate antibodies to block whatever is causing your reaction.

Instant relief

Want pain relief faster than you can say gesundheit? Try a few of these suggestions.

A warm, wet towel against your face. The steam will help open your sinus passages.

Horseradish. Mix 1 teaspoon of horseradish with ½ teaspoon of olive oil and 1 tablespoon of lemon juice. Eat ¼ teaspoon at a time until you feel your sinuses begin to drain. Have it with some bread or rice if it's too strong for your mouth or stomach.

Jumping jacks. Exercise stimulates the flow of mucus.

Your pain toolbox

In addition to steam baths and decongestants, here are other strategies at your disposal.

A saltwater rinse. Washing out your sinuses with a nonprescription saline solution or one you make yourself can clear out mucus and moisten mucous membranes. It can counter that annoying post-nasal drip. To make your own saline solution, mix one teaspoon of table salt in 475 millilitres of water at body temperature. Fill a bulb syringe, available from pharmacies, insert into a nostril, and squeeze *gently*. Repeat on the other side. Wait a few minutes and blow your nose *gently*. Repeat several times per day. Alternatively, use a neti pot, a small teapot-like container with a tapered tip at the spout. It's important to keep these devices clean, use clean water (boil it beforehand if the water supply is dubious) and be gentle when inserting the fluid and when blowing your nose—despite the temptation to blow the blockage away.

Liquids. Drink plenty of water or herbal tea throughout the day; it can help thin the mucus. Pass up the cocktails; alcohol can increase the swelling in your sinuses.

Antihistamines. If your sinusitis stems from allergies, nonprescription antihistamines can help prevent nasal congestion. Ask advice from the pharmacist.

Nonprescription mucus thinners. Guaifenesin, which is available in a range of nonprescription preparations, can thin mucus, speeding sinus drainage.

 Serious help

When chronic sinusitis persists despite medicines and home treatment, you may require surgery. The blockage could come if the septum has a bone spur or if the septum itself is crooked. You might also have a cyst or polyp blocking your sinuses. Your doctor may refer you to an otolaryngologist—an ear-nose-throat (ENT) doctor, who performs sinus surgery. The surgeon, using local or general anaesthesia, can straighten the septum, remove the blockages or make drainage holes in your sinuses.

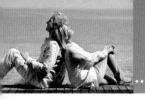

Temporomandibular disorder (TMD)

If you have pain that has been there some time when you open and close your mouth, you may have temporomandibular disorder (TMD), a name that sounds more like a dinosaur than a dental condition. TMD exhibits itself in a broad range of painful symptoms. The condition can be acute (lasting less than 3 months) or chronic (lasting more than 3 to 6 months). The best analogy is to think of a sprained ankle: the jaw joint and the surrounding muscles have been 'sprained'.

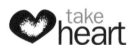

Ninety per cent of TMD patients **improve on their own** or with minimal treatment, such as anti-inflammatories, softer food and a mouthguard.

The disorder, which affects almost one in six people, most of them women, causes pain and tenderness in the joint by each ear where the lower jawbone joins the temporal bone at the side of the head and the muscles around the joint and face. It's the busiest joint in the body. Its flexibility allows your jaw to move up and down, side to side and backwards and forwards. When the joint is out of sorts you may experience not only pain and tenderness but earaches, ringing in the ears, headaches, toothaches, nausea, dizziness and difficulty opening your mouth as far as you used to.

It is not clear what causes TMD but it can be related to an injury to your jaw, such as in a car accident or from a sporting injury; stress; prolonged jaw opening, such as a long dental appointment or may have no apparent cause. You can also develop TMD if the joint's cartilage is damaged by osteoarthritis or rheumatoid arthritis, the joint is injured or the joint muscles give out from clenching and grinding. Of course, the cause determines how your doctor or dentist will address your pain. Treatment often includes a trip to the dentist, with the simplest treatment often the most effective. Surgery to the jaw joint is not indicated for TMD.

✔ Best first steps

When pain stabs you in the jaw or face, it's hard to think about much else. To attack the pain, follow these steps.

1. Quit jawing so much.
You don't have to stop talking, but it will help if you protect your jaw when yawning so you don't overstretch and strain the muscles. Your dentist can teach you how to protect your jaw and muscles when yawning. Eat softer foods, cut food into smaller pieces and skip the chewing gum, crunchy toast and raw vegetables such as carrots. In other words, give your jaw muscles a break. This is not forever but just while you are experiencing the painful episodes. You should not be scared to return to eating these food in consultation with your dentist.

2. Take anti-inflammatories.
Taking nonprescription anti-inflammatories, such as ibuprofen and naproxen, every 4 to 6 hours can bring relief.

3. Find out what's driving your pain.
If you have ongoing symptoms of TMD, see your doctor or a dentist who specialises in TMD.

🩺 Doctor's bag

Your doctor or dentist will first ask about you and your pain: how long have you had it? What kind of pain is it? Have you had an injury

🕐 Instant relief

When pain stabs you in the jaw, try these tricks.

A warm, wet face washer. Hold a warm, not hot, face washer on your cheek for 15 minutes to relax your jaw. If you are at work you can even hold a coffee cup with warm water against the side of your face for a few minutes to give you some relief. Repeat as needed. A warm shower first thing in the morning is also useful and can provide great relief.

Deep breathing. Breathe in deeply through your nose and release the air slowly through your mouth for 10 breaths. If your TMD is related to stress, doing this exercise several times a day will help relax you *and* your jaw.

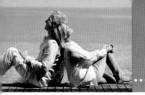

to your jaw or recent dental treatment? Dental work can sometimes trigger TMD pain because procedures can place too much pressure on the jaw or because the mouth has to be wide open for long periods. Your dentist will also check your teeth and bite and listen for clicking noises when you move your jaw. He'll even inquire about your stress levels. Once he knows the answers, he may suggest one or several of the following.

Mouthguard. If your pain does not resolve after 4 to 6 weeks with simple home management tools then your dentist may prescribe a plastic bite guard (also called a mouth splint) for a short time. It slips over your top or bottom teeth and is worn only at night. The teeth may feel a bit sore when you take the splint out in the morning but this should not last more than an hour. The splint should not restrict your jaw movement in any way and should be regularly adjusted and checked by your dentist. Under no circumstances should your teeth or bite be adjusted in an attempt to correct your bite. There is no evidence for this as an effective management tool and it causes irreversible changes to your teeth. Studies regarding the effectiveness or mechanisms of the action of splints vary but splints can be quite useful for some people. The best analogy of a mouth splint is like a crutch or walking stick that is used when you sprain your ankle. If the splint is uncomfortable or causes your pain levels to increase then you must stop using it and contact your dentist immediately.

Tricyclic antidepressants. It is well recognised that low-dose tricyclic antidepressant medications, such as amitriptyline (Endep), can be beneficial. They work by increasing levels of neurotransmitters, which reduce pain signalling.

Your pain toolbox

Many cases of TMD are caused by stress-related clenching, posture problems or a prolonged dental procedure. Attack those problems with these approaches.

Stretching your jaw and neck muscles. This can help them relax and can relieve pain. Try the following exercises several times a day. Hold your mouth open and insert two or three stacked fingers, resting them on your upper teeth without letting them touch your bottom ones. Hold for 5 to 10 seconds. Close and relax. Repeat four to five times.

Next, bend your head to one side as if trying to touch your ear to your shoulder. Hold for 5 seconds, then repeat on the other side. Then lean your head forwards, holding for 5 seconds. Repeat several times.

Good posture. Poor posture can contribute to TMD pain. When you're seated, remind yourself to have an arch in your lower back. Then, keeping your chin level, lift your breastbone and shift your shoulder blades back and down. At night, avoid sleeping on one side only, or on your stomach, which strains jaw and neck muscles. If possible, sleep on your back; you're less likely to clench and grind.

Cognitive behavioural therapy. If your TMD is stress related, your doctor may refer you to a therapist who can help you look at what's causing your tension and help you develop skills to deal with stress more effectively. The therapist may also teach you relaxation techniques such as deep breathing or progressive muscle relaxation, in which you tighten and relax different sets of muscles throughout your body. Researchers at the University of Washington in Seattle found that TMD pain improved by 50 per cent in people who had just four sessions of cognitive behavioural therapy.

Speaking up at the dentist's surgery. If you face a lengthy dental procedure that requires you to hold your mouth open wide for a long period or in which the dentist will apply a lot of pressure, ask your dentist if he can work in shorter sessions, allowing you to relax your jaw in between.

Serious help

Most of the time fairly simple, reversible approaches clear up TMD. Surgical repair, joint replacement and Botox are not recommended by Australian experts. It's better for you to put up with the pain of TMD than to have an unhelpful procedure that can cause you harm.

Pain management strategy. Ask your dentist to refer you to a pain management centre. There you will be taught techniques to help manage your pain on a day-to-day basis.

Surgery. Surgery to the temporomandibular joint and associated muscles is not indicated unless there is evidence of serious disease such as a tumour or anklyosis. In this case your dentist should refer you to an oral and maxillofacial surgeon.

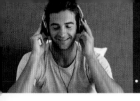

Diverticulitis

You have a monster pain on the left side of your abdomen that comes on suddenly, reminding you of the birth scene from the movie *Alien*. Or you have mild pain that fluctuates or gets worse by the day. Your stomach feels tender, you're feverish and nauseated. You may have the runs, or else be constipated. If any of that sounds familiar, you may have diverticulitis, an infection of tiny pouches called *diverticula* that form in the lining of the colon.

Many of us develop these pouches after age 40, without even knowing it, probably because the elasticity and strength of the bowel wall change. Here's how it happens: weak spots in the lower colon are created by increased intestinal wall tension from hard stools and strained bowel movements. At some point they give way, creating marble-sized pouches that protrude through the colon wall. Real trouble starts if some of the pockets become infected, resulting in diverticulitis—usually an acute illness, coming on over a few hours or days, but occasionally it can be more chronic.

Researchers at the University of Maryland Medical Center say that they are seeing increasing numbers of younger patients who have diverticular disease as a result of obesity.

'Once you have an episode, you are much more likely to have another one', says Eamonn Quigley, MD, professor of medicine and human physiology at University College Cork in Ireland. 'There's a suggestion that chronic symptoms may be related to a low-grade inflammation.'

If your case is mild, antibiotics, rest and a temporary soft diet usually do the trick. However, a severe infection can require hospitalisation, even surgery.

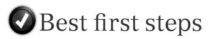 Best first steps

Diverticulitis can be serious, even life threatening. So, once you feel unexplained abdominal pain, it's important to act fast. Here's how.

1. Have your symptoms checked.

If you have pain on your left side, fever, nausea, constipation or diarrhoea, you should call your doctor. Less common symptoms include vomiting, bloating, rectal bleeding and excessive or painful urination.

2. Calm your diet.

Until you can see your doctor, eat only soft foods and drink plenty of liquids.

3. Take nonprescription pain relief.

Paracetamol or ibuprofen may temporarily decrease your pain.

Doctor's bag

The first thing your doctor will do is determine if your pain is related to diverticular disease. Diverticulitis symptoms can resemble other conditions, such as appendicitis, pelvic inflammatory disease or irritable bowel syndrome. Your doctor will check you for stomach tenderness and will probably give you a blood test to check your white blood cell count, a sign of infection. She may also order a CT scan of the abdomen.

Antibiotics. Once the doctor confirms that you have diverticulitis and that the infection is mild, she may send you home with a prescription for antibiotics to take for 7 to 10 days. She may also suggest you continue nonprescription pain relievers.

A liquid diet. To give your colon a rest, she may put you on a liquid diet for a few days.

Instant relief

Nobody wants to live with abdominal pain for even a minute. Here are ways to get relief fast.

A heating pad. A British study found that heat therapy can reduce abdominal pain for up to an hour. Lie down with a hot-water bottle or heating pad next to your skin, and you'll feel not only comforted but in less pain.

A warm bath. For the same reason, a warm bath may help, and will also relax you.

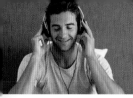

Your pain toolbox

What you do about your pain besides taking a nonprescription pain reliever depends in part on how serious the pain is. Here are a few suggestions.

Soft foods. Along with antibiotics, your doctor will want you to pamper your colon with liquids and/or soft foods that will keep your stool soft, easing any pressure on your intestinal walls.

Better bathroom habits. If you let stool sit around in your body, it dries up; dry stool is harder to eliminate, putting pressure on the infected pockets. Make it a habit to head to the toilet within half an hour after each meal, especially if you're prone to constipation.

More fibre, eventually. Once you're healed, the memory of pain will motivate you to keep diverticulitis at bay. The best way: get more fibre from foods such as whole grains, fruit and vegetables. Aim for at least 25 to 30 grams a day.

Liquids. Sip more fluids as you add fibre; fibre without liquid will dry your stools. When you're in pain, avoid coffee, tea and alcohol, which can act as irritants.

Exercise. After you're healed, work up to 30 minutes of exercise per day. Exercise helps keep your colon functioning normally and also reduces pressure.

Serious help

In rare cases, your doctor may suggest the following.

Hospitalisation. If your infection is severe and your doctor believes you're at risk of serious complications, she may put you on intravenous antibiotics in the hospital.

Surgery. If you have a fistula, an abnormal passageway in your intestine or you have had repeated attacks of diverticulitis, the doctor may suggest surgery to remove the diseased part of your colon.

Haemorrhoids

The word haemorrhoid tends to raise a snicker, but the resulting pain, inflammation, and itching are no laughing matter. Haemorrhoids, also called piles, which affect half of us by the time we're 50, are inflamed veins inside or outside the anus. They're often triggered by too much straining on the toilet, but they can also crop up because of constipation, which of course leads to straining, or diarrhoea. Getting older and heavier, or being pregnant, increases the risk as well. Simply sitting on the toilet too long (finishing that last chapter, for instance) can make haemorrhoids worse.

The most common sign of haemorrhoids is bright red blood on your toilet paper or stools, or in the toilet water. You may also feel aching or itching after a bowel movement. External haemorrhoids can cause a painful swelling or a hard lump around the anus. They can be painful, itch, crack and bleed. An internal haemorrhoid may slip through the anus, causing a painful condition called a protruding or prolapsed haemorrhoid. Sometimes a protruding haemorrhoid can be pushed back inside, but surgery may be necessary.

Fortunately, most haemorrhoids and the related pain will clear up with a little care: warm baths, cleaning well after each bowel movement, applying ice, eating more fibre, drinking more water and exercising regularly all help prevent them. However, you may need to see a doctor for medication or even surgery if the haemorrhoids persist. Remember, not all bleeding is haemorrhoidal. If you see obvious blood in the toilet bowl, especially if you are over forty, discuss it with your doctor. *Bowel cancer and other serious bowel conditions also cause bleeding, so don't take any chances!*

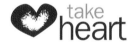

Most people treated for haemorrhoids won't ever need to undergo surgery.

✅ Best first steps

Initially, you can make a few changes that should clear up your haemorrhoids and relieve your pain.

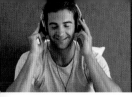

1. Try anti-inflammatories.
Nonprescription pain relievers such as ibuprofen, paracetamol or aspirin taken every 4 to 6 hours can temporarily tackle your pain and inflammation.

2. Apply soothing agents.
A variety of soothing creams, ointments and suppositories is available. Ask your pharmacist for advice on what to use.

Doctor's bag

If your haemorrhoids and their pain persist, there's plenty a doctor can do. He'll start by giving you a rectal examination and maybe even a sigmoidoscopy or colonoscopy—procedures that use a lighted instrument to examine your colon—to rule out more serious conditions. Once he's certain you have haemorrhoids, he may suggest one of the following remedies.

Rubber band ligation. In this office procedure, the doctor places two to three rubber bands around the haemorrhoid to cut off the blood supply, which causes the haemorrhoid to fall off.

Sclerotherapy. Your doctor will inject a chemical (phenol, a caustic compound in almond oil) or saline solution around the haemorrhoid, causing it to shrink and drop off within 10 days.

Infrared coagulation. The doctor applies a 1–2-second burst of infrared light to the haemorrhoid, causing its blood to clot, shrinking the haemorrhoid.

Your pain toolbox

Perhaps the most important way to deal with the pain of haemorrhoids is to prevent them in the first place. The following will help you.

Fibre. Eat at least 25 to 30 grams a day of stool-softening fibre, including whole grains, fruit and vegetables. (Half a cup of baked beans has 6 grams; an apple or half a cup of spinach, about 3 grams.) The softer your stool, the less you'll have to strain when you go to the toilet. If you can't down so much fibre, consider taking a fibre supplement such as psyllium husks (Metamucil).

Berries. Some research suggests these nuggets of inflammation-fighting flavonoids may reduce the pain, bleeding, itching and even recurrence of haemorrhoids. Tuck into about ¾ cup of blackberries, raspberries, blueberries, strawberries or cherries every day.

Fluids. Drink plenty of water or other fluids every day, especially as you add more fibre, to prevent dry stool.

Prompt evacuation. Postponing a bowel movement allows stool to dry up making it harder to pass, leading to straining when you finally go.

Exercise. Exercising just 10 to 15 minutes per day accomplishes two things: first, it speeds up the movement of food through your large intestine. By raising your breathing and heart rate, it also stimulates your intestinal muscles, speeding up the exit of your stools.

Moist toilet paper. After you go, wipe up with moist towelettes or wet toilet paper. It causes less friction than dry toilet paper.

Serious help

If your haemorrhoids are severe or extensive, your doctor may recommend one of the following.

Haemorrhoidectomy. If other treatments don't work or if you have very large haemorrhoids, your doctor may suggest having a haemorrhoidectomy, which surgically removes them.

Stapling. The process of stapling around the haemorrhoid works by cutting off its blood supply. Although stapling involves less recovery pain and itching than surgery, it also carries greater risk that the haemorrhoids will reappear or protrude through the anus.

Instant relief

For fast relief, try the following in addition to a haemorrhoid cream or pad.

Warm baths or sitz baths. Soaking for 10 minutes in warm water several times per day will relax your muscles and soothe and clean the painful, irritated haemorrhoids and rectum. Adding Epsom salts to your bath pulls fluid from the blood trapped in the haemorrhoid, reducing swelling and inflammation.

Ice packs. Putting an ice pack on your bottom will help decrease the swelling.

Cold black tea. Soak a cloth in the brew and apply the compress to the painful area. Tea's astringent properties reduce inflammation.

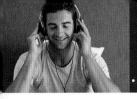

Heartburn and GORD

Heartburn hurts. You have a heavy meal, and later that night you feel a fierce burn in your oesophagus, low in your chest. That's the result of acid spilling back through the opening between your oesophagus and stomach. A band of muscle near the bottom of your oesophagus called the oesophageal sphincter relaxes to let food and water through, and then it squeezes shut again. However, if the muscle weakens or relaxes too often, you suffer from acid backup. The pain may get worse when you bend over, lie down, eat and when you go to bed.

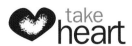

Lose 5 to 7 kilograms, say Boston University researchers, and you can **cut your risk of heartburn** by 40 per cent.

Most people have an occasional bout of heartburn. However, if you have heartburn more than twice a week, you likely have GORD, or chronic gastro-oesophageal reflux disease. Over time, the ongoing backflow of acid can inflame and damage the oesophagus, leading to a condition called reflux oesophagitis. In a small number of cases, this damage can lead to further changes in the cells. This is called Barrett's oesophagus, which occasionally leads to cancer. About 5 to 10 per cent of GORD patients may develop Barrett's and, very occasionally, Barrett's may lead to cancer. So while GORD is usually just a nuisance problem, it can occasionally be more serious.

You're at increased risk of developing heartburn if you're overweight or have one of a number of conditions including hiatal hernia (a protrusion of part of your stomach into your chest), pregnancy, asthma, diabetes, stomach blockage and connective tissue disorders, such as scleroderma. Certain medications, such as opioids and some antidepressants and antihistamines, can also slow the emptying of your stomach, which can cause acid backup.

Fortunately, most heartburn is mild and easily treated, perhaps with nonprescription medications and a few changes in diet. People who suffer heartburn several times per week may need prescription medications, and some may even need surgery.

✔ Best first steps

When you first feel the burn, it's time to take action.

1. Don't eat another bite.

If you suspect your pain is from heartburn, don't eat while you still have pain. Overeating increases the pressure on the oesophageal sphincter, upping the risk that it will loosen and let more acid spill back into the oesophagus.

2. Take an antacid.

Nonprescription brands such as Mylanta or Gaviscon work by neutralising stomach acid. However, take too many, and, over time, they can lead to diarrhoea or constipation. Make sure your antacid contains magnesium hydroxide and aluminium hydroxide, which together will help your bowels function normally. Don't take aspirin or ibuprofen, which can make your heartburn worse.

3. Get medical answers.

If you still have heartburn after the antacid wears off or if the pain wakes you up at night, call your doctor. You should also call if you have heartburn several times per week. Note: don't confuse heartburn with angina (heart pain). Angina can sometimes mimic heartburn, but it usually causes a feeling of fullness, pressure or squeezing in the chest, and may lead to a heart attack if not treated. *So, if you're not sure it's heartburn, immediately seek medical advice or call an ambulance if it persists.*

🩺 Doctor's bag

If your doctor suspects GORD, he'll confirm the diagnosis by looking at your oesophagus with a small lighted instrument called an endoscope and, in some instances, by monitoring the pH level of the oesophagus using a tiny probe passed through a nostril. He also may prescribe one of the following.

Acid blockers. Also called H2-receptor blockers, medications such as Tagamet and Zantac work by reducing acid levels in the stomach, so there's less acid to back up into the oesophagus. Half-strength versions of these drugs are available without a prescription. If you know which foods or situations make your heartburn flare

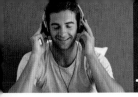

up, taking an H2-receptor blocker in advance may help you avoid discomfort better than taking an antacid afterwards.

Proton-pump inhibitors. These drugs reduce the amount of acid your stomach makes by about 90 per cent. Doctors often prescribe PPIs (such as Losec, Nexium, Pariet, Somac or Zoton) if H2-blockers don't bring relief or if you have severe heartburn or oesophageal damage. After about 8 weeks, your doctor should check to see if your oesophagus is healing and cut back on your dosage if it is. Some of these drugs are also now available without a prescription in a lower dose. There is a suggestion, however, that long-term use of PPIs may result in bone thinning (osteoporosis) and that some, at least, may interact with the blood thinner clopidogrel (Plavix, Isocover), which is often used by heart patients. If you're pregnant, talk to your doctor before taking either acid inhibitors or blockers.

Your pain toolbox

You can decrease the pain by taking a number of short- and long-term steps, including:

Weight loss. Extra weight pushes your stomach up, which causes acid to flow back into the oesophagus.

Portion control. Large meals can trigger heartburn by stretching the stomach, which in turn stretches the oesophageal band.

Quitting smoking. Smoking may increase stomach acid, and it's been linked to increased risk of oesophageal cancer.

Instant relief

Relieve the burning pronto with these strategies.

Water. Drinking a glass of water will wash acid back where it belongs.

Gum. All the saliva you produce when you chew gum helps wash acid away. Research has shown that chewing can help neutralise stomach acids for up to 3 hours after a meal.

Sitting up. Lying down will increase your pain.

A loose belt. Uncinching will lessen the pressure on your oesophageal sphincter and let gravity do its work.

High-fibre diet. A recent study found that people who ate fibre regularly—from whole grains, fruit, vegetables, beans—were 20 per cent less likely to have GORD, regardless of what they weighed.

A food diary. Although little evidence links heartburn to specific foods, doctors often recommend giving up chocolate, spicy and fatty foods and coffee to lessen symptoms. Keep track of which foods and drinks seem to spur your pain, and drop them from your menu.

Better work hours. People who work the night shift are three times more likely to have GI symptoms, including heartburn, possibly because of disturbed sleep and eating schedules, and stress.

Early dinners. Like to get to bed by 10.30 pm? Then make sure you've eaten dinner by 6.30 pm. According to a Japanese study of 441 people with GORD, those who hit the hay within 3 hours of dinnertime were seven and a half times more likely to have acid indigestion than people who went to bed 4 or more hours after eating.

Raising the bed. Although some GORD patients with night-time reflux find relief by placing the head of the bed on bricks or blocks, it is generally not necessary if the other measures are taken.

Becoming a lefty sleeper. Lying on your left side reduces the pressure on the muscular valve between your stomach and oesophagus. In a study published in the *Journal of Clinical Gastroenterology,* right-side sleepers had double the reflux of people who slept on their left side.

Serious help

People who have GORD but who don't respond to nonsurgical therapies may need more serious measures.

Laparoscopic surgery. This minimally invasive surgery tightens the oesophageal sphincter or repairs any protrusion through that band of muscle tissue.

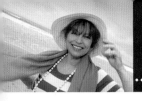

Inflammatory bowel disease

Is that a Clydesdale stomping around in your gut? The cramps, pain, bleeding and diarrhoea may mean you have inflammatory bowel disease (IBD), a catch-all name for disorders that inflame the intestines. Two of the most common are Crohn's disease and ulcerative colitis.

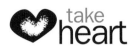
take
heart

According to a recent Canadian study, a majority of patients with **ulcerative colitis** improved or went into remission **after 6 weeks** of taking probiotics, supplements of beneficial bacteria that live in our guts.

Crohn's disease causes ulcers throughout the small and large intestines, and sometimes around the rectum. Its inflammation may spread to other neighbouring organs such as the bladder or vagina through an abnormal connection called a fistula. Other calling cards of Crohn's are reduced appetite and weight loss. Although no cure yet exists for Crohn's, medications can help relieve the pain and sometimes even cause a remission.

Ulcerative colitis affects only the lining of the large intestine and the rectum. There are several types. Ulcerative proctitis, signalled by rectal bleeding and a feeling of urgency even when you don't have to go, is confined to the rectum. Left-sided colitis (only from the rectum up the left side of the sigmoid and descending colon) and pancolitis, which affects the whole colon, have symptoms of bloody diarrhoea, cramps and weight loss. No one knows what causes IBD, although doctors are coming closer to an answer. A recent study found that mice without a certain signalling molecule that helps gut cells deal with stress developed IBD. When that molecule is missing, the intestine can grow inflamed, allowing bacteria to invade the intestinal wall, which, in turn, activates the immune system. The result: chronic inflammation. Heredity plays a part as well.

Although IBD can be serious, even life threatening, if not controlled with medications and lifestyle changes, both the disease and its pain can be treated.

✅ Best first steps

The discomfort and pain of IBD will make you want to act fast, and you should. Here's what to do.

1. Take a pain reliever.
Most people with IBD occasionally get mild diarrhoea, wind and cramping. If your pain is mild, you can try taking paracetamol every 4 to 6 hours to help relieve inflammation and discomfort.

2. Try a fibre supplement.
Taking psyllium husks (Metamucil) can help relieve mild diarrhoea and cramping by adding bulk to your stool. Check with your doctor first, and start slowly to see how your body will react. Don't take antidiarrhoeal medications, such as loperamide (Imodium, Gastrostop) or diphenoxylate with atropine (Lofenoxal, Lomotil), unless you have seen your doctor and she has recommended it.

3. Call your doctor's surgery.
If the change in your bowels lasts more than 10 days, see your doctor. If you have stomach pain, blood in your stools or fever, go sooner.

🩺 Doctor's bag

Your doctor will do a series of tests including some of the following: blood tests to check for low red blood cell count and infection; a stool sample to test for blood and infection; X-rays with a barium enema, which uses a white liquid that displays the ulcers on imaging; a sigmoidoscopy and/or a colonoscopy, both tests that allow the doctor to look with a lighted instrument at part or all of your colon; computerised tomography (CT), a kind of X-ray that provides more detail than a standard X-ray. Once he determines that you have IBD, he may prescribe several of the following.

Anti-inflammatory drugs. There is a range of options, including sulfasalazine (Salazopyrin), aminosalicylates and corticosteroids (Prednisone). You may have to try several, depending on what other medications you take and what kind of side effects and relief each provides.

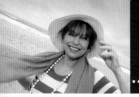

Immune-system suppressors. These are used for more severe disease, reducing inflammation by suppressing the immune system. Some, such as azathioprine (Imuran) and 6-mercaptopurine (Puri-Nethol), can take 3 to 6 months to take effect, so they're often taken with corticosteroids for more immediate relief.

Biologics. These new compounds are antibodies against molecules involved in sustaining the inflammation that is the hallmark of IBD. Infliximab (Remicade) and adalimumab (Humira) are examples of this class of compound, which can be very effective in controlling acute flare-ups.

Antibiotics. Your doctor may prescribe antibiotics, particularly if you have Crohn's disease. They can help heal abscesses, reduce harmful bacteria and stifle the part of the immune system that is kicking up inflammation.

Probiotics. These 'good bacteria' may have a role in some patients with IBD, especially ulcerative colitis as suggested in a recent Canadian study. We are likely to hear a lot more about probiotics, prebiotics and symbiotics in treating gut diseases in the coming years, so watch this space!

Your pain toolbox

You are a partner with your doctor in treating the symptoms of your disease. Here are steps you can take to diminish your pain and discomfort.

Instant relief

To anyone with IBD, the idea of relief in any form is welcome, but faster trumps slower. Here are some tips for speedy relief.

Deep breathing. Part of the distress of IBD is the anxiety it arouses. Take a few minutes to do deep breathing exercises. Not only do they lower stress, but they help relax your stomach muscles, which can help with cramping and make your bowel movements more normal. Simply spend a few minutes in your garden, or do something else that relaxes you.

Warm soothing baths. Soaking in the tub will also lower stress. The warm water will help relax your muscles.

Stop smoking. There is evidence that stopping smoking reduces recurrence of Crohn's disease.

Fibre supplements and laxatives. Diarrhoea medicines such as fibre supplements or loperamide (Imodium) and laxatives for constipation can be helpful, depending on your symptoms. Check with your doctor before taking them, because even these drugs may be too strong for your system or they may make your symptoms worse.

A low-fibre diet, for now. To an intestine affected by IBD, bran (the outer shell of many grains) may feel as irritating as whiskers on a soft cheek. Your best bet: when your IBD flares up, skip whole grains, nuts, seeds and corn, which can increase cramps. When the bout is over, slowly reintroduce these foods; they are important for the production of butyrate, a fatty acid that quells inflammation and helps keep the intestinal lining healthy.

Exercise. Regular exercise can lower stress, lift your spirits and help make your bowel movements more normal. A Canadian study found that walking for 30 minutes just three times per week improved symptoms and overall wellbeing.

Hypnosis. It's worth asking your doctor if this therapy might help. Some evidence suggests that hypnosis, in which a therapist guides you to a relaxed state, can reduce stomach pain and bloating.

Avoiding fatty foods, lactose and sweets. Obviously, food affects your gut, some helpfully and some not. It may pay to avoid fatty foods, which can make you crampy and gassy. Researchers at the Newcastle University in England found that people with ulcerative colitis who ate the most red meat, such as steaks, and processed meats, such as sausage, were five times more likely to have painful relapses than those who ate few of these foods. You may also want to avoid lactose, which can increase diarrhoea, cramps and gas. Look for low-lactose dairy products and make sure you take a calcium and vitamin D supplement, as people with IBD are at greater risk of osteoporosis. If you crave something sweet, pass on the lollies and instead have some fresh fruit, which can cut your risk of IBD. Several studies have shown that refined sugary desserts triple the odds of developing Crohn's disease and ulcerative colitis.

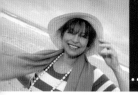

Cutting down on soft drinks and chocolate. Dutch researchers found that indulging in these doubled the risk of both ulcerative colitis and Crohn's disease in 688 people with IBD and in 616 people without it.

Serious help

If medications and other lifestyle changes don't relieve your symptoms, you may need one of the following.

Strictureplasty. This procedure for Crohn's disease involves widening a part of the intestine that has narrowed because of built-up scar tissue.

Laparoscopic surgery. This minimally invasive surgery for Crohn's disease allows a surgeon to remove the damaged part of the intestine, reconnecting the other healthy sections.

Ileoanal anastomosis. After removing the entire colon the surgeon creates a pouch from the end of your small intestine and connects it to your anus. It eliminates ulcerative colitis, but you will have frequent soft bowel movements throughout the day as a result. Fortunately, medical therapy is usually successful in controlling ulcerative colitis, so surgery is rarely needed.

Irritable bowel syndrome

At the mercy of unpredictable bowels? That's something that most people don't want even to whisper about. However, the cramping, diarrhoea and/or constipation, bloating, gassiness of irritable bowel syndrome (IBS) are miseries that afflict one in five people, and twice as many women as men. Fewer than half of those people affected ever seek treatment.

What causes irritable bowel syndrome isn't certain, although it clearly involves a conversation between the brain and the gut: people with high levels of anxiety and stress are much more likely to develop IBS than their more sanguine counterparts. One related factor may be altered levels of serotonin, a neurotransmitter affecting mood that's found in both the GI tract and the brain.

In some people, however, irritable bowel syndrome appears to stem from a stomach infection that revs up the immune system, which never returns to a normal state, stoking a chronic inflammatory response. 'What's new is the idea that with IBS you can have a low grade of immune dysfunction or inflammation, which leads to the activation of the pain pathways', says Eamonn Quigley, MD, professor of medicine and human physiology at University College Cork in Ireland. People with IBS may also have particularly sensitive stomachs that overreact to stress and certain foods such as milk, chocolate or alcohol. Because more women than men have IBS, hormonal changes may also be involved. Genes may play a part as well.

Although irritable bowel syndrome can be disabling, it doesn't damage the intestinal tract or lead to other serious diseases. In most cases of IBS, simple changes in diet and stress management can diminish the pain.

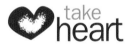
take heart

In studies involving 644 IBS patients, **hypnosis relieved symptoms** in 80 per cent.

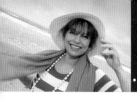

✅ Best first steps

IBS symptoms aren't pleasant companions. Here are some ways to start getting relief.

1. Talk to your doctor.

Some change in bowel habits can be a sign of a more serious disease, such as colon cancer or inflammatory bowel disease. Talk to your doctor to rule out other conditions and to plan a course of treatment, including diet changes, stress relief and medications.

2. Avoid suspicious foods.

Some foods are more likely to trigger gut problems in IBS. These include alcohol, caffeine, fatty foods, lactose and the artificial sweeteners sorbitol and mannitol. Food allergy and intolerance can also be associated with IBS. If you suspect that any foods are making your symptoms worse, try keeping a symptom diary. For more comprehensive help, your doctor can refer you to a dietitian specialising in IBS.

🩺 Doctor's bag

First, your doctor will verify that you have IBS by eliminating other possible causes of your distress, such as coeliac disease, an autoimmune disease in which grain proteins, such as gluten, damage the lining of the small intestine. Expect a blood test, a sigmoidoscopy or colonoscopy and screening for lactose intolerance, which can cause similar symptoms. Although there's no cure for IBS, your doctor can suggest treatments along with changes in diet and lifestyle that will help.

Medications. Many medications have been tried in the treatment of IBS, with variable success. These include antispasmodics such as Colofac and Buscopan, and even low-dose antidepressants.

Counselling. Your doctor may refer you to a psychologist, psychiatrist or hypnotist to help you deal with stressful situations that worsen your symptoms. Cognitive behavioural therapy, which focuses on changing attitudes and ways of dealing with difficulties, can be effective, as can hypnosis, which focuses on imagery aimed at taming your digestion.

Your pain toolbox

Soothing your restless bowels is something you can do lots about on your own. Here are some suggestions.

Chamomile tea. This herbal tea may calm the irritated bowel by increasing levels of glycine, which is an amino acid associated with relief of muscle spasms. This also makes chamomile a natural for soothing menstrual cramps. Since irritable bowel syndrome often worsens during menstruation, drinking the tea may do double duty. If you have the constipating form of IBS, the extra fluid can help that as well.

Caraway seeds, fennel seeds, cardamom and coriander. Ever wonder why Indian restaurants often set out a bowl of fennel seeds for after-dinner treats? Both fennel and caraway seeds help lessen gas and bloating. Cardamom and coriander help quell intestinal spasms that can jump-start diarrhoea. Add them to soup, stir-fries and other dishes to help quiet your intestinal traumas.

Enteric-coated peppermint-oil capsules. Peppermint oil helps to relieve gas by relaxing the smooth muscles in the digestive tract and may also discourage growth of bacteria in the small intestine. A Taiwanese study of 110 people with irritable bowel syndrome found that taking one capsule three or four times daily, 15 to 30 minutes before meals, reduced stomach pain by 79 per cent and bloating by 83 per cent.

Exercise. Regular exercise such as walking or yoga can help you feel more relaxed and deal more effectively with stress. It also stimulates more normal contractions in your intestines.

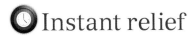 Instant relief

To help symptoms fast, try these steps.

Deep breathing. When pain strikes, spend a few minutes breathing in deeply, allowing your belly to expand, then exhaling slowly from your mouth. The movements will help relax your abdominal muscles, which may help your cramps and pain and make your movements more normal.

A warm, candlelit bath. The warm water will help relax your stomach muscles, and the ambiance will help stress to buzz off.

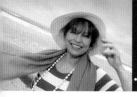

Drink lots of water. If you have diarrhoea, replenish your fluids. Drinking water will also ease constipation.

Eat small, frequent meals. Large meals can increase diarrhoea and cramping, so try eating small meals more frequently to keep these symptoms under control.

Do you have IBS?

Everyone has stomach discomfort from time to time. How do you know if you really have IBS?

Here are the main criteria doctors use to make a diagnosis.

You have had stomach pain for 12 weeks (these do not need to be consecutive) in the past year.

You have experienced at least two of the following:

• relief when you go to the bathroom
• a change in frequency of your stools (three bowel movements a day or fewer than three per week)

• a change in the appearance of your stools (lumpy and hard, or loose and watery)

Other symptoms such as urgency, bloating, straining or passing mucus are also common.

Ulcers

Gastrointestinal ulcers announce themselves with burning pain that simmers between your belly button and breastbone. A gastrointestinal ulcer can wake you at night, with pain lasting for minutes or hours. The pain can worsen with food— or also if your stomach is empty. It can make you vomit or feel bloated. However it manifests itself, it's never pleasant.

Ulcers are irritated areas along the gastrointestinal tract. They are mostly caused by the bacterium *Helicobacter pylori*, which humans have carried, largely harmlessly, in their intestinal tracts for more than 60,000 years. About half the people in the world carry their own *H. pylori* colony, but most have no symptoms. Other causes of ulcers include excessive use of pain relievers such as aspirin and nonsteroidal anti-inflammatories (NSAIDs), such as ibuprofen and naproxen, which can irritate the stomach lining. Smoking and alcohol can have a detrimental effect too by raising acid levels, which increase your risk of an ulcer. Although stress and fiery foods don't actually cause ulcers, they can aggravate them and prevent them from healing.

Most ulcers do heal and return; you may notice symptoms for days or weeks that disappear, only to reappear just when you thought you were in the clear. How ulcers make you feel depends on where they are in your gastrointestinal tract. Duodenal ulcers (in the duodenum, the first part of the small intestine), the most common, tend to be dormant when you wake up, only to gnaw at you by midmorning. They also may wake you up in the middle of the night. Gastric ulcers, which occur along the upper curve of the stomach, may result in bloating, nausea or vomiting after eating. Stress ulcers, which are the result of illness or trauma, occur in the stomach and duodenum.

Eliminating ulcer pain is relatively easy. Some ulcers heal themselves within 6 to 12 months, but with medication most ulcers can clear up within several weeks. Of course, the way you treat your stomach can reduce your pain and hasten healing as well.

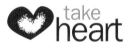

take
heart

Less than 10 per cent of people with ulcers who are treated for *H. pylori* bacteria **have a recurrence**.

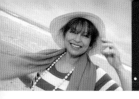

✅ Best first steps

You suspect that the gnawing pain that wakes you up at night is an ulcer. What should you do?

1. Stop smoking.
This is the single most important health decision you can take, not only for the sake of your stomach, but also your heart, lungs and several other organs.

2. Do you really need those nonprescription pain relievers?
Review your need to take aspirin or NSAIDs. Remember several nonprescription pain relievers are actually NSAIDs (Nurofen, Advil). Check with your doctor or pharmacist if in doubt.

3. Try nonprescription antacids.
Until you can see your doctor, antacids such as Quick-Eze or Mylanta can relieve pain temporarily by neutralising stomach acids. Liquid forms may act more quickly than tablets. Antacids can interact with other medications such as certain NSAIDs, tetracycline (an antibiotic) and oral corticosteroids, so check with a pharmacist who knows the medications you're taking before adding antacids.

4. Enlist medical help.
An ulcer isn't something you can clear up on your own. Even if antacids relieve your pain, they will not heal an ulcer.

🩺 Doctor's bag

To find out if you have an ulcer, your doctor will probably insert a small lighted tube, called an endoscope, into your GI tract and, if she sees ulcers, take a tissue sample to rule out cancer. She may also take an X-ray of your gastrointestinal tract as you swallow a white liquid that will help reveal any ulcers. Other tests may include blood or breath tests or stool samples, all to detect *H. pylori*. Depending on what she finds, she'll suggest several of the following.

Antibiotics. You may be prescribed 1 to 2 weeks' treatment of two to three antibiotics to quash *H. pylori*. Some antibiotics include an acid suppressor.

Acid blockers. Also called histamine or H2-receptor blockers, medications such as cimetidine (Magicul, Tagamet) and ranitidine work by reducing the amount of acid in your gastrointestinal tract.

Antacids. Your doctor may prescribe antacids or suggest nonprescription versions for you to take in conjunction with other therapies.

Proton-pump inhibitors. These drugs include Losec, Nexium, Pariet, Somac and Zoton. They reduce the amount of acid your stomach makes by blocking the cellular pumps that secrete acids.

Cytoprotective agents. Sucralfate (Carafate, Ulcyte) and misoprostol (Cytotec) work by making your stomach more resistant to acid and the enzyme pepsin.

 ## Your pain toolbox

Small changes you make can help heal your ulcer and shift pain out of your life. Give these a try.

Smaller meals. Eating smaller, more frequent, meals, and sipping fluids often, can help to protect your stomach lining from acid.

More broccoli. Cruciferous vegetables, such as broccoli, broccoli sprouts, brussels sprouts, cauliflower, cabbage and kale, contain sulforaphane, a compound that appears to squelch *H. pylori*. In one study, 78 per cent of infected patients who ate half a cup of broccoli sprouts twice a day for a week tested negative for the bacteria.

Cabbage. The amino acid glutamine in cabbage may help heal ulcers. Glutamine helps to strengthen the mucous lining of the intestinal tract and improve blood flow to the stomach, which can also speed healing of sores. Use cabbage to make salads, coleslaw and wraps. Or add cabbage when you are juicing fruit and vegetables.

 ## Instant relief

Cracker biscuits. Depending on what kind of ulcer you have, eating a few cracker biscuits can help buffer stomach acid, soothing the burning.

Slippery elm tea. Available in health and natural foods stores, slippery elm contains a mucilage, a substance that becomes slick and gel-like when you mix it with water. The tea coats the gastrointestinal tract, protecting it from acids and giving you some relief.

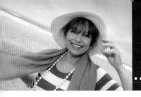

Yogurt with live bacteria. Foods such as yogurt and kefir, both cultured milk products, that contain so-called good bacteria may inhibit *H. pylori* and speed healing. In a Swedish study, people who ate such milk products at least three times a week were much less likely to have ulcers than people who ate them less often. A cup of yogurt per day may help.

Oatmeal and fruit. In a Harvard study of more than 47,000 men, those who ate seven servings of fruit and vegetables per day had a 33 per cent lower risk of developing ulcers than those who ate fewer than three servings per day. Large helpings of soluble fibre, found in beans, barley, apples and oatmeal, cut the risk by 60 per cent. Why? It's possible that soluble fibre turns into a protective gel in your digestive system, protecting the small intestine from damaging digestive juices.

Serious help

If your symptoms don't improve with antibiotics and acid reduction, your doctor may suggest the following.

Endoscopy. This procedure involves inserting an endoscope, which is a tiny camera on the end of a thin tube, into your mouth and down into your stomach and duodenum while you are sedated, so as to inspect the area and biopsy the tissue.

Surgery. You may need surgery if an ulcer is bleeding, is cancerous or causes a perforation in your digestive tract, or if you develop a blockage because of an ulcer's scarring—all rare occurrences.

Cluster headaches

Cluster headaches aren't for sissies. One of the most painful kinds of headaches, these monsters appear suddenly without warning on one side of the face, often starting behind or around one eye and reaching a peak within minutes. They disappear just as abruptly as they started. They usually last up to 90 minutes, but can occur many times per day for weeks, months or even a year, then disappear for months or years. This is called the cluster period. Although cluster headaches tend to stay on one side throughout the cluster period, they do sometimes switch sides.

Lying down often seems to increase pain that is characterised as sharp and burning. Many people prefer to stand, walk around or even exercise. The headaches often begin after several hours of sleep, during the dream, or REM, sleep cycle, revving up the autonomic nervous system, which regulates blood pressure, heartbeat and body temperature. As a result, you may sweat, have a stuffy nose and tearing, red eyes. Many people try to forestall the headaches by staying awake, which compounds the problem by creating chronic fatigue, which can then spiral into depression.

Although many doctors believe that cluster headaches are related to migraines, what causes them is unclear. Some doctors think they may result from a burst of histamine (a chemical released during allergic reactions) or serotonin, a brain chemical that constricts blood vessels. The hypothalamus, the part of the brain that operates the body clock, may also be involved, which may explain why the headaches tend to occur at the same time each day. Triggers include heavy smoking, drinking and drugs such as nitroglycerine, a heart medication. Some people find that the headaches recur at about the same time each year, so seasonal or weather factors may play a role.

The headaches are rare, striking less than one half of 1 per cent of adults and five times more men than women, usually between ages 20 and 40. Fortunately, medication and prevention can help reduce both frequency and severity.

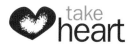

take heart

Sumatriptan (Imigran), a triptan medication, **helps** relieve at least 74 per cent of acute cluster headaches **within 15 minutes**.

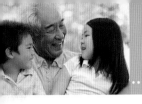

✅ Best first steps

Anti-inflammatories are too slow to be much help at relieving the pain of cluster headaches, but you can begin taking steps that will help cut the headaches' effects.

1. Create a treatment plan with your doctor.
It's especially important to see a doctor or go to the emergency department if the pattern of your cluster headaches suddenly changes; if you have fever, a stiff neck, rash, confusion, weakness or double vision with your headache; if your pain worsens with movement; or if your headaches start after age 50.

2. Keep a diary.
Note what time your headaches strike, how long they last, what you did, such as smoking or sleeping and what you ate and drank within the previous 24 hours. This information will help your doctor.

🩺 Doctor's bag

Your doctor can help you control both how often you get the headaches and the level of pain once they arrive. He will start by asking about the pattern of your headaches and doing a physical examination, checking for neurological signs such as a drooping eyelid or constricted pupil, common symptoms during and between attacks. He may also order imaging tests such as an MRI to rule out other conditions. Once he is certain you have cluster headaches, he will likely offer medications for stopping the attack (acute medications) as well as preventive drugs.

For attacks

Oxygen. Inhaling 100 per cent oxygen for 15 to 20 minutes will often stop an attack, although it may simply delay it. Your doctor may prescribe an oxygen cylinder for you to keep at home and/or a smaller, more portable unit.

Triptans. These migraine drugs—especially those in nasal spray form—may bring relief to cluster headaches by shrinking swollen blood vessels in the head and inhibiting the release of the inflammatory chemicals. Triptans can be very effective in cluster headaches, but because of the fast onset and short duration of the headaches the drugs need to get into the bloodstream quickly; therefore giving an injection or nasal spray of sumatriptan (Imigran) may work better than tablets. However, these drugs are not suitable for use several times a day for weeks on end and hence should be used sparingly.

For prevention

Calcium channel blockers. These medications, which relax and widen blood vessels, may also help. Of them, verapamil, taken three times daily from the start of the attack to several weeks following the last attack of the cluster, appears to be the most effective at reducing headache frequency. However, your doctor must check that it doesn't excessively slow your heart rate nor lower your blood pressure.

Antiseizure drugs. The anticonvulsant drug topiramate (Topamax) is effective against cluster headaches when taken daily. It may work by blocking signals from overactive nerves.

Lithium. Also used to treat bipolar disorder, lithium can be particularly helpful for cluster headaches that are chronic and unremitting.

Prednisone. Although doctors aren't clear why this works, taking a high dose by mouth or intravenously, then tapering off the dosage over several days, seems to result in fewer cluster headaches.

Instant relief

Nobody wants to wait for medication to kick in when a headache is raging. Here are some tips for getting relief while you wait.

Ice. A bag of ice, a cold pack or even a cold soft drink wrapped in cloth and held against your throbbing eye and face for 10 minutes can dull the pain. Repeat every 20 minutes until the attack is over.

Oxygen. Ask your doctor if he can prescribe an oxygen cylinder that you can keep on hand at home. Breathing pure oxygen for 15 to 20 minutes can stop an attack.

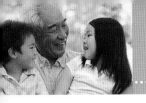

Your pain toolbox

Although dealing with the immediate pain of a cluster headache is tough without a doctor's help, you can act to prevent the headaches with the following steps.

A regular sleep schedule. Interruptions in your regular sleep patterns can bring on an attack. Even if you want to crawl under the covers for a nap, don't.

Avoiding smoking and drinking. Cigarettes and alcohol may give you a buzz, but they can also trigger attacks.

Magnesium. This mineral helps regulate how your blood vessels work, reduces pain and soothes the nervous system. With your doctor's okay, take 400 milligrams per day for at least 2 months.

Migraines

Migraines come on like a bushfire, forcing you to retreat until the worst is over. Sometimes a migraine smoulders and can flare up, and sometimes it gets out of control and has to burn itself out. After the headache fades, you can feel wiped out.

A migraine may announce itself with an aura affecting sight. Scientists aren't sure why; it could be that an electrical or chemical wave moves across the visual parts of the brain, causing hallucinatory disturbances such as squiggly lines or a small blind spot that gradually gets larger. Migraine pain pulses or throbs on one or both sides of your head. The pain may last, if untreated, for hours, even days. Symptoms associated with migraine are nausea, queasiness, lack of appetite and sensitivity to light and sound.

According to one theory, if you have migraine, then all your headaches—even the little ones—are probably a form of migraine. Although all of us have headaches from time to time, those who develop the more severe pain of migraines may simply have a lower threshold for their triggers, such as strong odours, too little or too much sleep, bright lights and hormone fluctuations, which can set off the trigeminal nerve, the largest nerve in the head. Once activated, the nerve releases chemicals that cause inflammation around the brain blood vessels and nerves, triggering pain, most often around one or both eyes, the forehead or one or both temples. The higher the trigger load (either more of one trigger or multiple triggers at the same time), the greater the likelihood of a migraine.

Although there's no cure for migraines, there are many medicines that can stop attacks dead. Lifestyle changes can also help and should be the foundation for managing your migraines.

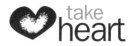

The vast majority of migraine patients **can find treatments** that reduce attack frequency by 50 per cent or more.

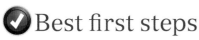 Best first steps

You're fed up with being at the mercy of migraines. You can take control by following these steps.

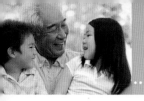

1. Use a nonprescription pain reliever.

A high dose of aspirin (600 to 900 milligrams) or a rapidly absorbed formulation of paracetamol or ibuprofen may be enough for many migraine sufferers. Medications also containing codeine might be effective, but these should be used no more than twice per week because they may cause rebound headaches.

2. Keep a migraine diary.

Note the time and severity of the migraine, how long it lasted, what helped relieve the pain, what foods you ate and drank in the day prior to the attack and how much you slept the night before. This information will help you and your doctor manage your migraines.

3. Develop a treatment plan with your doctor.

It's especially important to seek medical care if the pattern of your headaches changes suddenly and significantly; if you have a sudden, abrupt (like a thunderclap) severe headache; if you have fever, a stiff neck, rash, confusion, weakness or double vision; or if you are over age 50 and have never had headaches before. If you experience weakness or numbness (not just tingling) on one side of the body or if an aura lasts more than an hour or is notably different from previous ones, you should promptly seek medical attention.

Doctor's bag

Your doctor will likely suggest several treatments, including medicine for addressing acute attacks, and another drug to relieve the pain if the first one doesn't work. Finding the right medicine or combination of medicines is a trial-and-error process. In general, if a medicine knocks you out or takes more than 4 hours to work, it isn't right for you. Abortive treatments, which stop attacks, work best when you take them as soon as a migraine begins. Depending on the frequency of attacks, your doctor may also prescribe a preventive medicine. If he does, be patient; although the right drug could halve the average number of headaches you have every month, it may take 4 or more weeks for you to improve and up to 6 months to know if a therapy is working. Many preventive medicines must be started at a low dose and gradually increased in order to minimise side effects.

Abortive treatments

Triptans. These drugs slow down the activated nerves, inhibiting the release of inflammatory chemicals, and shrink swollen blood vessels, all of which play a role in causing your migraine. Triptans available in Australia are sumitriptan (Imigran), zolmitriptan (Zomig), rizatriptan (Maxalt) and naratriptan (Naramig). Triptans and most other abortive medications can cause rebound headaches if taken consistently twice per week or more.

Ergotamine medications. Two older active ingredients—ergotamine (in Cafergot) and dihydroergotamine—have some effectiveness in migraine but these are now very difficult to access in Australia as they are not marketed there anymore. Cafergot is available in New Zealand. Dihydroergotamine (Dyhydergot) given by injection may be very helpful.

Oestrogen replacement. Women whose migraines are triggered by changing levels of oestrogen during their menstrual cycle may benefit from timed hormonal treatments. However, too much oestrogen may act as a trigger, so talk to your doctor about appropriate doses. Birth control pills are another option.

Antinausea medications. If you have nausea or vomiting with your migraines, you may benefit from medications such as metoclopramide (Maxolon) or prochlorperazine (Stemetil). These work by altering chemical messengers in the brain that affect nausea and vomiting. These drugs may cause drowsiness or dizziness.

Opioids. Opioids such as codeine, hydrocodone and oxycodone relieve pain but can be habit forming, and are associated with a high risk of progression to chronic daily headaches. Opioid pain relievers should be used only if other treatments are not effective and only under specialist supervision.

Medications for prevention

Cardiovascular drugs. The beta-blockers propranolol (Inderal), atenolol (Noten) and metoprolol (Betaloc) are effective in reducing the frequency of migraines. Two other blood pressure-lowering drugs, candersartan (Atacand) and lisinopril, are also effective, but, in general, other blood pressure-lowering drugs are not effective.

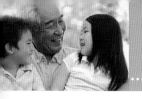

Anti-epileptic drugs. Some anti-epileptic drugs reduce the frequency of migraine attacks. These are topiramate, valproate (Epilim, Valpro) and gabapentin. The latter is expensive because it is not on the Pharmaceutical Benefits Scheme Australia or PHARMAC in New Zealand. This class of medicine is thought to work by stabilising the hypersensitive, overactive nerves in the brain.

Antidepressants. The tricyclic antidepressant, amitriptyline (Endep), is effective in reducing the frequency of migraine attacks. There may be some weak effect from fluoxetine and venlafaxine, but other antidepressants have not been shown to be effective.

Botox. Botox is not generally effective in migraine but it might have a small effect in people who have very high-frequency migraines, that is, more than 15 days per month.

Your pain toolbox

Migraines may make you miserable, but you can fight back with your own arsenal of nondrug weapons.

Biofeedback. Biofeedback is essentially relaxation therapy involving special equipment to monitor physical responses, such as heart rate and muscle tension. A review of 55 studies found that biofeedback decreased the frequency of migraines and improved people's sense of control over their headaches for an average of 17 months. Health insurance rarely covers this therapy, so you may have to pay out of your own pocket.

Instant relief

When you feel a migraine coming on, you need to act fast to get relief. Try these measures.

Try a cup of coffee. At the first sign of an attack, have a cup of coffee. Caffeine may make other pain medicines more effective and may help them get into the bloodstream. However, skip caffeine if you are already taking a painkiller that contains caffeine or have been told by your doctor to avoid it. You should not try this more than twice per week.

Darkness and ice. Sit or lie down in a dark room. Put a cold compress or ice pack on your head or at the back of your neck, and massage the painful parts of your scalp and temple.

Relaxation exercises. Meditation, yoga and progressive muscle relaxation (tightening and releasing one muscle group after the other) help by relieving stress and loosening tight muscles. Other therapies include visual imagery, in which you imagine yourself in a relaxing setting.

A good night's sleep. Lack of sleep may trigger a migraine, as can sleeping too much. A regular sleep schedule is a must. Keeping a regular schedule for meals and exercise can also reduce headaches.

Exercise. A recent Swedish study found that headaches are linked to inactivity. Regular exercise may help by releasing endorphins, brain chemicals that help block the mechanism that jump-starts headaches. Daily exercise also reduces stress. Don't start off at a sprint, since intense exercise can trigger a migraine.

Weight loss. A number of studies have suggested a link between migraines and obesity. If you are overweight or obese, follow a healthy diet, including more fruit, vegetables and whole grains and fewer sugary or fatty snack foods to get as close to your ideal weight as possible.

Butterbur. This herbal anti-inflammatory supplement has been tested for safety and effectiveness more than almost any other supplement. According to a study of 245 people at the Albert Einstein College of Medicine in the Bronx, New York, 68 per cent of those who took a butterbur product called Petadolex cut the number of migraines they had by at least 50 per cent.

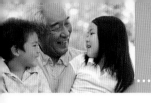

Tension headaches

If you feel as though a steel band is tightening around your head, you probably have a tension headache. Tension, in this case, refers to muscle tension or tightness rather than emotional stress. It can also come on as a dull ache or even as tightness and pain at the back of your neck.

Scientists believe tension headaches are caused by changes in brain chemicals, such as serotonin and endorphins, which activate pain pathways and may contract the muscles around the neck, head and face. The trigeminal nerve, originating in the brain stem and carrying sensory impulses to and from the face, may also play a role. Any number of triggers, including stress, depression, anxiety, fatigue and hormonal changes, can stir up trouble, as can long hours at the computer or detail work that keeps your head in one spot for a long time. Smoking, drinking too much alcohol or coffee and the wrong neck position during sleep can also do you in.

✅ Best first steps

When a tension headache strikes, relief can be less than half an hour away if you do the following.

Take a painkiller.
Ibuprofen, naproxen, aspirin and paracetamol all bring relief. For fastest relief, take ibuprofen in liquid gel capsules, which, in one study, brought relief in 24 minutes for volunteers. Paracetamol took 29 minutes, which is a small difference, but every second counts when your head hurts.

🍴 Your pain toolbox

What you do every day may have far more effect on your tension headaches than medications. Here are ways to get on top of your pain.

A firm press. Try massaging the web of flesh between your thumb and forefinger. According to Chinese medicine, this point links to the energy channel that runs to your head and around the eyes.

Heat or cold. Either one of these can help relieve pain. Place a heating pad or warm compress over painful spots to reduce muscle tightness. If you prefer cold treatment, try an ice pack wrapped in a cloth. The ice numbs the pain and takes your attention from the headache.

A foot soak. Soak your feet in hot water. This is a simple way to distract your mind from your headache. Try to focus on your feet and the pleasant sensation of warmth.

Water. Sometimes a headache is a sign of dehydration. Drink a large glass of water.

Exercise. Exercise such as walking, swimming or yoga can cut both the frequency and the intensity of headache pain. Exercise also relieves stress and relaxes tense muscles.

Biofeedback. This technique involves using special equipment with a therapist who will teach you to monitor and control physical responses to stress such as heart rate and muscle tension.

Cognitive behavioural therapy. Working with a therapist, you'll learn ways to change stressful behaviours and thoughts. Even a few weekly sessions can be helpful.

A lavender- or peppermint-oil massage. Each of these has calming effects on the body that, linked to a head and neck massage, can help quieten your headache.

Worst headache ever?

See your doctor immediately if your pattern of headaches changes; if the headache is sudden and severe; if you have a rash, stiff neck, confusion, double vision or numbness; or if the headache arrives after an injury. Such symptoms may be signs of something more serious, such as a stroke or tumour.

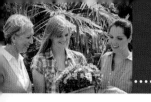

Bursitis

Yesterday you raked the front yard, arms sawing back and forth for hours, and today your elbows feel like they're on fire. Or you went dancing last night and this morning the cha-cha is gone from your hips. It may be that you've inflamed the tiny fluid-filled sacs or pouches that are called bursae. These sacs allow the many different structures in the body to move easily over each other. They are most commonly found between structures that move such as between muscles and tendons, and between muscles or tendons and bones or skin. The fluid in the sacs lubricates the area to allow smooth, friction-free movement between these structures.

Bursae can cause problems if there is excessive or abnormal movement in the surrounding muscles or tendons. This applies particularly if you have been doing repetitive work. The bursae can become inflamed and swollen. Then they are painful when the muscles and tendons around them move, so movement in the joint near the bursa becomes painful. There are at least 150 bursae in the body but only a small number commonly cause problems. These are the bursa between the skin and bone at the elbow (the olecranon bursa), the bursae around the shoulder or hip joints and their muscles and tendons and the bursa over the front of the knee cap, or at the back of the heel.

Bursae can become inflamed in some types of inflammatory arthritis, particularly rheumatoid arthritis and gout. You're also at risk if you have an occupation or hobby in which overusing your joints is common: a gardener, for example, is kneeling his way towards bursitis; a shop assistant who stands 8 hours a day may be more susceptible than an office worker.

You can suspect bursitis if you feel tenderness and aching that get worse when you move. The area over the bursa may be swollen, warm, even red. You may not even remember doing anything in particular to tax your joints.

Most of the time, simple remedies such as rest, ice and anti-inflammatories resolve bursitis within a week or two. If they don't, be sure to see your doctor. Untreated bursitis, especially in the shoulder, may lead to progressive stiffness and may cause a permanent lack of mobility in the joint.

✅ Best first steps

Maybe you were a little ambitious in pulling all the weeds in one day. Luckily, you can begin improving with a few easy steps.

1. Rest.
Stop doing whatever you think was irritating your bursae. You might even want to go to the pharmacy for an elastic bandage or brace that will limit some of the joint motion until the inflammation is gone.

2. Get out the ice pack.
Apply an ice pack or a bag of ice wrapped in cloth to the painful area for 15 to 20 minutes every 4 to 6 hours for 3 or 4 days, until the swelling has gone down. Thereafter, moist heat is generally helpful.

3. Start taking anti-inflammatories.
Pain-relieving NSAIDs such as ibuprofen and naproxen can help relieve pain and inflammation. Follow the dosage instructions on the label unless your doctor tells you otherwise.

🕐 Instant relief

If bursitis threatens to ruin your day, you're eager for fast relief. Here are a few suggestions to ease pain quickly.

Heat. If your joint's no longer inflamed but still painful, apply a warm, wet towel or a heating pad (preferably with moist heat) to the spot for up to 20 minutes at a stretch. That will ease both pain and stiffness.

Elevation. By raising whatever joint's affected, you help reduce the swelling, which in turn reduces your discomfort.

Anti-inflammatory cream. Head to the pharmacy for a cream containing an anti-inflammatory drug. It will help relieve pain and dilate the blood vessels, allowing more blood to reach the site. You might also try a capsaicin cream; they're made from the ingredient that gives chillies their heat.

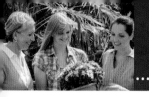

4. Make an appointment.

Call your doctor if the pain and swelling don't diminish in a week, or if you have an unusually large amount of swelling. Don't fool around with a fever or sharp, shooting pains. If you already have a condition such as rheumatoid arthritis or gout, or take medications that may make you more vulnerable to infection, seek medical attention early.

Doctor's bag

Sometimes home remedies such as anti-inflammatories, rest and ice may not be enough to treat bursitis. If so, your doctor can check out the problem joint, ask what you've been doing and perhaps take X-rays or blood tests to rule out other causes of your discomfort. Then she may offer the problem solvers here.

Corticosteroid injections. An injection of a corticosteroid into the painful bursa will often relieve the inflammation, usually easing your discomfort pronto.

Drainage. If the bursae are excessively swollen and filled with fluid, your doctor may drain them using a needle and syringe. She may send some of the fluid to a laboratory for analysis to see if infection or gout is the cause.

Antibiotics. If your bursitis stems from an infection, your doctor will prescribe a course of antibiotics.

Your pain toolbox

You have more solutions at your disposal than you might think. Here are a few things to do at home to relieve the pain and prevent a recurrence.

Pads and cushions. Now's the time to sink into plump chairs, kneel on foam-rubber pads or use knee pads if you're gardening, or buy elbow pads if you have to lean on your elbows. If you've been thinking about buying a cushy mattress pad, do it. Memory and latex foam are good choices because they conform to the body's shape, reducing pressure. If your feet, knees or hips are affected, wear comfortable, well-padded shoes, not tight ones with worn heels.

Movement. Don't sit in one place for a long time. Get up and move your joints.

Frequent breaks. Anytime you're doing a repetitive task such as vacuuming or raking, or a prolonged one such as kneeling, stop and rest frequently, or switch to another kind of task for a while.

Strength training. Once your pain and inflammation subside, think about working with a physical trainer to strengthen the muscles around the affected joint. Strong muscles are like bodyguards for your joints.

Stretches. Gently stretching the muscles around the affected joint helps ease pain by taking pressure off the joint and also helps you maintain the joint's range of motion.

Smart ergonomics. From now on, ease the burdens you place on your joints. For instance, if you're using a heavy tool, support it with both hands. Get someone else to lift heavy objects.

Black cherry juice. This old-time folk remedy contains an anti-oxidant plant pigment called quercetin, which works as an anti-inflammatory. Aim to drink two small glasses of the juice per day just for a short time to see if it helps.

Serious help

Occasionally a doctor may have to resort to more invasive measures. Here's what she may try.

Intravenous antibiotics. If your problem is a serious infection within the bursae, you may need intravenous antibiotics to prevent the infection from spreading throughout your body. The therapy might require that you stay in the hospital for a few days. It would likely be followed by oral antibiotics as well.

Bursectomy. Although this step is rare, if your doctor can't sufficiently drain the bursae or if you have recurrent infected bursitis, your doctor may choose to drain and surgically remove the infected bursae.

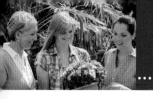

Gout

Long associated with overindulgent eating and drinking, gout was once called the 'disease of kings'. But this painful condition doesn't require a crown and throne, only an excess of uric acid. Uric acid is formed from purines, compounds found in our bodies and also in many foods. Produce too much of it, and the acid forms crystals that build up in joints and tissue around the joints, particularly the big toe, causing intense pain, swelling and inflammation. The crystals can also land in other spots: the foot, ankles, knees, hands and wrists.

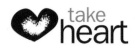

Several studies have shown that **soy foods** such as tofu and edamame **lower uric acid**. Soy foods are a **low-kilojoule protein option** that can be used to reduce intake of red meat.

The pain often starts at night. A bout can last 1 to 2 weeks, affecting one joint or several. At particular risk are people who drink excessive amounts of alcohol; people with untreated high blood pressure, diabetes or obesity; people taking some medications such as diuretics for high blood pressure; those with a family history of gout; men in their forties and fifties and women after menopause.

What triggers an attack? A meal rich in organ meats such as liver and kidneys, a boozy evening, a recent injury or surgery or an infection. All of these are prime candidates.

Fortunately, you and your doctor can address the pain with medications, diet and other lifestyle changes. Preventing the circumstances that cause excess amounts of uric acid is key to avoiding its pain.

✅ Best first steps

If a throbbing big toe wakes you at night, here are a few tips for short-circuiting it right away.

1. Take nonprescription pain relievers.
Ibuprofen and naproxen taken as directed on the package can help ease both pain and inflammation.

2. See your general practitioner.

Let your doctor see it. He can confirm that the condition is gout and not an infection (the two can present in a very similar fashion) and offer medications to lower the levels of uric acid in your blood. Untreated gout can damage the joint and lead to more pain.

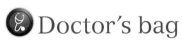 Doctor's bag

Your doctor will examine the joint and may draw some fluid to examine for uric acid crystals. He may take blood to measure uric acid levels. However, some people can have high levels of acid without having gout. Once he confirms that you have the condition, he may suggest one or several of the following treatments.

Prescription nonsteroidal anti-inflammatory drugs (NSAIDs). NSAIDs, such as indomethacin (Indocid, Arthrexin) and naproxen, can control pain and inflammation. However, taken long term, they carry a risk of gastrointestinal bleeding and sometimes an increased risk of heart disease.

Colchicine. This drug, taken orally or injected, tamps down the inflammation of gout. However, its side effects can be unpleasant, including nausea, vomiting, stomach pain and diarrhoea. In some people, it can lower white blood cell counts, which raises the risk of infection.

Steroids. Oral steroids, such as prednisone or those injected directly into the affected joint, can also lessen inflammation and pain.

Instant relief

Here are some measures to take when gout pain seems too much to bear.

A walking stick. This can help lighten the load on painful joints if a lower limb is affected. Hold the stick in the hand opposite the affected limb.

Ice packs. Put a bag of frozen peas, a bag of ice or a gel pack on painful joints for 15 to 20 minutes. The cold will numb the pain. Always wrap the cold object in a towel or face washer to avoid cold damage to the skin.

A bed cradle. Taking the weight of the sheets and blankets off the sore joints at night can help relieve the pain. You can use a bed cradle, made out of pillows or cushions beside the legs.

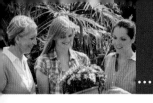

Medications that lower uric acid levels. If you have at least four attacks of gout each year, you will need treatment to reduce the amount of uric acid in your blood to normal. This will stop the attacks of gout occurring. The main drug that is used is allopurinol, which works by stopping the formation of uric acid. Another drug, probenecid, is occasionally used. It works by making the kidneys remove more uric acid from the blood; it should not be used if there are any kidney problems. Allopurinol or probenecid can trigger an acute attack of gout when you start taking them. To stop this happening they are started in a low dose, which is slowly increased until the uric acid is at the correct level. To stop an acute attack of gout you also have to take a low dose of prednisone, colchicine or a nonsteroidal anti-inflammatory drug until the uric acid has been reduced to the correct level. The allopurinol (or probenecid) should be continued. The uric acid comes out of the joint over the next 1 to 3 years, so that there are no more attacks of gout.

Your pain toolbox

You have many ways to prevent and address the pain of gout.

Dietary tweaks. Cut back on rich foods, especially meat, offal, seafood, gravy and foods containing a lot of yeast such as Vegemite and yeast supplements. They're high in purines, the compounds that form the troublemaker uric acid. Instead, eat more plant-based protein foods as well as fruit, vegetables and whole grains such as brown rice. Because all meat, poultry and fish contain purines, eat no more than 120 to 170 grams per day.

The right drinks. Alcohol, especially beer, makes it tougher for your body to get rid of purines. Sugary soft drinks and fruit juice may also be linked to an increased risk of gout. Quench your thirst with water instead: staying hydrated is also a key to keeping painful attacks at bay by eliminating uric acid from your body. Some studies suggest that coffee may lower gout risk in men. Low-fat dairy foods, such as skim milk and yogurt, also seem to reduce the risk of a gout attack.

Weight loss. Being overweight can make gout attacks more frequent. Work on losing weight by changing your diet, as discussed previously, and by adding 30 minutes of exercise to your calendar most days of the week. Skip the crash diets, though: losing too quickly—in most instances, more than 1 kilogram per week—can also trigger gout attacks.

Citrus fruit. Load up on oranges, red capsicums, broccoli and other fruit and vegetables packed with vitamin C. In a Tufts University study, those who ate two bowls of gazpacho loaded with high-vitamin-C vegetables, such as tomatoes and green capsicums, reduced their uric acid levels by as much as 18 per cent. Try to get about 72 milligrams of the vitamin per day, which is about the amount in one orange or half a red capsicum.

Cherries. Dive into a bowl of cherries; they may lower uric acid levels. A University of California study showed that women who ate generous serves of cherries experienced significantly lower levels of uric acid in their blood and higher levels in their urine.

Pineapple. Bromelain, a protein-digesting enzyme derived from pineapple, may help lower inflammation and pain. Eat half a cup per day during an attack.

Olive oil. Sure, you've cut the butter and fatty meats out of your diet, but not all fat is bad. You can get healthy richness from olive, avocado and canola oils, all unsaturated fats that research suggests may lower uric acid levels. You need about 30 per cent of your kilojoules from fat; at least 20 per cent of those should come from unsaturated fat.

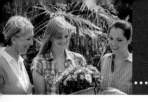

Knee pain

Knee pain is common and has a variety of causes: mechanical causes such as tears of the cartilage or ligaments, or unstable kneecaps; degenerative causes such as osteoarthritis and inflammatory causes such as rheumatoid arthritis or gout.

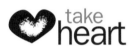

A Tufts University study of more than 700 people found that just 20 to 30 minutes of daily leg exercises using elastic bands **significantly reduced knee pain** and **stiffness**.

Almost one in three people over age 45 experience knee pain. The knee, after all, is a complicated joint that sees a lot of action. It includes the main knee joint, where the thighbone and shinbone meet, and a secondary joint between the kneecap and the thighbone. These joints bend and straighten, twist and rotate. Wrapped around the knee, giving it stability and strength, is a series of ligaments. Between the joints is a thick cartilage called the meniscus that absorbs the pounding of every step you take.

Aside from pain, the signs that something's amiss vary, depending on which part of your knee is affected. If something's wrong with a ligament, you may hear popping sounds when you move, be unable to put your weight on your leg or feel that your knee is about to buckle. If the tendon or kneecap is affected, you may have swelling, be unable to straighten your knee or feel like your knee is about to give way. If the meniscus is torn, you may have slow swelling and your knee may feel frozen in place. Bursitis or infection may show up with swelling, redness and fever. Fortunately, in most cases, you have many ways both to manage the pain and to get your knee back up to speed.

✔ Best first steps

Attending to knee pain fast will help contain it as well. Here's how.

1. Get out the ice.
If there's swelling, hold an ice bag on your knee for 20 minutes at a time to help relieve both swelling and inflammation. Use three to four times a day.

2. Elevate your feet.
This also helps reduce the swelling.

3. Take some inflammation fighters.
Ibuprofen and naproxen can help relieve the pain. Follow the dosage instructions on the label unless your doctor tells you otherwise.

4. See a doctor or physiotherapist.
If this is a new problem, and your knee doesn't get better within 3 to 7 days, get professional attention. Go to the doctor or physiotherapist immediately if you can't stand on or bend your knee, if you have a lot of swelling or pain, if your knee looks deformed or if you have a fever.

Doctor's bag

Your doctor is going to ask you a lot of questions, such as when your knee started hurting, if the pain started suddenly or slowly, if you've had knee pain before and if the pain is in one spot or several. He will want to know if you can stand on or bend your knee, if the pain comes and goes, if you've been doing anything that stressed your knee, such as playing sport or beginning a new exercise program. He'll want to know what makes the pain better or worse, and he'll check for bruising and swelling. He'll ask you to move your leg in different ways. He may also do imaging tests such as X-rays or an MRI, checking for damage, and he may perform blood tests or draw fluid from the injured joint to check for infection or other sources of inflammation. Once he understands what's going on, he'll likely recommend one or more of the following.

Prescription anti-inflammatories. If you find that nonprescription anti-inflammatories aren't enough help, your doctor may prescribe stronger NSAIDs.

Corticosteroids. Another option is an injection of cortisone into the knee, which reduces inflammation. This steroid is used sparingly because of its side effects, including an increased risk of infection. Injections of steroids should be given at intervals of not less than 3 months to avoid suppressing the natural activity of the adrenal gland.

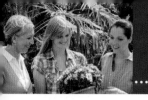

Arthritis drugs. If a condition such as rheumatoid arthritis or psoriatic arthritis is causing your pain, your doctor may prescribe disease-modifying antirheumatic drugs (DMARDs), such as methotrexate. He may also prescribe injectable proteins called biologics, such as etanercept (Enbrel) or adalimumab (Humira), which alter aspects of the immune system to reduce inflammation.

Hyaluronic acid. This acid is found naturally in our joints. A single injection into aching, arthritic knees may provide lubrication and pain relief, perhaps by easing inflammation. The effects can last up to a year and can be repeated.

Your pain toolbox

In addition to your doctor's help, you have other avenues of relief. Here are just a few.

Compression. If your knee is swollen, wrapping an elastic bandage around it or pulling on some compression tubing such as 'Tubigrip' will reduce swelling and help support your knee.

Instant relief

Knees get a lot of use, and even if you're doing everything right, some days you're going to hurt. Here are some quick ways to get relief.

Knee stretches. Once you've established a stretching and strengthening routine with your physiotherapist, doing a few of the stretches when you're in pain can loosen the tight muscles, stimulate the nerves and lower stress. For instance, stretch the muscles behind your knee by placing your foot on a step or low stool in front of you. Place your hands at the top and front of your knee and gently bend forwards pressing with your hands to straighten your knee. Make sure you are safely balanced when you try this stretch.

Pain-relieving creams and gels. NSAIDs such as ibuprofen are available in gel, cream or spray form. Research indicates they can be as effective as pills without the risk of stomach upset or heart disease.

Creams containing capsaicin (the fiery ingredient in chillies) can also provide relief.

Ginger and orange essential oils. Try a little self-massage using a mix of aromatic ginger and orange essential oils (available at health and natural foods stores or online). Add three drops of orange and two drops of ginger essential oils to one cup of jojoba or sesame seed oil, shake and apply. A 3-week Chinese study found that people with knee pain who had six massage sessions with ginger and orange essential oils had less pain and more functionality 1 week after the study's end than people massaged with olive oil only.

Breaks. Simply stop what you're doing and rest, elevating your legs a bit.

Knee support. Orthotics are footwear inserts, such as wedges on the inner or outer part of your shoes, which may help change where pressure lands on your knee. Elastic knee braces can also help stabilise the knee. Ask your doctor or physiotherapist what to try. At the very least, switch to comfortable shoes with good arch supports.

Physiotherapy. Depending on the cause of your knee pain, your doctor may recommend physiotherapy that will focus on building up the strength of the muscles around your knee and maintaining the knee's range of motion. Not only will the therapy help you recover more quickly, but it will help prevent knee pain from recurring. With your doctor's okay, try this simple stretch: standing, put your leg with the aching knee behind your other leg. Lean to your healthy side until you feel a stretch on the outside of your thigh. Hold for 30 seconds; repeat five times. This stretches the muscle running from your thigh to below the knee.

Swimming. Getting in some low-impact exercise such as swimming, hydrotherapy (doing exercises standing in water) or riding a stationary bike (keep the seat high to avoid too much knee bend) can loosen tight muscles, lubricate joints and increase healing blood flow to the area. These exercises can get you going early by relieving the weight from your knee joints while making the muscles work and maintain their strength and endurance.

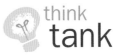

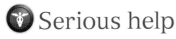 Serious help

When simpler measures don't work to relieve your knee pain, your doctor may suggest one of the following.

Arthroscopic surgery. A surgeon can operate inside the knee joint without making a big cut. By inserting a thin telescope and special thin tools into a few small incisions, the doctor can repair ligament injuries or remove cartilage tears, helping relieve the pain. Although the damage to surrounding tissue and muscles is minimal, some people may still need physiotherapy afterwards.

Knee replacement. Joint replacements are becoming more advanced, and the surgery itself is now less invasive, as instruments and incisions grow smaller. Depending on the amount of damage present, you can opt for a partial or full knee replacement. These days, replacement metal and plastic parts may last 20 years.

'The two key things for knee pain are to have good thigh muscles and a normal weight.'

—Rheumatologist Rodger Laurent, MD, ChB, MMedEd, FRACP, Head of Rheumatology, Royal North Shore Hospital, Sydney, NSW

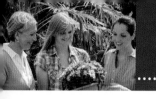

Osteoarthritis

You're not bounding out of bed in the morning anymore. How can you? You feel as stiff as a wind-up toy, and you wouldn't mind a wind-up to get you going. If you're over 40, that morning creaking could be a sign of osteoarthritis, a wearing away of the cartilage that lines your joints. The painful condition can affect any joint, but especially affects hips, knees, hands and spine.

It's not just achy morning stiffness that tips you off to the condition. You may notice that a joint is tender or swollen, or that you can't bend it as well as you used to. You may even feel a grating sensation from roughened cartilage or even bones rubbing together. On X-rays, your doctor may see bone spurs (hard bony extensions that form around the joint) and narrowing of the joint space.

Certain factors increase the risk of osteoarthritis: age, gender (many more women than men have osteoarthritis), obesity, deformed bones or defective cartilage, joint damage (that old sports injury coming back to haunt you) or other diseases that affect the joints, such as gout or rheumatoid arthritis.

There's no cure for osteoarthritis, but you can ease the ache and get back to doing the things you love, from playing fetch with the dog to playing tennis. 'The biggest thing is lifestyle modification', says Theodore W Parsons III, MD, chairman of the Department of Orthopaedic Surgery at Henry Ford Hospital in Detroit, Michigan. 'If you exercise, take anti-inflammatories and lose weight, you can have a positive impact on the pain of osteoarthritis.'

✅ Best first steps

When you feel the pain and stiffness of osteoarthritis creeping in, try one or several of these measures.

1. Take a break.
If a joint's aching, avoid taxing it. As much as possible, give the joint a 24-hour hardship break. Just be sure to get up and move around

gently for 10 minutes every hour, giving your joint and surrounding muscles a change of pace and position.

2. Alternate cold and warm packs.
Hold a cold pack or ice bag to your sore joint for 20 minutes several times per day to relieve pain and muscle spasms. Alternate with 20 minutes of a hot-water bottle, a heating pad or warm bath to relieve pain and stiffness.

3. Try a pain-relief rub.
Creams and gels containing anti-inflammatory medications, such as salicylates or diclofenac, can help relieve pain and inflammation. Creams containing capsaicin (which gives chillies their kick) help reduce pain—give them a few weeks to achieve full effect. Another option is creams that contain ingredients such as menthol, winter-green or eucalyptus oil, whose icy or hot sensation temporarily relieves pain. Only use the amount prescribed on the package, and don't use the creams with ice or heat packs.

4. Get the joint checked out.
If you've had pain, stiffness or swelling around a joint for more than 2 weeks, your doctor should examine you to find out what's going on.

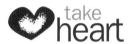 Doctor's bag

If initial self-help measures don't provide enough pain relief, your doctor can offer more powerful options. Before he prescribes any-thing, he'll examine the joint, possibly taking X-rays to check for narrowing space within a joint, which is a sign of cartilage erosion, and for bone spurs, the bony outgrowths around a joint. He may take samples of the fluid in the joint to rule out other conditions such as rheumatoid arthritis or gout. Once he confirms osteoarthri-tis, he may prescribe one or several of the following and should go over all their risks and benefits with you.

Prescription nonsteroidal anti-inflammatory drugs (NSAIDs). If life-style changes and nonprescription pain relievers aren't enough, your doctor may prescribe one of these. Long-term use and large doses can cause stomach ulcers and bleeding, and may even increase the risk of heart disease.

take heart

In studies of women with spine and hip joint pain, the Center for Gerontology at Virginia Polytechnic Institute and State University in Blacksburg found that **small lifestyle changes**, such as stretching before doing any physical activity, rolling out of bed instead of sitting up, and carrying a seat cushion to soften hard seating **helped** them most in **managing pain**.

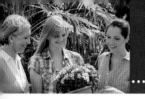

Hyaluronic acid. This acid is found naturally in our joints. A single injection into aching, arthritic knees may provide lubrication and pain relief. The effects can last up to a year and can be repeated.

Corticosteroids. A cortisone injection in the joint reduces inflammation. Cortisone is used sparingly because of its side effects, including an increased risk of infection. Injections should be given at intervals of not less than 3 months to avoid suppressing the natural activity of the adrenal gland. Prolonged high doses may damage the joint.

Opioids. For severe pain that doesn't respond to lesser measures, your doctor may prescribe opioids such as buprenorphine (Norspan), fentanyl (Durogesic), hydromorphone (Dilaudid, Jurnista), morphine (Anamorph, Kapanol, MS Contin), oxycodone (Endone, OxyContin, OxyNorm, Targin). These drugs do not change inflammation; they are powerful pain relievers. For osteoarthritis pain, often they are best used as an oral slow-release, or as a skin patch, formulation to provide a fairly constant background of pain relief. They should be combined with other pain management measures. Their side effects include tiredness, poor concentration and memory, nausea and constipation. They can be habit forming. You must be careful if you drive when using these medications.

Your pain toolbox

If you're like most people with osteoarthritis, your best bet for relief will be the everyday measures you take yourself. You'll have the condition for life, so it's important to put in the time and effort to discover which combination of approaches works best for you. Don't rely on pills alone. Be active. And keep your weight under control.

Instant relief

When it hurts, reach for an anti-inflammatory—and for these helpers.

A tennis ball. Take a tennis ball and, applying some pressure, roll it back and forth over the sore spot.

Tight-fitting gloves. If you have arthritis in your hands, put these on before you go to bed to prevent swelling. You can find gloves designed specifically for arthritis at medical supply stores and online.

A face washer. Soak it in hot water, then apply to the stiff joint.

Nonprescription pain relievers. These are very helpful to many people with arthritis. Paracetamol can help relieve pain but not inflammation. A safe dose spread over the course of one day is no more than 4 grams, taken as directed on the package. More than that, or the day's dose taken all at once, can be harmful to your liver, especially if you drink alcohol. In contrast to previous medical opinion, recent research suggests that there may be some inflammation in osteoarthritis. Nonsteroidal anti-inflammatory drugs (NSAIDs) such as ibuprofen and naproxen can help relieve both pain and inflammation. Follow the dosage instructions on the label unless your doctor tells you otherwise. Taken long term and at high dosages, NSAIDs can increase the risk of stomach upset and even heart disease.

Walking, cycling or swimming. Moving when you're in pain seems counterintuitive. But exercise is the best thing you can do to relieve pain and to keep the muscles around your joints healthy and strong. 'People who are physically fit sleep better and deal with pain better than people who are not fit', says Theodore W Parsons III, MD, chairman of the Department of Orthopaedic Surgery at Henry Ford Hospital in Detroit. See your doctor first and start slowly, working up gradually to at least 30 minutes per day. If you choose walking, keep it brisk. If you're in a lot of pain, it may be easier to pedal a recumbent bike or to swim or do water exercises, especially in a heated pool.

Physiotherapy. Physiotherapists are experts in the amount and type of activity appropriate to your situation. They can show you specific stretching and strengthening exercises for your type of arthritis.

Weight loss. Excess weight puts increased pressure on your joints. In one major study of arthritis patients, it took only about a 10 per cent weight loss to significantly improve participants' knee and hip function and to lessen pain. Aim to lose a half to 1 kilogram a week by cutting out fast foods and sugar, eating more vegetables and whole grains, serving yourself smaller portions and increasing your exercise to at least 30 minutes a day.

The Arthritis Self-management Program. This program is available through hospitals and Arthritis Australia (http://www.arthritisaustralia.com.au). It teaches you how to manage your disease. One study found that after 4 years in the program, participants had far less pain, made fewer visits to the doctor and spent fewer days in the hospital than those who weren't in the program.

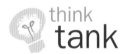

think
tank

'Losing weight is probably the most important thing you can do to treat your osteoarthritis of the hip and knee. It will reduce your pain and make it less likely that you will need joint replacement surgery.'

—Rheumatologist Rodger Laurent, MD, ChB, MMedEd, FRACP, Head of Rheumatology, Royal North Shore Hospital, Sydney, NSW

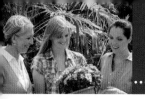

Sunshine. Low vitamin D levels were implicated in knee pain osteoarthritis, according to a study at Tufts University. Because sunlight cranks up the production of vitamin D in your skin, you can get your daily dose (and exercise) by a taking a 15-minute stroll with at least some of your skin exposed (dark-skinned people will need more time). You can also take a vitamin D supplement (at least 1000 IU a day).

Omega-3 fatty acids. Oily fish such as trout, anchovies and salmon, along with walnuts, linseeds and pumpkin seeds, and olive and canola oils, contain omega-3 fatty acids that act as powerful anti-inflammatories. Eat fatty fish at least twice a week or consider taking a daily omega-3 fatty acid supplement of fish or linseed oil. They need to be taken for 2 to 3 months before you know whether they are going to help reduce your pain.

Devil's claw. Devil's claw is a plant that may relieve your pain. A review of 14 studies found that devil's claw appears to work well on all aspects of osteoarthritis. One study of 75 people with knee and hip osteoarthritis who took 2400 milligrams of devil's claw daily for 12 weeks showed a 24 per cent improvement in pain, 22 per cent in stiffness and 23 per cent in physical function. It should not be taken with warfarin or some heart drugs—check with your doctor or pharmacist.

Glucosamine and chondroitin. Glucosamine and chondroitin sulfates are as effective as some of the nonsteroidal anti-inflammatory drugs in relieving the pain. They need to be taken for about 2 months before you know if they are going to help. There is no good evidence that they stop the arthritis from getting worse. Glucosamine and chondroitin can be taken separately or together; generally they are sold together in the one tablet.

Serious help

Sometimes lifestyle changes and medications aren't enough to manage the pain. In those cases, an orthopaedic surgeon may recommend one of the following.

Joint replacement. Joint replacement surgery is less invasive than it used to be, and the metal and plastic substitute joints can last for up to 20 years before they need to be replaced. Although hip and knee replacements are the most common, you can also replace shoulder, elbow and sometimes even ankle joints. Joint replacement usually provides very good pain relief.

Joint clean-up. Occasionally, pain may come from loose or torn pieces of cartilage in the joint. Your doctor may suggest removing those pieces by inserting an arthroscope (a small surgical telescope) and surgical tools through small incisions to clean out the joint, although this may provide only partial relief.

Bone realignment. If knee replacement isn't an option, as it may not be for young people with osteoarthritis, since they would have to have the part replaced at least once more, the doctor might suggest osteotomy, surgery in which he cuts off part of the bone above or below the knee so that the force of your weight no longer falls on the damaged part of the knee. It's not a procedure to undertake lightly—the recovery time can be extensive.

Bone fusion. Again, this may be an option if you can't have joint replacement surgery. Fusing a painful joint in a procedure called arthrodesis decreases pain and stabilises the joint. The major downside is that you will no longer have movement in that joint. If it's your knee, your gait (walking style) will be abnormal and may cause pain elsewhere. If it's your elbow, use of that arm is limited.

Make everyday life easier

Tweaking a few of your daily habits can help you cope with your arthritis.

Make use of arthritis aids. From jar openers and doorknob grabbers to key turners, devices made for people with arthritis can make many of life's tiny tasks less troublesome. Check online or head to a medical supply store or seek help from an occupational therapist.

Consider a walking stick. Okay, it may irk you to use one. However, at painful times, using a stick takes the pressure off a painful hip or knee. Be sure to hold the stick in the hand opposite the painful side.

Ask for paper, not plastic. When you head home with the groceries, instead of carrying plastic bags with handles, which stresses the joints in your hands, elbow and shoulder, ask for paper bags that you can hold in both arms close to your chest, or better yet, bring your own shoulder bag or backpack.

Switch to a backpack. Instead of putting strain on your fingers by clutching a purse by the handle or hoisting it on one shoulder, use a backpack or a backpack purse.

Use a chair in the kitchen. Many jobs, such as loading and unloading the dishwasher or preparing food, can be done just as easily from a seated position.

Turn on the tap water. Instead of wrestling with hard-to-open jars, hold the lid under hot running water for 15 seconds or tap the lid firmly on the benchtop and it should open more easily.

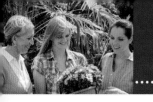

Rheumatoid arthritis

Rheumatoid arthritis is a painful inflammatory form of arthritis that can affect anyone, though it's most common in people between the ages of 40 and 60. Women are affected two to three times more often than men. Usually, if the disease affects a joint on one side, it also affects the corresponding joint on the other.

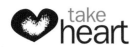

A British study found that 87 per cent of people with rheumatoid arthritis who did water exercises for 30 minutes once per week for 6 weeks **felt physically** and **mentally better** or very much better (a rating of 6 or 7 on a 7-point scale) at the program's end.

Unlike osteoarthritis, which is caused by wear and tear on your joints, rheumatoid arthritis is triggered when your body's immune system mistakenly turns on itself. Antibodies, designed to attack foreign invaders, instead attack your joints, causing swelling, pain, stiffness and warmth in the joint lining. Cells on the lining divide, causing the lining to thicken. Soon, the inflamed cells release enzymes that start to destroy the bone and cartilage. Genetics may increase your risk, as may smoking or infections. Along with pain, swelling and stiffness, rheumatoid arthritis announces itself through fatigue, fever, weight loss and bumps of tissue, or nodules, under the skin on your arms. The disease can strike system-wide, affecting the heart and lungs as well as joints.

Although there's no cure, early treatment to control the inflammation will stop or reduce joint damage and deformities. The newer medications, the disease-modifying antirheumatic drugs (DMARDs), must be started as soon as the diagnosis has been made. They are more likely to stop the inflammation if started early. This change in the approach to treatment means that many more people with rheumatoid arthritis can lead normal active lives.

The commonly used DMARDs are methotrexate, sulfasalazine and leflunomide (Arava). If these are not effective there is a new class of drugs, the biological response modifiers, which may be able to be used. It's also important that you work on lifestyle changes such as exercise, healthy eating and relaxation that ensure you have more energy, a better mood and less pain.

✅ Best first steps

If you begin to notice pain in several joints on both sides of your body, here are some steps to ease your pain, and your worry.

1. Get a diagnosis.
This is by far the most important first step: See your doctor. The sooner you are on prescription medication, the less damage you'll have to your joints and the more control you'll have over your pain.

2. Reduce pain with nonprescription anti-inflammatories.
Anti-inflammatories, such as ibuprofen or naproxen, can both ease inflammation and lower pain. Don't take more than directed on the package unless your doctor advises you to.

3. Try heat and ice.
A 20-minute hot bath or 20 minutes with a heating pad can ease stiffness and pain by relaxing your muscles. Alternate heat with a cold pack, an ice bag or even immersion in a cold bath, if you can stand the goose bumps. Cold lessens pain and muscle spasms. Limit cold treatments to 20 minutes as well.

🩺 Doctor's bag

Getting your doctor's help is essential. He'll begin by asking about your symptoms and giving you a physical examination. He will also likely draw blood looking for antibodies called rheumatoid factor and anti-cyclic citrullinated peptide (anti-CCP) that are commonly found in people who have, or go on to develop, RA. The doctor may also draw fluid from your joints to check for other conditions, and may take X-rays to check for joint damage and establish a basis for comparison over time. Once he confirms RA, your doctor may recommend one or several of the following.

Disease-modifying antirheumatic drugs (DMARDs). These are the most important drugs used in the treatment of rheumatoid arthritis because they can stop the inflammation that causes damage to the joint. They include methotrexate, sulfasalazine, leflunomide, azathioprine and hydroxychloroquine. These drugs modify or suppress the parts of the immune response that cause inflammation.

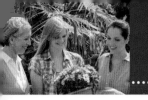

The TNF-alpha inhibitors (see below) are also DMARDs. All the DMARDs are used with NSAIDs and corticosteroids. They take at least 4 weeks to work and you will require regular blood tests to check for any side effects.

Corticosteroids. Your doctor may prescribe a short course of prednisone, which reduces inflammation and limits the damage of RA. Used long term, corticosteroids become less effective and can have side effects such as bone thinning, bruising, cataracts and diabetes. If needed long term, your doctor will aim to limit the dose of prednisone to 5 milligrams or less per day to minimise these side effects.

Prescription NSAIDs. Nonprescription ibuprofen or naproxen can help, but your doctor can offer stronger versions. Like their non-prescription cousins, they can cause stomach bleeding and raise the risk of heart disease, so discuss their pros and cons. They mostly relieve pain rather than having a major effect on the course of RA.

TNF-alpha inhibitors. Also called biologic response modifiers, these medications work by inhibiting a protein called TNF-alpha that fires up the inflammation in RA. The inhibitors, given by subcutaneous or intravenous injection, mimic natural substances already

Instant relief

Stopping pain fast is always the goal. Here are some speedy pain busters.

Ice and heat. Try putting some crushed ice in a plastic bag, wrapping it in a towel and giving yourself an ice massage on painful spots. Or, if you can stand it, give yourself a 20-minute soak in cold water. Cold eases pain and muscle spasms. Alternate cold treatments with 20-minute heat treatments such as a hot bath or shower. You may also use a heating pad. Heat relaxes tense muscles and relieves pain.

Rice. Take inexpensive white rice, pour some into a pillowcase, heat it in the microwave for several minutes, and you've got a reusable mobile heating pad that adjusts to your body shape. A bonus: for the first few heat-ups, the rice will provide moist heat, the most soothing kind.

Range-of-motion exercises. Get relief by slowly and gently moving each achy joint as far as it can go. For instance, sitting down, turn your head slowly to the right, then to the left. Feel the stretch, but stop if you feel pain.

Relaxation. Shake off muscle-tightening stress by finding a quiet spot. Close your eyes and breathe in through your nose, picturing relaxation entering your body. Breathe out through your mouth and picture stress and tension leaving. Repeat for 5 minutes.

A massaging showerhead. If you don't already have one, splurge. Pulsing hot water on sore joints and muscles can feel like a quick trip to spa heaven.

present in the immune system, which help decrease inflammation and joint damage. Some of the more common ones include etanercept (Enbrel), infliximab (Remicade) and adalimumab (Humira). These drugs may increase the risk of infection.

Your pain toolbox

Yes, you have to take medicine for RA, but there's a lot more you can do to feel better.

Swimming, cycling and tai chi. You'd probably rather take a saw to your hip, but moving is one of the most important things you can do to strengthen muscles around the joints and keep them flexible. Swimming or water aerobics in a heated pool not only feels good but allows you to exercise without putting too much pressure on your joints. Walking and cycling are good choices, too. If you cycle, try a stationary bike with a recumbent seat; these bikes are easier to get on and put less strain on your joints than upright bikes. Tai chi involves slow, graceful movements and is best done in a class. Check with your doctor before you begin exercising, start slowly, and work up gradually to at least 30 minutes per day most days of the week.

Anti-inflammatory foods. Oily fish such as salmon, trout and anchovies, along with walnuts, linseed and pumpkin seeds, and olive and canola oils, contain omega-3 fatty acids that act as powerful anti-inflammatories. Eat fatty fish at least twice a week or consider taking a daily omega-3 fatty acid supplement of fish or linseed oil. They need to be taken for 2 to 3 months before you know whether they are going to help reduce your pain.

A healthy weight. Eating lots of whole grains, fruit, vegetables and lean proteins, such as fish, will give you a lot more healthy nutrients for fewer kilojoules than soft drinks and chips. And eating those foods in combination with exercise can help you take kilograms off, unburdening damaged joints.

Devices that ease joint stress. At painful times, you'll find that using a walking stick can take the pressure off a painful hip or knee. Other devices, from easy-to-grip jar openers to electric can openers, long-handled sock pullers to rubber-grip pens, can make tasks easier and less painful.

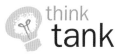
think
tank

'Early treatment of rheumatoid arthritis is essential to stop joint damage and deformities. Rheumatoid arthritis treated early often requires fewer drugs to control the arthritis than if treatment is delayed.'

—Rheumatologist Rodger Laurent, MD, ChB, MMedEd, FRACP, Head of Rheumatology, Royal North Shore Hospital, Sydney, NSW

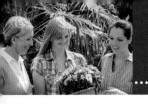

Music. Sleep is often a problem for people with RA, and fatigue can exacerbate pain. A Taiwanese study of older adults found that people who listened to their choice of soothing music for 45 minutes at bedtime got a better night's sleep, stayed asleep longer and had greater function the next day than those who didn't. Several studies have also shown that listening to music every day reduces both pain and depression, and helps people feel they have more control over their pain.

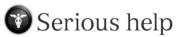 Serious help

When there is severe damage to joints or tendons, surgery may be necessary.

Joint replacement. If joints, especially the knees or hips, become badly damaged, your doctor may suggest replacing them. Replacement surgery is not as invasive as it once was, and the plastic and metal parts may last 20 years, if you take care of them by keeping your weight down and avoiding pounding exercise such as running and jumping. Although hip and knee replacements are the most common, you can also replace shoulder, elbow and sometimes even finger and ankle joints.

Removing the joint lining. If the joint lining is inflamed, enlarged and painful, your doctor may perform a synovectomy, removing the lining.

Tendon repair. Sometimes RA damage can loosen or even rupture tendons around the joint. A surgeon may be able to repair them.

Joint-soothing diet

No food will cure RA, but the right diet can help ease your symptoms and protect your joints.

Vitamin-C-rich foods. Citrus fruit, capsicums, strawberries and dark leafy greens are all rich sources of vitamin C, which helps the body produce collagen, a major part of the cartilage that surrounds joints. Vitamin C also acts as an anti-oxidant, protecting you from free radicals that attack joints.

Ginger and turmeric. Many spices fight inflammation, especially these two. Use fresh ginger liberally in cooking. Turmeric gives curry powder its yellow hue. In one study, turmeric extract was found to work like prescription DMARDs, targeting a process that turns on a gene for inflammation.

Olive oil. Toss salads with extra virgin olive oil. Whenever possible, substitute olive oil for butter or corn oil. Olive oil contains anti-oxidants called polyphenols that, according to several studies, help fight arthritis-related inflammation by blocking pain and swelling. Corn oil, however, may make inflammation worse.

Tendon pain

Tendons are the fibrous structures that connect muscle to bone. Some are long, for example the Achilles tendon, others are short, such as the ones connecting forearm muscles to the elbow. Normally, whenever muscles move, tendons move easily as well; but prolonged use, or a period of intense use, can cause problems. Tendinopathy is the term that is now used to describe painful, irritated tendons.

You may have heard of tennis elbow, swimmer's shoulder or even jumper's knee. These problems usually start out as tendinitis (inflamed tendon) but over a period of time become tendinosis (wear and tear in the tendon but no true inflammation). These conditions can occur in any tendon but most commonly affect the shoulder, elbow, knee and heel.

It is a normal part of ageing that your tendons start to fray and lose their rubber band-like elasticity, making you more susceptible to tendon problems when you repeat motions continuously, as you do when you're playing tennis, gardening or painting your house. It can also happen after a sudden injury. Having a condition such as rheumatoid arthritis or psoriatic arthritis can make you more susceptible. Sometimes, even poor posture or overstretching can strain tendons. In a common scenario, a new, eager exerciser starts a workout without warming up or goes overboard fast. The tendons can't take the sudden overuse, and become painful. If the condition grows severe or is ignored, you may tear or rupture a tendon.

Regardless of how you get tendinopathy, the key is to rest and then gradually build up again.

✔ Best first steps

You don't have to be miserable. Try some of the steps here.

1. Stop moving.
Whatever activity you were engaging in, stop and rest.

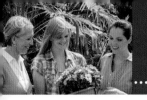

2. Break out the ice.

Place a bag of ice or an ice pack on the sore spot for 20 minutes to ease the pain and swelling.

3. Pull out the pain relievers.

It's time for some paracetamol, ibuprofen or naproxen. Follow the dosage instructions on the label.

4. Try moist heat.

If the swelling is gone but the area's still painful, place a heating pad or warm wet cloth on the spot for 20 minutes. The heat opens the blood vessels, increasing blood flow to the area, which speeds healing. Try massaging the area or gently stretching after you apply the heat.

Doctor's bag

Your doctor or physiotherapist can check for a tendon problem by having you perform certain movements and determining where it hurts. He may order X-rays or an ultrasound or an MRI to rule out a tear and to view any changes to the tendon. In more difficult cases, the doctor may recommend the following.

Corticosteroids. Your doctor may suggest corticosteroid injections, which reduce inflammation and pain. However, repeated injections can weaken the tendon. Corticosteroids should not be used around some tendons (in particular the Achilles tendon) because of the risk of rupture.

Physiotherapy. A physiotherapist can provide you with a suitable exercise program and also may give ultrasound treatment to the affected area to decrease pain.

Novel therapies. There is limited evidence supporting the use of low-level laser therapy (LLLT) for tennis elbow and Achilles tendinosis,

Instant relief

Your shoulder (or elbow, wrist or heel) feels tender and sore, and you want the pain to stop. Here are some fast pain busters.

Breaks. Whether you're at your desk or getting physical, schedule regular breaks.

Stretches. Gently stretching the area can help relieve the pain. You are pushing too hard if the stretching hurts.

and for shock-wave therapy for patella tendinosis (the tendon of the kneecap) and Achilles tendinosis. Also injection of blood or blood derivatives near the painful tendon may be helpful in some situations. The place of all of these therapies is yet to be defined.

 ## Your pain toolbox

Unless the pain is severe or the tendon is injured, relief is pretty much up to you. Here are suggestions for your pain and prevention arsenal.

Rest. Avoid putting any stress on the inflamed tendon, even protecting it from motion by using a sling, brace or elastic wrap. When you can, elevate the body part that hurts to reduce the swelling. Don't go for total immobility: careful stretching and gentle activities such as swimming may be fine.

Compression. If swelling is present and the injury is new, wrap the inflamed area in an elastic bandage. This should help to limit the swelling, which in turn helps the tendon to heal faster. Don't wrap the bandage so tightly that it feels uncomfortable or restricts blood flow.

Ergonomics. Examine the way you do things, such as sitting, holding books, leaning on your elbows, and so on, that may stress your muscles and tendons. Practise giving your body a scan, relaxing the muscles that feel tense. Try to change the load you place on them. For instance, instead of holding up a heavy book with bent wrists, prop it on your lap while you read. Review the activity that caused the tendon pain: it may be that you were doing it in a way that inappropriately stressed the tendon. If it was associated with a sport, get a coach to check you.

Strengthening and stretching exercises. Once the swelling has gone down and healing has begun, work with a physiotherapist to strengthen and stretch the involved tendons and nearby muscles; this can help heal the tendon and return it to normal.

 ## Serious help

If the pain and limitation are severe enough, your doctor may have to take more serious measures.

Surgery. Although surgery is not often necessary, in some cases it's important to remove some excess tissue around the tendon. If the tendon is ruptured or torn, your surgeon may also repair it, easing pain and allowing you to use that part of your body again.

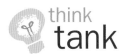
think
tank

'A first episode of tendinopathy is a signal to initiate RICE (rest, ice, compression and elevation). Do this for a few days, then build up your activity gradually by slowly increasing your repetitions and then the difficulty of the activity. If the pain doesn't go away after a few weeks it's time to change strategies. Check in with your physiotherapist.'

—Anne Daly, D Clin Physio, M Manip Physio, BAppSc (Physio), Musculoskeletal Physiotherapist, Pain Service, Austin Health, Melbourne

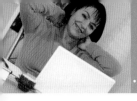

Achilles tendon pain

Overdo it on the walking track last week? Or playing cricket in the backyard with the kids? The Achilles tendon, the large swathe of tissue connecting your calf muscles to your heel bone, may be protesting. Every time you step, you may feel a dull ache or tenderness, or notice a swelling at the back of your calf and stiffness after you've been sleeping or sitting. The tendon may hurt when you touch it, even responding with a creaking sound when you move.

Achilles tendinopathy is the payback for overdoing it, especially if you're athletic. It can also strike the weekend warrior, particularly one who decides to get some exercise after months or years of enjoying the couch. Your muscles may not be strong or flexible enough to handle so much activity, particularly if it involves sudden stops and starts such as tennis or basketball. If the arches of your feet have flattened over the years, you'll be even more prone to injury. Each of these scenarios stresses your Achilles tendon, which then becomes inflamed from the small tears that come from too much activity too fast. Often Achilles tendinopathy sneaks up on you, with increasing increments of pain after physical activities.

Although some cases can be stubborn, rest and simple pain relievers will usually fix your Achilles tendinopathy, if you act quickly.

✅ Best first steps

Achilles tendinopathy is definitely a party pooper. To get yourself on the mend, use the RICE recipe for the first few days.

1. Rest.
Stop whatever activity hobbled you and any other activity that causes calf pain.

2. Ice.

Apply ice to the painful area every few hours for a few days.

3. Compress.

Compress the painful tendon with an elastic bandage, taking care not to have it painfully tight.

4. Elevate.

Keeping your foot higher than your heart, especially at night will help relieve swelling.

5. Dial a doctor.

If pain in the low calf or tendon is moderate or severe, see your doctor or physiotherapist without delay to make sure there is not a partial or complete rupture: recovery is much better when these injuries are treated immediately.

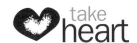

Doctor's bag

Your doctor or physiotherapist will examine your foot and calf, checking for tenderness and inflammation along your Achilles tendon. You may be asked to stand on your toes to see if it hurts. He will ask what kinds of physical activity you've been doing lately. He may order an ultrasound and/or X-ray of your foot; in special circumstances an MRI might be ordered. However, often no tests are needed. He may then suggest one or several of the following.

A shoe insert. He may suggest that you wear an insert, or orthotic, in your shoe to keep your heel elevated, relieving the strain on your Achilles tendon; he also may suggest that you wear a splint on your foot at night to keep the Achilles tendon stretched.

Although some cases can stubbornly persist, **rest** and **simple pain relievers** will usually fix an acute Achilles tendinopathy.

Instant relief

Your calf doesn't have to be a throbbing pest. Here are some ways to get instant relief.

Ice. Apply an ice pack to the tendon, holding it there for up to 20 minutes at a time several times a day.

The medicine chest. Take an anti-inflammatory, such as ibuprofen, following the directions on the pack.

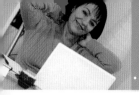

A boot, cast or brace. If your Achilles tendon is severely inflamed, the doctor may suggest you wear one of these for 2 to 3 weeks to keep the foot immobilised until the pain and inflammation subside.

Physiotherapy. A physiotherapist can guide you through gentle stretches and range-of-motion exercises to keep the ankle joint and muscles flexible. A program of specialised exercises will be prescribed for you and progressed once you are able to complete each step without pain.

Your pain toolbox

You have much more up your sleeve to help you out than you may think.

Goody two shoes. Buy some shoes that cushion your heel and have good arch support. Make sure you get rid of shoes that are ground down at the heel.

Stretching. Do the classic runner's stretch: stand a metre from a wall. Place your hands on the wall, keeping the affected leg straight and bending the other. Lean forwards until the Achilles tendon is stretched. Do this three to four times per day.

Heel raises. Rise on your toes, then lower your heels slowly. Do this a few times to start and gradually build up the repetitions.

Serious help

When simpler measures such as rest and physiotherapy don't work, or if the injury worsens, you could consider the following options.

Shock treatment. Despite the off-putting name, this just means therapy with strong sound waves. There is some evidence that this may relieve pain in persistent cases of Achilles tendinopathy.

Surgery. Your doctor may suggest surgery to remove the injured tissue from around the joint and to repair any tears. Afterwards, you may need to wear a cast temporarily and go through physiotherapy to strengthen your leg.

Bunions

Bunions are not only unsightly, they *hurt*. The triangular bony bump at the base of the big toe is not, as many people believe, formation of new bone. It's the abnormal protrusion of the bone and the bursa of the joint between the big toe and the first metatarsal bone of the foot. The main cause seems to be an inherited tendency to bunions. Experts debate the role of footwear, but, once the process of bunions is present, footwear that has a high heel (over 6 centimetres) or is tight is considered to aggravate the condition by causing the big toe to deviate further towards the other toes. As the toe joint rotates, the sesamoids, the two small bones under the toe, become dislocated, causing pain. The big toe's deformity means it's less able to bear weight.

Bunions are often progressive, and as they get worse from day-to-day loads on the foot they can also cause arthritic changes, adding to your pain. The initial symptoms are swelling, redness or soreness, as well as a thickening of the skin, at the big-toe joint. You may also develop corns or calluses where your first and second toes overlap. You'll begin to feel pain and may even notice less flexibility in your big toe. Wearing low-heeled (under 6 centimetres) shoes that are roomy at the front will keep the condition from getting worse and definitely make it less painful.

✔ Best first steps

One day, you're looking at your foot, and you notice a bulge, swelling or redness at the base of your big toe. Here's what to do.

1. Change your shoes.
Place your shoe beside your foot while you are standing barefoot. If the width of the toe box is narrower than the front of your foot, take the shoe (and all your other shoes) to a shoe repair shop and ask to have the toe box stretched. That will immediately relieve the

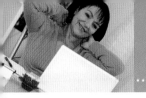

pressure on your big toe. Save the heels over 6 centimetres high for special events that include gawking but very little walking.

2. Consult a specialist.
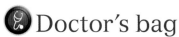

Bunions can't reverse themselves, but early assessment and treatment by a physiotherapist or podiatrist can help keep the condition from getting worse and can stem the pain.

Doctor's bag

Your doctor, podiatrist or physiotherapist will examine your foot and ask about the kind of pain you are feeling and where it's located. She will also ask about your and your family's history of foot difficulties and your history of injuries. You will be asked about your shoes and may have your foot X-rayed. Once the foot specialist has the information needed, she may suggest one or several of the following.

Taping. Using sports tape to partly correct your resting foot posture may help relieve your pain. This is usually only a short-term fix.

Shoe inserts. Being fitted for custom-made orthotics may help stabilise the big toe joint and help keep the bunion from getting worse. You can try a nonprescription version, sold in pharmacies and running stores, or have them custom-made. But they work only if you keep them in your shoes and those shoes on your feet!

Cortisone injection. If the area around your bunion is inflamed, your doctor may suggest a cortisone injection at the site to relieve the inflammation, which will in turn diminish the pain temporarily.

Your pain toolbox
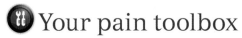

You don't have to be a bunion victim. Here are several measures that can ease the pain.

Anti-inflammatories. Ibuprofen or naproxen can help lower pain and inflammation. Take as suggested on the bottle.

Arch support. Arch supports are available online and at most pharmacies, shoe stores and running stores. Add them to all your shoes to take the pressure off your bunion. Arch supports can also be custom-made, but these are pricey.

Toe separator. Another aid is a toe separator, available online and at pharmacies, to keep your first and second toes from overlapping.

A good shoe store. Ask your health care clinician to recommend a shoe store whose employees are accustomed to fitting feet with special problems. Ask them to stretch your shoes out over the bunion. Buy shoes made of a soft, stretchable material.

 # Serious help

Bunions can be severe and more painful than simple measures can address.

Surgery. A variety of surgeries is possible, partly depending on the severity of your bunions and your level of physical activity. Your doctor may recommend a bunionectomy. A surgeon will remove the swollen tissue around the joint, then straighten the joint by removing part of the bone. Recovery can take up to 8 weeks. If you don't wear roomy, supportive shoes thereafter, your bunion could return.

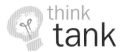

think
tank

'No one should live with chronic foot pain, especially from a bunion. With advanced surgical techniques, almost all bunion problems can be made much better with outpatient surgery—especially if people limit their use of very high-heeled shoes following the procedure.'

—Glenn B Pfeffer, MD, director of the Foot and Ankle Center, Cedars-Sinai Medical Center, Los Angeles; past president, American Orthopedic Foot and Ankle Society

 # Instant relief

If you have bunions, a day on your feet can be murder. Besides slipping off your shoes, here are some ways to get relief fast.

Ice. Place an ice pack over the painful spot for 10 minutes at a stretch, several times a day. It will tamp down the pain and inflammation.

Sandals. Around the house, wear sandals with good arch support. They'll relieve pressure on your toe.

Topical pain reliever. Rub on a painkilling gel.

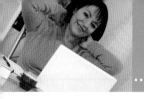

Foot and ankle arthritis

Inexplicably, the top of your foot hurts. Or your ankle aches. You may notice that your big toe hurts whenever you push off. If you experience these annoying pains regularly, you may have osteoarthritis in your feet and ankle.

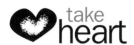

A study by the Arthritis Research Institute of America found that **regular exercise** for people with foot osteoarthritis did not increase foot pain or damage.

Midfoot arthritis strikes the top of the foot, where nine tiny bones bear the enormous loads of being upright and walking. Sometimes an injury can lead to this form of osteoarthritis, or it can simply develop from years of strain. Although it's common, it often goes unrecognised, partly because it may not show up on routine X-rays.

Ankle arthritis can be caused by wear on the joint between the shinbone, the tibia and the ankle bone. However, ankle arthritis more often results from a prior fracture, multiple sprains or occasionally an infection. It can also be the result of rheumatoid arthritis, a more serious form of arthritis that can affect the entire body.

Another common foot arthritis, great-toe arthritis, may sound funny, but something that hurts that much is anything but. The cartilage on the joint of the big toe where the toe meets the foot can wear away, and a spur may develop on top of the toe bone. The result is stiffness and pain every time you take a step, which may discourage you from doing much walking. You may also notice swelling at the joint and a bump or callus on top of the toe at the joint.

As painful as foot and ankle arthritis is, you can address it with some simple steps, such as changing your shoes and taking nonprescription pain medications.

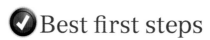 Best first steps

No need to suffer. In fact, the sooner you address the pain, the easier it is to treat.

1. Try a pain-relief cream or gel.
Creams and gels containing salicylates, an ingredient in aspirin, can help relieve pain and inflammation. Creams containing capsaicin, which gives chillies their kick, help kill pain over time. Another option is creams that contain ingredients such as menthol, wintergreen or eucalyptus oil, whose icy or hot sensation temporarily relieves pain. Use as directed, and don't use the creams with ice or heat packs.

2. Take nonprescription painkillers.
All three kinds of foot arthritis will respond to pain relievers such as paracetamol and anti-inflammatories such as ibuprofen. Take at the lowest dose that relieves your pain.

3. Modify your activities.
It's important to stay active but switch to things that minimise weight-bearing, such as cycling or swimming in place of running or jogging, and aquarobics rather than aerobics.

4. Get professional help.
See your physiotherapist or doctor. It may not be possible to remove the problem, but knowing the cause can help to stop it getting worse.

5. Cushion your shoe.
Choose new shoes that have cushioning in them or can easily accommodate a nonprescription soft foam or sheepskin insole.

Doctor's bag

Your doctor, physiotherapist or podiatrist will examine your foot, asking about when the pain occurs and about past foot injuries. He may X-ray the toe to assess the joint damage. He may also order a

Instant relief

On days when foot pain haunts you, try these fast fixes.

Foot baths. Fill a foot-sized container with very cool water and another with very warm water. Put your foot in the cool water for 30 seconds, then submerge it in the warm water for 30. Alternate from cool to warm for 5 minutes.

Relaxation. Some moderate activity is a good thing for arthritis and your overall health. But when your feet are hurting, prop them up and read a good book.

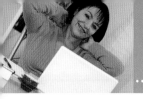

bone scan that can show evidence of arthritis or other problems not seen on X-rays. He may then suggest one or several of the following.

Shoe inserts. For both midfoot and great toe arthritis, custom-made orthotics (inserts, braces or splints) may be recommended to help reduce stress on the foot if nonprescription insoles have not helped. In the case of ankle arthritis, the doctor may fit you for a brace or splint to limit joint movement.

Cortisone injections. Steroid injections, usually not more than one or two, can help reduce inflammation.

Your pain toolbox

You too can be aggressive about pain by trying these measures.

New shoes. Choose shoes with stiff soles that will limit how much you can bend your feet, which can lessen your pain. If your big toe's the problem, make sure that the toe box is big enough, putting no pressure on the toe.

Fewer kilos. If you're overweight, foot arthritis may give you more incentive to shed the extra kilos. Less weight translates to less stress on your foot.

Serious help

If simple measures don't keep you walking with a spring in your step, your doctor may recommend surgery. Here are some options.

For big-toe arthritis, your doctor may suggest a procedure called cheilectomy. The surgeon cleans away scar tissue and bone spurs, which will help return some flexibility to the big toe. Or, in severe cases, he may suggest arthrodesis, or bone fusion, reducing the pain movement causes. Joint replacement remains very controversial and is rarely necessary.

For midfoot arthritis, if spurs have formed, you may need surgery to remove them. If the condition is severe and nothing else has worked, the doctor may want to fuse the joints. They don't normally move much anyway.

For ankle arthritis, the doctor may replace injured cartilage with cartilage from another part of your body, or he may fuse or replace the joint.

Peripheral vascular disease

You're the person who ambles along in an airport or on a shopping trip, stopping every hundred metres because your legs hurt. You may dismiss it as arthritis or age, but it might be peripheral vascular disease (PVD), a blockage of the blood vessels beyond the heart and brain. It's a form of arteriosclerosis (hardening and narrowing of the arteries). Affecting as many as 20 per cent of people aged 65 and over, it is the most common disease of the arteries. It results when fatty deposits stick to artery walls and harden, eventually restricting blood flow to the kidneys, legs and feet and to the bowel.

When blood flow drops, so does the supply of oxygen. When the same process happens in coronary or brain vessels, a heart attack or stroke can occur. You may not have symptoms. Or you may develop what's called intermittent claudication: cramps, pain or fatigue in your legs, buttocks, hips or feet when you're walking that stops when you stand still. In severe cases, your leg pain may be worse at night, when you're lying down and your feet are elevated. Your toenails may look cloudy and thicker, your legs a little blue, white or pink, and you may lose your leg hair, all symptoms of a circulation problem. Without treatment, sores that don't seem to heal may pop up on your toes or feet and the tissue may eventually die (gangrene), so amputation is required.

You're vulnerable if you're overweight, a smoker and a couch hugger. People who have high blood pressure, high cholesterol, diabetes or a family history of heart disease or stroke are more at risk as well. Although you may be worried about your legs, your real concern should be that PVD increases by 30 per cent your risk of dying from heart attack or stroke within 5 years.

If the condition isn't too severe when you address it, you can diminish the pain by stopping smoking, increasing your walking range and medication.

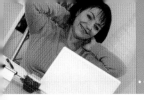

✓ Best first steps

There are several things you can do immediately that will make you safer and more comfortable.

1. Get evaluated.

If you have any of the symptoms of peripheral vascular disease, make an appointment with your doctor. If you also feel chest or throat pain, numbness, confusion, dizziness or a sudden headache, call for emergency help. *These could be the early signs of a heart attack or stroke.*

2. Lower your legs.

If you have pain in your toes or feet while you are asleep, lower them over the side of the bed and let them hang. This will increase blood circulation and help decrease the pain.

Doctor's bag

To help him diagnose you, your doctor will probably do pulse tests to measure the strength of the arteries behind your knees and in your feet, check your cholesterol and measure the difference between the blood pressure in your arm and ankle. He may also order tests of blood flow such as Doppler studies or an angiogram—the latter involves an X-ray imaging of blood flow while dye is injected. Once the doctor makes a diagnosis, he may offer one or several of the following.

Cholesterol medications. Cholesterol contributes to the fatty build-up blocking your arteries, so statins, medications that lower cholesterol, help reduce the chances of a heart attack or stroke. Your aim is an LDL (bad) cholesterol reading of less than 2.6 mmol/L.

Blood pressure medications. If your blood pressure is high, your doctor may recommend beta-blockers or ACE inhibitors to bring it down.

Clot busters. PVD raises the risk of blood clots, so your doctor may suggest taking a low-dose aspirin (100 milligrams) daily or a clot-preventing medication such as clopidogrel. Both prevent the platelets in blood from sticking together and forming a clot.

Artery openers. Cilostazol (Pletal) may reduce pain by dilating the blood vessels, increasing the blood flow to your legs. 'It's the only drug that will help people walk with less pain', says cardiologist Gary Ansel, MD, FAAC, director of the Center for Critical Limb Care, Riverside Methodist Hospital, Columbus, Ohio. 'In half the patients, it will double their walking distance without pain.' It has the added benefit of preventing blood clots. It can take 3 months for the effects to kick in. (Unfortunately, this medication is not suitable for people with heart failure.)

Medication for high blood glucose. If you have diabetes, which increases the risk of PVD, it's even more essential to control your blood glucose levels with diet and medication.

 # Your pain toolbox

Changing your habits may be the most important thing you can do to help prevent increasing pain and the risk of amputation from PVD.

A smoke-free life. Tossing your cigarettes can have a dramatic effect on your pain, says Dr Ansel. 'You may have cut back to three a day, but until you get to zero, it won't make much of a difference. Just one cigarette a day knocks out the body's ability to dilate its blood vessels for 24 hours.' Dilated blood vessels mean greater blood flow, less pain.

Supervised walking. Walking until you have pain, stopping, then walking again for at least 20 minutes a day on most days will reduce

 # Instant relief

Who doesn't want the drone of pain to stop? Below are some quick pain relievers.

R and R. Take a 10-minute break in a chair, keeping your legs lower than your heart. That will help blood flow and stop the pain.

A warm (not hot) bath. Staying warm keeps circulation going, and soaking in a warm bath also takes the edge off stress.

Loose-fitting wool socks. Cold constricts blood vessels, so staying warm with loose-fitting wool socks on cold days will lower your pain. Skip the hot-water bottles and heating pads; PVD can desensitise your feet, so you may get burnt and not realise it.

Bricks under your bed. Your blood flow is better when your legs are lower than your heart. So, with help, raise the head of your bed by placing bricks under its base.

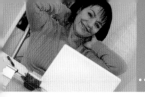

your pain. Exercise increases the number of tiny collateral blood vessels that help keep blood moving around a blockage. Of course, the more you push, the better condition you'll be in.

A better diet. Eating more fruit, vegetables, whole grains and lean proteins such as fish and chicken, and chucking high-fat fast food, will help keep the disease, and hence the pain, from progressing. Eating fatty fish, such as salmon, tuna, halibut and sardines, at least twice a week may be particularly smart: some research shows that omega-3 fatty acids, found in fatty fish as well as linseeds, walnuts, soya beans and canola oil, may improve the health of blood vessel walls.

Pampered feet. Because you have reduced blood flow to your feet, injuries will be slower to heal and vulnerable to infection, especially if you have diabetes. Wear shoes all the time, even slippers for late-night bathroom visits. Protect your feet by washing them and applying moisturiser to prevent cracks. Wear thick, dry socks, examine your feet regularly, and call your doctor at the first sign of injury.

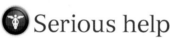 Serious help

In some cases, lifestyle changes and medications aren't enough to treat the pain and other symptoms, and your doctor may suggest more invasive steps. What you choose will depend on your symptoms, how advanced your case is and what other conditions you have.

Angioplasty. Your doctor may perform this procedure, passing a thin tube through your artery from the groin or arm to the blocked spot, where a balloon is inflated, pushing back the accumulated plaque, or fatty build-up.

Stent. If the angioplasty isn't enough, your doctor may, during the angioplasty, insert a stent, or synthetic tube, covered with a material that tissue can't grow through. The stent keeps the artery open the way scaffolding keeps a mine shaft open.

Bypass surgery. Using part of one of your veins or a synthetic tube, your surgeon creates a new blood vessel that he attaches below and above the blocked spot on your artery. Like cars on a highway bypass, your blood can now flow around the blocked portion.

Plantar fasciitis

One morning, when you swing your legs over the side of the bed and plant a few steps towards the shower, you suddenly feel like your foot is on fire. That pain in your heel, which can feel like stabbing or burning, may be plantar fasciitis, inflammation of the plantar fascia, the thick, tough tissue that runs along the bottom of the foot, connecting heel bone to toes.

The scourge of dedicated exercisers everywhere, plantar fasciitis usually results from too much stress on your heel bone and tissue while you're doing the right thing, such as jogging and walking regularly. Factors that increase your chances of pulling up lame include flat feet or high arches, obesity, weight gain (including pregnancy) or a tight Achilles tendon, which connects the calf muscles to the heel. You don't do your foot any favours by wearing stiletto heels or flimsy shoes that don't absorb the shock of each footstep. You're more likely to get the condition if you're a woman or between the ages of 40 and 70.

The pain usually develops gradually but may come on suddenly. It's definitely worse in the mornings or after sitting because the plantar fascia tissue tightens up at rest. Usually, though not always, it affects only one foot at a time—a small blessing. Untreated, the condition can become chronic, interfering with your daily activities and also with other parts of your body as you alter the way you walk in order to avoid pain.

Most of the time, however, you can recover and relieve the pain with at-home remedies such as rest, anti-inflammatories and stretching. A few sessions of physiotherapy, custom-made orthotics and even nonprescription arch supports can be of some help. Chances are greater than 90 per cent that your sensitive feet will respond, but be patient: it can take months.

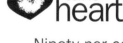

take
heart

Ninety per cent of people with plantar fasciitis improve after **2 to 3 months** of treatment.

 Best first steps

Don't hobble through the day. To lessen your pain and get recovery started, try the following.

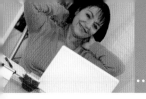

1. Stop.

Stop the activity that may have triggered the inflammation, letting your foot get some rest.

2. Relieve the inflammation.

Nonsteroidal anti-inflammatory drugs (NSAIDs) such as ibuprofen or naproxen can help. If your stomach doesn't tolerate NSAIDs, you can use paracetamol to relieve the pain, but paracetamol does not have an anti-inflammatory action.

3. Stretch.

Do it before you even get out of bed. Stretch your arch, Achilles tendon and calf muscles by slowly extending your ankle and pointing your toes towards your chest.

4. Pad your feet.

Use a nonprescription heel cushion of rubber or gel in your shoes.

Doctor's bag

If the condition fails to settle with standard treatment, your doctor or physiotherapist will examine your foot. She may order tests such as an X-ray, ultrasound, bone scan or MRI to confirm the diagnosis or exclude other causes. She may then recommend one of the following.

Splints. This device fits on your calf and foot while you sleep, holding the plantar fascia and the Achilles tendon in a lengthened position, augmenting your stretching routine.

Corticosteroids. To relieve continuing pain, your doctor may suggest injections of corticosteroids at the heel, always a temporary measure.

Instant relief

When pain is pinching your heel, relief can't come fast enough. Try a few of these speedy pain relievers.

Ice. Put your foot on ice for 20 minutes at a time. This will numb the pain and relieve the inflammation. Try placing a bottle of frozen water on the ground and rolling the sole of your foot across it.

Heat. Alternate ice with heat, which increases blood flow to the heel, speeding healing.

Keep your feet off the ground. Weight on your foot adds to inflammation. If you work standing up, try to take sit-down breaks as often as possible. Standing on a cushioned mat may also help.

Your pain toolbox

You have lots of weapons in your home arsenal to attack and prevent this kind of heel pain. Here are a few things to try.

Avoid walking barefoot. Walking barefoot only puts more stress on your plantar fascia.

Stretching exercises. Stretching is a mainstay of recovery and prevention. As well as stretches on waking, add this to your routine: sit with your legs crossed and, with your hand, pull your toes and ankle back towards your shin for 10 seconds. Repeat 10 times, three times per day.

Better shoes. Supporting the arch of your foot is critical. Mothball your high heels, ditch the flip-flops and get a pair of sturdy lace-up shoes with good arch support and a well-cushioned sole.

Warm-ups. Once your pain has subsided and you start exercising again, warm up with a few heel stretches before you get going.

Weight loss. The more you weigh, the greater the stress on your plantar fascia.

Orthotics. These shoe inserts, which can be off the shelf or custom-made, can help distribute the pressure on your foot more evenly, taking some burden off your heel.

Serious help

Sometimes even the best self-care measures and simple doctoring may not be enough to get your foot back on track. Here are several options for more stubborn cases.

Shock treatment. The doctor directs sound waves at the heel, which slightly traumatise the tissue, triggering a healing response by the body. Early studies showed uncertain results but more recent studies are more encouraging—worth trying before having surgery.

Plantar fasciotomy. Ninety per cent of people with plantar fasciitis improve without surgery. For the few who don't, a surgeon can detach the plantar fascia from the heel, which often relieves the pain. There are risks: your arch can drop slightly, which can cause other foot problems. Discuss potential side effects with your orthopaedic surgeon or podiatrist before you agree to surgery.

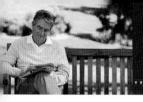

Mystery pain

Most of the time, pain has an obvious cause, but sometimes doctors can't find it, at least not for a while. The clinical term for such mystery pain is idiopathic pain, a way for a doctor to say, 'I don't know why you're hurting'. Some people hurt all over for seemingly no reason, or they have, say, back or pelvic pain, where it's hard to define exactly what tissue is involved in generating the pain signals. That doesn't mean that the pain is any less real, but it can make it harder to accept.

Sometimes, even the best medical tests are poor at detecting the sorts of changes in the intervertebral discs (of the spine) that cause pain. Perhaps our neural pathways have become hypersensitive and are sending signals that the brain interprets as pain. When we're depressed, our nerve centres that suppress pain are less effective at damping down pain signalling. If we're anxious or if we've had a traumatic experience, our minds may become over-vigilant, causing increased transmission of signalling that our brains interpret as pain.

Most of the things we do for any state of chronic pain apply whether we have a diagnosis or not. There are many things you can do to feel better. In fact, many of the measures may be even more useful than the prescription drugs your doctors prescribe.

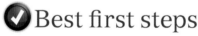 Best first steps

The first thing to do is get your life going again.

Look for a diagnosis.

Of course you should try to get a diagnosis. But once you've seen one or two specialists who can't give you an exact reason for your pain, respect their training and competence. You're not the first patient to be told that your pain lacks a clear explanation and you won't be the last. It's not in your best interests to keep looking for that elusive diagnosis: that just exposes you to more tests or surgery (which risks causing incidental damage to your body) when you would be better off focusing your energy and time on managing your pain. It can also lead to false hope and great disappointment.

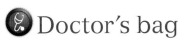 Doctor's bag

Your doctors may not have been able find the exact cause of your pain but they, with other therapists such as a psychologist and a physiotherapist, have an important role helping you plan your pain management strategy. Your doctors can also trial medications with you to see whether they provide useful alleviation of your pain. Remember that where chronic pain is the problem, an assessment has to be made whether any side effects caused by the medication are justified by the medication providing sufficient improvement, not just in pain relief, but in helping you to achieve the things that give you quality of life.

Antidepressants. You may ask why your doctor would suggest a drug for depression to ease your mystery pain. In fact, tricyclic antidepressants such as imipramine (Tofranil, Tolerade), nortriptyline (Allegron) and amitriptyline (Endep) increase neurotransmitters in the spinal cord and brain that reduce pain signals. As well, taken before bed, they may help you sleep better. Serotonin-noradrenaline reuptake inhibitors (SNRIs) such as venlafaxine (Effexor) and duloxetine (Cymbalta) also lessen pain by modifying pain signalling. The pain-relieving effects of tricyclic antidepressants occur at low doses, which means that some of the more troublesome side effects of these medications can be avoided—things such as dry mouth, constipation, difficulty emptying your bladder—but an actual antidepressant effect may not occur. If your doctor considers you would benefit from an antidepressant effect as well as a pain-modifying effect, venlafaxine or duloxetine would be appropriate.

Opioids. If your pain is chronic and severe, your doctor may prescribe opioids. There are many opioids on the market: buprenorphine (Norspan), fentanyl (Durogesic), hydromorphone (Dilaudid, Jurnista), morphine (Anamorph, Kapanol, MS Contin), oxycodone (Endone, OxyContin, OxyNorm). Codeine, found in many preparations, is converted to morphine and this is considered the main way that codeine brings about pain relief. Using codeine preparations is commonly thought to avoid exposure to significant amounts of opioid but really it is a matter of dosage. For example, taking eight tablets of Panadeine Forte per day is approximately

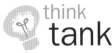
think
tank

'A study at Kaiser Permanente Medical Center in Santa Clara, California, found that depression contributes more to sleep difficulties in chronic pain patients than the pain itself.'

—Rochelle Cairns, BAppSc (Psych), GradDip (Psych), PhD (Psych), Senior Health and Clinical Psychologist, Pain Service, Austin Health, Melbourne

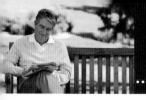

equivalent to 30 milligrams of morphine. The long-term benefits and risks of opioids are uncertain. Although they have been shown to decrease pain scores, they do not seem to improve function. In other words, you might feel better, but still find yourself sitting on the couch rather than getting up and about. If opioids are used, they should be as part of a pain management strategy with a focus on achieving the activities that are important to you.

Sleep medications. Your doctor may prescribe a temporary sleep aid to break the sleepless cycle while you also improve your sleep habits. The key to achieving long-term improved sleep is not to rely on medication but to undertake good sleep practices—see 'More sleep' opposite. Benzodiazepine sedatives such as temazepam and oxazepam are suitable for occasional or short-term use. Beware: they can be habit forming; they should not be used for more than a week or two at most. Non-benzodiazepine alternatives include zolpidem and zopiclone (Imovane, Imrest). These drugs also can be habit forming and should be limited to short-term use only, that is, 4 weeks or less.

 # Your pain toolbox

Now's the time to go back and read Parts One and Two of this book and discuss them with your partner and your health team—your doctor and your other therapists.

Instant relief

Here are some tips to help you manage your pain.

Music you love. Even if you like earsplitting rock, listening to it—or any music that sets your foot tapping—may lessen your pain, lift your spirits and make you feel more in control, according to a study at Cleveland Clinic Foundation. Chronic pain patients who listened to music on a headset for an hour a day over 7 days had a 12 to 21 per cent reduction in pain; nonlistening groups had a pain decrease of just 1 to 2 per cent. Listeners also felt less depressed.

A yoga class. Not only does yoga help keep muscles from tightening up in response to pain, it also helps ease depression and anxiety, two things that often go along with pain. According to a Boston University study, yoga raises levels of a neurotransmitter called gamma-aminobutyric acid (GABA). Low levels are associated with depression and anxiety. After each hour-long yoga session, GABA levels rose an average of 27 per cent.

A bag of peas. You've probably heard of using a bag of frozen peas wrapped in a cloth to chill your aching spots for 15 to 20 minutes. You can also microwave the bag and let it double as a heating pad, again wrapped in a cloth and held on an aching place for 15 to 20 minutes.

Psychologist. A psychologist can help you work out strategies to manage situations related to chronic pain. These strategies can supplement medication or reduce the reliance on medication. Examples of these strategies are relaxation and good sleep practices. Psychologists can help you decide what areas to focus your energies on to best deal with the challenges of chronic pain, and to help you decide what steps to take to achieve what's meaningful in your life. Psychologists are experts at helping you develop ways of dealing with fellow travellers of chronic pain—depression and anxiety.

Physiotherapy. Chronic pain can leave you wanting to curl up on the couch. A physiotherapist can work with you to stretch and strengthen tight muscles, which can help relieve pain. They also can create a regular routine of aerobic exercises to accompany the stretching and strengthening ones. Physiotherapists are experts in helping you plan and achieve physical activities appropriate to your situation. Physical activity, even when you've got pain, is important: it improves mood, promotes release of endorphins—the body's natural pain-relieving agents—and helps you sleep.

More sleep. Chances are you're not sleeping well, a situation that compounds your pain and drags down your spirits. In fact, a recent study at Johns Hopkins University found that disturbed sleep alters some pain control mechanisms, making chronic pain worse. Tidy up your sleep habits. Get up at the same times every day. Use the bed only for sleep and sex: the bedroom is not the place for the laptop or the TV. Try a warm (not too hot) bath before bed: the warmth will relax you and ease your transition into sleep.

Partnering with your partner. Most patients don't tell other people about their pain, or they tell them in hidden ways by being grumpy or withdrawn. 'But your friends and family need to know what's going on', says Dr Maine, Director of the Center for Interventional Pain Medicine, Mercy Medical Center, Baltimore. 'That's what family is for. Take your partner to your medical evaluations. That's part of empowering yourself to feel better.' If one of the things you want to do is to increase your activity, enrol your partner in this; get them to come with you for walks; and ask them to encourage you when they notice you are feeling a bit down.

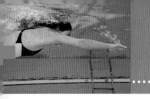

Complex regional pain syndrome

Complex regional pain syndrome (CRPS) is a painful condition that affects mostly the arms or legs and occasionally the face. The pain is intense, often a sensation of burning and aching. The symptoms may also include skin sensitivity, changes in skin temperature and colour, changes in hair and nail growth, joint stiffness or swelling, muscle spasms and a limited range of motion in the affected limb. Women, usually between the ages of 40 and 60, are most commonly affected.

The syndrome is rare, affecting 26 people out of 100,000. Two forms of CRPS are recognised. Type one (previously known as reflex sympathetic dystrophy) occurs after an illness, some surgeries or an injury, sometimes of a minor nature. Type two (previously known as causalgia) springs up after an injury that involves a nerve.

Symptoms can range from mild to severe and may last months or years. The cause of CRPS is not clear, but treatment aims to relieve symptoms and restore limb function (movement and activity). Most people almost completely recover, but the condition can recur and, for a small group of people with CRPS, symptoms may be severe and persist for years. Early treatment seems to improve your chances of a good result.

✅ Best first steps

This pain syndrome requires fast action. Here's what to do.

1. See your doctor pronto.
If you're experiencing ongoing severe pain in one limb, see your doctor straightaway. Managed within the first months, CRPS can improve dramatically.

2. Join the team.

CRPS is a complicated condition and that means that a single type of treatment probably won't be enough. Adopting a multi-disciplinary approach to managing CRPS is usually best. This may include seeing a physiotherapist, an occupational therapist and a psychologist and participating in both individual and group-based programs. Meeting up with other people who have CRPS can help you to feel less isolated and give you some tips on helpful ways to manage your condition.

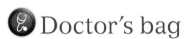 Doctor's bag

There is no diagnostic test for CRPS. Diagnosis is based on your medical history and symptoms. Recovery of movement is critical to achieving improvement in CRPS. The role of medical treatment is not simply lessening pain, but lessening pain so that more movement is achieved. Sometimes your doctor may order blood tests, bone scans, X-rays, CT scans or MRI scans to rule out other conditions that have similar symptoms.

He may then offer one or more of the following medications. All of these medications have side effects that may include poor concentration, impaired memory, drowsiness and impaired balance. Some of these medications were developed for other conditions that involve the nervous system, but have been found also to be helpful for 'neuropathic' pain, which is a name for the type of pain associated with CRPS. It helps to remember this when you get the medication home and start reading the patient information leaflet.

Antidepressants. Tricyclic antidepressants such as amitriptyline (Endep) and nortriptyline (Allegron) are very effective for relieving neuropathic pain. The dose required is much lower than that used for treating depression. Some of the newer antidepressants such as duloxetine (Cymbalta) and venlafaxine (Effexor) may also be beneficial.

Opioids. Studies show that highish doses of opioids—such as fentanyl (Durogesic), morphine (Kapanol, MS Contin), oxycodone (Endone, OxyContin, OxyNorm, Targin)—can relieve nerve pain. The drugs have drawbacks, including sleepiness, constipation and nausea. Used over long periods, opioids may cause an increase in sensitivity to pain, a problem called opioid-induced hyperalgesia. Long-term use may also lead to dependence.

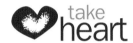

In an Australian study, **pain and disability improved** in patients with CRPS **after 6 weeks** of graded motor imagery and the results were **still evident 6 months later**.

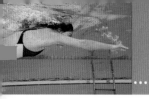

Anticonvulsant medications. Drugs such as gabapentin and pregabalin (Lyrica) sometimes help relieve this neuropathic pain. Unfortunately, the gabapentinoids are not currently on the Pharmaceutical Benefits Scheme in Australia or PHARMAC in New Zealand so they are expensive.

Topical medications. Topical lignocaine or compound creams and gels may be useful in reducing any skin sensitivity. A chemical compound called DMSO (dimethyl sulfoxide), widely used in Europe as a topical pain reliever, can sometimes be accessed in Australia and New Zealand by a compounding pharmacy making the cream for you.

Bone-loss medications. Your doctor may also recommend osteoporosis medications such as alendronate (Fosamax) and calcitonin (Miacalcin). It is unclear how these agents work in CRPS.

A nerve block. Your doctor may inject an anaesthetic that will block the pain. Not everyone responds to this treatment but in those that do, it can be very beneficial. Usually a course of injections over several months is required.

Your pain toolbox

You can add to your doctor's orders with pain weapons of your own. However, as with all medical treatments for CRPS there is no guaranteed cure, and there is no single treatment that, used in isolation, will make you better. That's why you will benefit from the involvement of a team of therapists.

Physiotherapy. There is good evidence that physiotherapy can help to reduce your pain and improve your function if you have CRPS. Treatment methods progress over time. Initially there is more emphasis on reducing your pain and swelling, but before too long the emphasis swings towards getting your movement and your tolerance of sensations (such as touch, pressure, hot and cold) under your control. After that, attention is given to functional activities and general fitness. Your physiotherapist will talk to you about ways to get things done despite your pain and about good strategies to prevent causing a flare-up of your pain.

Occupational therapy. The primary goal of occupational therapy is to enable you to participate fully in the activities of your everyday life. For people with CRPS, specific activities are used to enhance your ability to participate. Sometimes modifications to your physical environment can facilitate this further. An occupational therapist can help you learn how to cope with demands, adapt to tasks and overcome challenges in your day-to-day life, at home, out in the community, driving your car and at your workplace.

Graded Motor Imagery (GMI). GMI is a relatively new approach to reducing pain and improving function in CRPS. It is based on scientific research conducted in Australia. Patients of all ages with CRPS of both short and long duration have had good results. But, like all treatments for CRPS, not everybody benefits. Ask your physiotherapist or occupational therapist about GMI, or go online and read about it for yourself.

Psychology. CRPS can lead to depression, which can heighten pain and make it more difficult to do the activities, such as physiotherapy. While not all people with CRPS develop depression, a psychologist can help you keep things in perspective and can offer you ways to ward off defeating thoughts. She may also be able to teach you exercises such as deep breathing or meditation that can help you relax, thus reducing pain. Talk to your psychologist about learning some relaxation techniques, practising mindfulness meditation and understanding your sleep (or more likely your lack of sleep) and what you can do to improve it.

Serious help

In some rare cases that don't respond to other treatments, your doctor may suggest more invasive steps. These are significant interventions and should be discussed thoroughly with your doctor before they are undertaken. Usually a trial with a temporary form of the therapy is performed before proceeding to the definitive procedure.

A spinal cord stimulator. The doctor places one or two thin cables inside the spinal canal where the nerves that serve the affected limb enter the spinal cord. The other ends of the cables connect to an electrical impulse generator that usually has been surgically

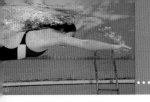

placed under the skin of the abdomen or above the buttock. This generator sends mild electrical signals to your spinal cord, scrambling and blocking pain messages. The patient can adjust the strength of the signals with an external control.

Intrathecal drug pump. Implanted under the skin of the abdomen, the pump delivers medications through a catheter to the fluid surrounding the spinal cord. The medications block the relaying of pain signals from the nerves of the affected limb to your brain. The advantage is that medications delivered directly to the spinal cord can improve the blocking action and can offer relief at lower doses than painkillers taken orally so that side effects may be lessened.

A sympathectomy. During this seldom-used procedure, the doctor will cut or chemically disrupt the sympathetic nerves that may be involved in the CRPS process. However, the relief may be only temporary because as months go by the nerves tend to regrow or develop alternative pathways that transmit pain signals.

Diabetic neuropathy

Diabetic neuropathy is the name for nerve damage in people with diabetes. About 70 per cent of diabetics suffer at least some neuropathy, commonly in their legs and feet. However, the disease can strike almost any part of the body, from the eyes to the bladder. The risk of neuropathy rises with age and with the duration of diabetes, with rates highest in people who have had diabetes for 25 years or longer.

Your risk is higher if you have trouble controlling your blood glucose, have elevated levels of the blood fats called triglycerides, have high blood pressure or are overweight.

Some people with diabetic neuropathy have no symptoms. Others may have pain, tingling or numbness, particularly in their limbs. They may also begin to have urinary tract problems, such as infections or incontinence; nausea, vomiting, indigestion or other problems in the digestive system; or blood vessel and heart troubles.

There are four types of diabetic neuropathy, and it's possible to have one or several. Peripheral neuropathy is the most common, damaging nerves in the limbs, primarily the legs and feet. Autonomic neuropathy affects the autonomic nervous system that controls the organs, leading to a wide range of difficulties from gastrointestinal and bladder problems to problems with body temperature. Proximal neuropathy causes severe pain in the hips, thighs or buttocks, and severely weakens the thigh muscles. Focal neuropathy usually involves only one nerve and usually goes away in weeks or months. It may make it difficult for your eyes to focus, cause paralysis on one side of your face or pain in your shin or foot.

Don't despair. A number of measures can slow the progression of the disease and manage the pain and complications that neuropathy causes.

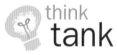

think tank

'Diabetes essentially starves the tiny nerves, so that the nervous system becomes confused about what is and what isn't painful. The hypersensitive nerves send signals to the spinal cord, where they're mistaken for pain.'

—Scott M Fishman, MD, co-author of *The War on Pain*

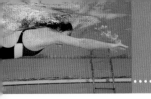

✔ Best first steps

The earlier you address diabetic neuropathy, the sooner you can slow its spread and banish its pain.

1. At the first tingle, give your doctor a call.
If you notice tingling, burning, weakness or pain in your hands or feet, head to your doctor as soon as you can. The same goes for dizziness, an increase or decrease in your sweating and changes in digestion, urination or sexual function.

2. Become the blood glucose police.
Monitor your blood glucose more closely than ever. Controlling it will slow the progression of the disease. Your doctor will likely recommend these goals: 5.0 to 7.2 mmol/L before meals; less than 10.0 mmol/L 2 hours after meals; and a haemoglobin A1c (the measure of control over several months) of less than 7 per cent.

℞ Doctor's bag

Your doctor will check out your symptoms and do a physical examination, monitoring your reaction to touch, temperature and vibration. He'll also check your muscle strength and reflexes, as well as your blood pressure and heart rate. He may do nerve conduction studies, measuring how quickly your limbs carry electrical signals, or an electromyography (EMG), which gauges how well your muscles respond to electrical signals. Once he's confirmed that you have diabetic neuropathy, he'll review steps you need to take to control your blood glucose. He'll also likely prescribe several of the following to relieve pain.

Antidepressants. It's likely that your mood will be affected by this kind of pain, but that's not why your doctor might suggest a tricyclic antidepressant such as amitriptyline (Endep) or nortriptyline (Allegron). The drugs help calm irregular nerve activity, which in turn helps stem pain. Another type of antidepressant, duloxetine (Cymbalta), has been approved specifically for diabetic neuropathy. In a recent study, 27 per cent of patients taking duloxetine had a 50 per cent reduction in pain within the first week of treatment.

Gabapentinoids. Anticonvulsant drugs such as pregabalin (Lyrica) and gabapentin work by decreasing pain signalling in neural pathways. Both of these drugs have been approved in Australia for neuropathic pain.

Opioids. Opioids such as buprenorphine (Norspan), fentanyl (Durogesic), hydromorphine (Dilaudid), morphine (Kapanol, MS Contin), oxycodone (OxyContin) offer some pain relief. Combinations of opioids with antidepressants or gabapentinoids often provide better pain relief with fewer side effects than occur when only one class of agents is used. Note that benefit from opioids should not require more than a low dose.

Lidoderm (lignocaine patches). Patches that deliver lignocaine, a local anaesthetic, placed over a painful area, reduce pain signalling from damaged nerves and limit pain for up to 12 hours. To prevent absorbing a dangerous level of lignocaine, not more than three patches should be worn at the same time and patches should not be worn for more than 12 hours daily.

ACE inhibitors. The ACE inhibitor class of blood pressure medications appears to have some protective effect against microvascular complications and organ damage from diabetes.

Lipid-lowering drugs. High blood levels of triglycerides, a type of blood fat, increase the risk of diabetic neuropathy, and drugs that lower triglycerides may help prevent damage to tiny blood vessels

🕐 Instant relief

Below are some ways to chase down pain fast.

A warm bath. Test the water with your wrist or a bath thermometer, as your feet may underestimate the heat. The temperature should be no higher than 40°C. The warmth will help relieve pain and loosen tightened muscles. Soak for no longer than 20 minutes.

A bed cradle. This device cradles your sheets, not you. Place this metal arc over the bottom of your bed, throw the bottom of the covers over it, and you can sleep without the sheets and blankets touching your painful feet and legs while you are cosily tucked in at the head of the bed.

Careful clothes. Wearing silk to bed and even under your clothes can help soothe sensitive skin. Various websites also sell shoes and socks designed to have a looser fit and more cushioning for painful feet.

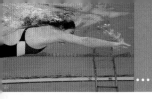

that often results in diabetic retinopathy. The lipid-lowering HMG-CoA reductase inhibitors (statins) may also help prevent nerve damage.

Aldose reductase inhibitors. Aldose reductase is an enzyme that may be important in the development of diabetic neuropathy, and blocking it may reduce the risk of diabetic nerve damage.

Your pain toolbox

You can take a number of steps to both relieve the discomforts and pain of neuropathy and to help prevent its progression.

Capsaicin cream. Capsaicin is the ingredient that gives chillies their heat. Creams that contain capsaicin, such as Zostrix, when used repeatedly over time, deplete compounds that carry pain signals to the brain.

Acetyl-L-carnitine (ALC). ALC is a form of the amino acid L-carnitine used as a dietary supplement and available in health and natural foods stores. Several large studies have found that 500 to 1000 milligrams of ALC taken three times a day for a year reduced pain in 27 per cent of patients with diabetic neuropathy, particularly patients in the early stage of the disease.

Omega-3 fatty acids. Alpha-linolenic acid, an omega-3 fatty acid in vegetable oils, such as canola oil, as well as linseeds, walnuts and soya beans, appears to lower the risk of diabetic neuropathy, according to a study by the Centers for Disease Control and Prevention. Suggested dose: 2200 milligrams per day, or almost half a cup of walnuts or soya beans.

Acupuncture and TENS. Several studies suggest that acupuncture reduces the pain of diabetic neuropathy. In a small Harvard study, weekly acupuncture sessions for 10 weeks cut pain scores by four to five points—from 18 to 19 at week one to 13 to 14 at week ten. TENS is transcutaneous electrical nerve stimulation. Electrodes placed on the skin provide a gentle electrical current, which can stimulate pain-blocking signals in neural pathways. There are some studies showing benefit from TENS in diabetic neuropathy. Both acupuncture and TENS avoid side effects such as drowsiness, which can be caused by medications.

Take charge of your bad habits. Smoking is a terrible compounder of the adverse cardiovascular effects of diabetes and should be stopped completely. Consult your doctor and use the help available from http://www.quitnow.gov.au. It might take a number of attempts but keep trying. Alcohol in excess worsens blood glucose and blood fat (triglycerides, cholesterol) levels: stay within recommended guidelines of not more than four standard drinks on any one occasion.

Exercise. Swimming is a particularly good choice if you have pain in your feet. Exercising at least 30 minutes per day most days can help you keep your blood glucose and weight down and your spirits up. It also improves blood flow and helps keep blood pressure under control.

Serious help

If your pain doesn't lessen with more moderate measures or the disease leads to a serious complication, your doctor may recommend one of the following.

Spinal cord stimulator. This device requires placing electrodes in the spinal canal. The electrodes are linked by a thin cable to a small impulse generator, which is commonly placed under the skin of the upper abdomen. The electrical impulses lessen the transmission of pain signals from the painful limb to the brain. These devices are reserved for use in situations of severe pain that is not responsive to other treatments. The patient can adjust the electrical signals with an external device. In a small Dutch study, the average pain score of patients who used the stimulator for 6 months dropped from 77 to 34.

Surgery. Diabetic neuropathy reduces the feeling in and the blood flow to limbs, especially feet. If an untreated foot ulcer becomes gangrenous—that is, if the tissue dies—the doctor will have to operate to remove the dead tissue and possibly even amputate the foot.

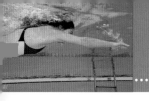

Shingles

Your skin feels as hot as a fireplace poker for days. Then, suddenly, a blistering rash breaks out. It may blaze a trail from the middle of your back to your breastbone, a band called a dermatome. Not only does it itch, it's so painful that even a light touch can hurt. Some people have nonspecific symptoms of infection—mild fever, headache, feeling vaguely unwell—but many have no symptoms other than pain or itch.

You have shingles, which is the same virus (herpes zoster) that causes chickenpox. Once you've had chickenpox, the virus may simply lie low for decades, reappearing as shingles for no apparent reason; or it may reappear triggered by stress, an immune-system deficiency (from chemotherapy or AIDS, for example) or cancer. People over age 60 are at most risk, although anyone who's had chickenpox can be a victim. Doctors believe the virus may migrate to nerve cells during chickenpox, then reactivate in the nerve fibres, affecting sensory cells, when it recurs as shingles.

Although the rash, when treated, can clear up within 3 to 5 weeks, the affected skin can remain painful for years, a complication called postherpetic neuralgia, which occurs in one out of five people who get shingles.

Fortunately, when caught early, shingles can be treated with antiviral drugs and self-care treatments.

✅ Best first steps

As with most painful conditions, the sooner you act the better.

1. Get to the doctor straightaway.

Call your doctor as soon as you suspect shingles, especially if the rash is near your eyes. Untreated, it can cause permanent eye damage. The sooner you get to a doctor for prescription meds, the better the chance that they'll work. You also need to hustle if you live with an infant, a pregnant woman or someone whose immune system has been weakened by cancer or a chronic illness, since this contagious condition poses a serious risk to them.

2. Nonprescription pain relievers.
Take paracetamol or an anti-inflammatory such as ibuprofen or naproxen. There is no clear evidence to show that one of these agents is superior to any other. Follow the directions on the package.

Doctor's bag

Your doctor will give you a physical examination, ask you about symptoms and may take a tissue sample to verify that you have shingles. Once that's confirmed, she will likely suggest several of the following.

Antiviral drugs. Aciclovir, famciclovir or valaciclovir can cut the severity and length of a shingles outbreak if you can take them within 72 hours of the first appearance of the rash. They also may help prevent postherpetic neuralgia. The antiviral is usually taken for a week.

Tramadol. This drug combines opioid and monoamine re-uptake actions. (Changing monoamine re-uptake is how antidepressants work in modifying depression and in modifying pain signalling.) It is available in both immediate release and slow-release preparations. Tramadol can be useful to relieve pain during the acute attack of shingles and afterwards if postherpetic neuralgia occurs.

Opioids. Sometimes the pain from either acute shingles or chronic postherpetic neuralgia requires strong pain relief. Generally slow-release preparations are preferable; in the acute phase immediate release may be required. Patches (transdermal) opioids are an alternative to oral slow-release preparations and may cause less constipation. When taking opioids, you're likely to need to deal with constipation proactively: that means taking preventive action before constipation occurs.

Corticosteroids. Used early, corticosteroids (for example, prednisone), taken orally or by injection, can reduce inflammation and pain. However, there are drawbacks: the drugs suppress the immune system and may cause overactive mood and insomnia.

Lidoderm (lignocaine patches). If you develop postherpetic neuralgia, your doctor may prescribe patches containing lignocaine, a local anaesthetic. Placed over a painful area, the patch

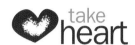

In 2006, the US adopted a varicella zoster virus vaccine (Zostavax) for people over 60, which **cut the number of shingles cases in half**. (In people aged 60 to 69, it cut cases by 64 per cent.) For people who got shingles despite the vaccine, the severity and length of the outbreak were greatly reduced.

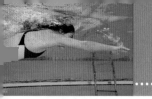

blocks nerve impulses, limiting pain for up to 12 hours. Up to three patches can be worn at the same time, but no patch should be used on a single area for more than 12 hours daily.

Antidepressants. Your doctor may suggest a tricyclic antidepressant such as such as amitriptyline (Endep) or nortriptyline (Allegron). These drugs lessen pain signalling and perhaps the irritability of the nerve damaged by the zoster virus. One study showed that taking amitriptyline during the blister phase helped lower the risk of postherpetic neuralgia.

Gabapentinoids. This class of anticonvulsant medications comprises gabapentin and pregabalin (Lyrica). In postherpetic neuralgia their effectiveness in reducing pain is similar to amitriptyline but with fewer side effects. Unfortunately, the gabapentinoids are not currently on the Pharmaceutical Benefits Scheme in Australia or PHARMAC in New Zealand so they are expensive.

Your pain toolbox

Here are nonprescription weapons you can use to ease the pain of shingles or postherpetic neuralgia.

Cool-water compresses. Applied for 20 minutes at a stretch several times a day when the blisters begin to weep and crust, these compresses help relieve pain and itching and also dry up the blisters and prevent infection. Stop the compresses once the blisters stop oozing.

Antihistamines. A nonprescription antihistamine can help relieve the itching and should help you scratch less; scratching increases the risk of scars and infection.

Medicated lotions. You won't be a beauty, but using medicated lotions containing calamine on the blisters can quell the pain and itching.

An oatmeal bath. Pulverise half a cup of raw oatmeal in a blender (or you can buy an already ground oatmeal product) and pour it into a cool bath. Soak for 20 minutes. Oatmeal helps soothe irritated skin.

Capsaicin creams. *Do not use these when you have shingles.* If you develop postherpetic neuralgia, creams containing capsaicin can help reduce pain. Capsaicin is the chemical in chillies that gives them their fire. Apply three to four times a day and, in 4 to 6 weeks, you should have some relief.

Trigeminal neuralgia

Suddenly, someone has jabbed a pencil in your face or poked it with an electric probe, or at least that's how you feel. The pain disappears as suddenly as it hits, only to return a few moments later. You may be suffering from trigeminal neuralgia, an intense pain caused by the irritation of the trigeminal nerve that has three branches on each side of the face. Trigeminal neuralgia usually strikes only one side of the face, often along the jaw. It begins with short, mild attacks, but those can become longer and more intense, triggered by something as simple as touching your face or brushing your teeth or they may just occur spontaneously.

You may have several attacks a day for weeks or months and then an interval when you have no pain at all. A less common form of trigeminal neuralgia causes a dull ache or a continuous burning sensation that is harder to treat.

The syndrome is usually caused by contact between the nerve and a major artery or vein at your brain's base. This puts pressure on the nerve, causing it to misfire. People over age 50, especially women, are most at risk. High blood pressure, multiple sclerosis or a tumour pressing on the nerve can also trigger the syndrome. There may also be a genetic component, or it may be the result of an accident involving the face. Fortunately, there are medications and self-care measures that can help diminish the pain.

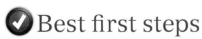 Best first steps

If your face feels like it is burning up, or you feel jolts of pain that make an electric shock seem tame, here's what to do.

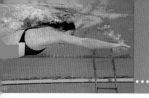

1. Take nonprescription pain relievers.
Take paracetamol or an anti-inflammatory such as ibuprofen or naproxen. These drugs work best when taken regularly through the day according to the directions on the package.

2. Get medical help.
As with all pain, the sooner you treat it, the better chance you have of controlling it. If you continue to have bouts of facial pain unrelieved by nonprescription medications, see your doctor.

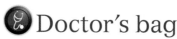 Doctor's bag

Your doctor will ask you to describe your symptoms as precisely as possible and perform an examination including testing your neurologic system. He may also use MRIs to rule out multiple sclerosis or tumours. Once he confirms that you have trigeminal neuralgia, he may prescribe several of the following.

Instant relief

These easy measures don't attack pain after it's arrived, but help prevent it.

Rinsing instead of brushing. When you're in pain, rinse your mouth with tepid water after meals. A vigorous brushing can jangle your nerves.

Chewing on the pain-free side. Avoid setting off fireworks by remembering to chew on your painless side.

Meditation. The pain of trigeminal neuralgia can be very stressful, and stress only exacerbates pain. Try sitting quietly for 15 to 20 minutes in a quiet room, breathing in deeply through your nose, and exhaling slowly through your mouth, clearing your mind of stressful thoughts.

A walk around the block. Okay, several blocks. The point is that exercising 30 minutes per day most days will help relieve stress, increase your output of pain-killing endorphins and help you sleep better at night, another important weapon in fighting pain.

Tepid food and drinks. Extreme temperatures can trigger an attack. The same goes for baths and showers, or even just washing your face: skip the extremes.

Softer foods. Let other people dive for the raw carrots or nuts. Hard, crunchy foods can set off pain. During bouts of pain, you may want to sip liquid meals.

Smelling something sweet. An Australian study found that people smelling sweet smells such as vanilla had increased pain tolerance compared with people sniffing simply pleasant (but not sweet) or unpleasant odours.

Anticonvulsants. Anticonvulsants such as carbamazepine (Tegretol, Teril) and oxcarbazepine (Trileptal) can help decrease pain by soothing the irritated nerve. Oxcarbazepine is the newer of the two and has fewer side effects, such as confusion or drowsiness, than the other. They can become less effective over time, so your doctor may have to increase the dose or switch to a different anticonvulsant. This might be a gabapentinoid. This class of anticonvulsant medications comprises gabapentin and pregabalin (Lyrica). Unfortunately, the gabapentinoids are not currently on the Pharmaceutical Benefits Scheme in Australia or PHARMAC in New Zealand so they are expensive.

Your pain toolbox

In addition to medication, you can try the following to relieve pain.

More whole grains and greens. Vitamin B is essential for healthy nerve function. In fact, in one Chinese study, when patients received three 2000-microgram injections of vitamin B_{12} over three sessions at an acupuncture site, 82 per cent experienced pain relief. To ensure that you have healthy levels of vitamin B, eat plenty of whole grains, fish, chicken, low-fat dairy products and vegetables such as spinach, beans and peas. Take a daily multivitamin that provides the minimum daily requirement of B vitamins.

Pumpkin seeds. These gems are loaded with magnesium, another nutrient essential for nerve function and for relaxing both nerves and muscles. Greens, beans and fish also pack a lot of magnesium.

More sleep. Too little sleep can worsen your pain and stress. Make sure you go to bed and get up at the same time every day, allowing for at least 8 hours per night. Don't work or watch television in your bedroom; use the bedroom for sleep and sex only. Sleep with a fan on: its steady drone will keep street clatter or other noises from waking you up.

Chilli creams. Creams containing capsaicin (Zostrix) can help reduce pain over time when used for several weeks. Capsaicin, the fiery chemical in chillies, reduces pain by eliminating substance P, a protein that causes pain by stimulating nerve endings. Be careful not to get the cream in or near your eyes.

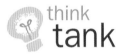

think tank

'Trigeminal pain is an abnormal firing or seizure of the largest sensory nerve in the face, the trigeminal nerve. It's both a sensory and motor nerve, so when it misfires, it causes pain and a physical reaction, such as twitching or muscle seizure. Hence its other name, tic douloureux.'

—Scott M Fishman, MD,
co-author of *The War on Pain*

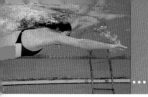

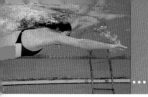 Serious help

If noninvasive measures don't help, your doctor may recommend one of several types of interventions. Surgery to perform microvascular decompression gives the best results with better relief, much longer duration of good relief and less disturbance of neuronal function (sensation of the face and motor function of the jaw). Unlike microvascular decompression surgery, radiation and needle-based procedures do not require general anaesthesia so these procedures can be performed in patients who are significantly unwell. Also they can be used if you are unwilling to have surgery that goes inside the skull.

Microvascular decompression. This procedure involves cutting through the skull to reposition the artery pressing on the trigeminal nerve and placing a pad between the nerve and artery. If the surgeon discovers that it's a vein rather than a large artery that's pressing against the nerve, he'll remove the vein. If neither appears to be causing pressure, he may cut the trigeminal nerve. The procedure can stop or greatly lessen the pain, although in 15 per cent of patients, the pain returns.

Radiation. This procedure, called gamma-knife radiosurgery (GKR), involves applying radiation to the trigeminal nerve root. This forms a lesion on the nerve that interrupts pain signals. The pain lessens after several weeks but can sometimes return. The attractive feature of the procedure is that it's not invasive and requires no anaesthesia.

Needle interventions. Using X-ray control (fluoroscopy), a needle is passed deep into the cheek and through one of the holes in the base of the skull to the origin of the trigeminal nerve. The needle is used to damage the irritable area of the nerve by delivering heat (radiofrequency ablation), or pressure (balloon compression) or a toxic chemical (glycerol or alcohol ablation). Because these procedures damage at least part of the trigeminal nerve, some disturbance of facial sensation is to be expected. Nerves are good at eventually recovering some function after damage and unfortunately this often means that pain recurs within months or a few years. However needle-based treatments can usually be repeated if this happens.

Carpal tunnel syndrome

You notice tingling, even numbness, in your hand and wrist, which makes you want to shake it out. Then a shooting pain hits that runs from your wrist right up your arm. The chances are you have carpal (from the Greek *karpos,* meaning 'wrist') tunnel syndrome (CTS). As the syndrome worsens, you may have trouble picking things up and be unable to distinguish hot from cold. CTS can affect both the sensory and motor parts of the nerve. If the motor part is affected, the muscles controlling the hand and fingers can become weak, or start to waste away.

On the palm side of your wrist is a narrow passageway, the carpal tunnel, surrounded by bones and ligaments. This passageway houses the median nerve, one of the main nerves in your hands and fingers. All sorts of things can trigger CTS. The most common cause is a swelling of the lining of the tendons in the carpal tunnel. When that happens, the passageway narrows, compressing the median nerve.

Other causes include bone spurs, health conditions such as rheumatoid arthritis, hormone fluctuations, fluid retention and abnormal protein deposits. Moving your wrist repetitively doing the same task, whether it's typing on a computer or working on a factory assembly line, can also set you up for the syndrome. It's also possible that you have a narrower carpal tunnel than other people. That's one reason why women have three times the risk of the syndrome than men do.

Your doctor can help you relieve the pain with medications, splints and perhaps surgery. You can also relieve your symptoms with nonprescription anti-inflammatories, rest and stretching.

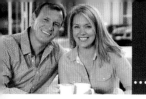

✅ Best first steps

Your wrist has been tingling and burning, and you want the pain to just go away. Here are immediate steps to take.

1. Try nonprescription anti-inflammatory drugs.

If the dosage on the label instructions isn't enough to ease the pain, talk to your doctor. He may advise that you can take up to 800 milligrams of ibuprofen three times a day or 600 milligrams four times a day or 500 milligrams of naproxen twice daily. If you take either of these for 10 days and it doesn't help your pain, stop taking it and let your doctor know. Don't take this much on your own and don't take high doses for longer than 10 days without first checking with your doctor.

2. Get an evaluation.

The sooner you have the problem diagnosed, the quicker you'll find relief. Your doctor can rule out other conditions and offer medications and suggestions to speed your recovery.

🩺 Doctor's bag

Your doctor will examine your hands, arms, shoulders and neck, testing them for feeling and strength to determine whether the pain is from a repetitive injury or another condition. He may also order a nerve conduction study, passing a current through surface electrodes to determine if the electrical impulse in the carpal tunnel has slowed. Once he diagnoses you with CTS, he may suggest:

Corticosteroid injections. In a study of 101 CTS patients, Spanish researchers found that the patients treated with a single injection of corticosteroids fared as well—20 per cent or better relief of night-time symptoms—as patients who had had decompression surgery for the condition. 'How long an injection helps depends on whether you continue to irritate the nerve', says Mara Vucich, DO, an osteopathic physician at the Maryland Spine Center at Mercy Medical Center in Baltimore. To improve the accuracy of the injection, your doctor may perform it with the aid of ultrasound imaging.

Your pain toolbox

You can take control of the pain by trying the suggestions below.

A nonprescription splint. Most of us sleep like cats, our hands bent and tucked under our chins, not a good contortion for people with CTS. A wrist splint with a hard plastic stay that doesn't allow the wrist to bend will give the wrist and its nerve a rest. 'I tell patients to wear the splint during the day too, if they can', says Vucich. They're available at most pharmacies. Wearing a splint may be most effective when combined with steroid injections, which will bring down inflammation in the wrist.

The telephone. Try giving your BlackBerry, iPhone and other hand-held toys a rest. Constant messaging can take its toll on your wrist and thumb.

Ergonomics. If you're at the keyboard all day, check your hand position, holding your wrist so it's in a neutral, unbent position. You may find that placing a wrist pad (available at office supply stores) under your wrist can help.

Frequent breaks. Every 15 or 20 minutes, pause whatever hand-taxing thing you're doing and gently stretch and bend your hands.

Stretching. From a seated position, raise your arms, interlace your fingers, turn your palms to the ceiling and hold for 10 slow deep breaths. This stretches the muscles in your arms and hands and increases blood circulation.

 Serious help

When simpler steps don't work and you have severe pain that lasts for more than 6 months, your doctor may suggest surgery, especially if the muscles begin to waste away.

Decompression surgery. The surgeon makes a small incision in the wrist to cut the ligament pressing on the median nerve, which relieves pressure on the nerve. The procedure is done with either general anaesthesia or a local anaesthesia. Studies show that, after 1 year, surgery reduces or eliminates pain in more than 90 per cent of patients with CTS.

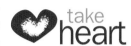

When it comes to carpal tunnel syndrome, **computers aren't the villains** we think they are. In a Swedish study of almost 2500 people, researchers found that of people who spent 4 or more hours a day on the computer, only 2.6 per cent had the syndrome compared with 5.2 per cent of people who didn't use a computer at all.

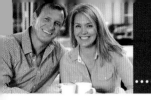

Muscle and tendon soreness

This time, you're determined to get fit: you run a kilometre and finish with a set of push-ups. Then, for the next several days, your arms and legs feel like they've been stretched on a medieval rack. That soreness is the result of two things: the build-up of lactic acid in the muscles and the true soreness culprits, tiny tears in your muscles. White blood cells, anti-inflammatory chemicals called prostaglandins, and nutrients and fluids rushing in to help repair the stressed muscles also cause them to swell. The swelling builds for several days, which is why you may still be hobbling down the staircase after 5 days. Such muscle soreness may also result from an injury or fall.

Whatever you do to make your muscles sore often affects your tendons, the tissue that connects muscle to bone. In fact, the difference between muscle and tendon soreness is so subtle that it's tough to tell them apart. But tendons are more likely to give pain around a joint—elbow, knee, hip, shoulder or heel.

Most soreness can be handled with rest and ice. The encouraging news is that when you repeat the exercise that affected you in the first place, you'll have less soreness and a speedier recovery. Your muscles may even be stronger.

✅ Best first steps

You had a great game of golf, but now your shoulders, arms and calves ache. Your treatment: RICE, which stands for rest, ice, compression and elevation.

1. Rest.
Lay off the parts that hurt for a little while.

2. Ice.

If you can stand it, soak the affected area in icy water for up to 15 minutes. Ice constricts the blood vessels, lessening swelling, plus it numbs your pain. If an ice bath is too much of a hurdle, apply ice packs wherever it hurts. A homemade recipe: put ice in a plastic zipper bag with a little water, wrap the bag in a cloth and apply. Or use a bag of frozen vegetables, such as corn or peas, which will mould to the area that hurts. You can refreeze and use these over and over but don't eat them once thawed and refrozen.

3. Compression.

Wearing a nonprescription compression bandage or brace for several days after you develop tendon pain, say, at the shoulder or elbow, relieves pain by taking pressure off the spot where the tendon attaches to the bone.

4. Elevation.

For muscle and tendon soreness in your legs, elevating them above your heart will help reduce swelling.

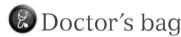
Doctor's bag

If the pain doesn't go away within a week, it's important to determine if it's something more serious than simple soreness. Your doctor will examine the painful spot and ask about your symptoms and activities. If the pain doesn't stem from a condition other than overuse, she may suggest the following.

Prescription nonsteroidal anti-inflammatory drugs (NSAIDs). If nonprescription anti-inflammatories haven't helped, the doctor may prescribe a stronger version.

Corticosteroids. If your muscle pain is actually due to tendon soreness and becomes chronic, your doctor may inject corticosteroids around the tendon to relieve the pain and inflammation.

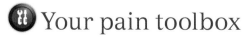
Your pain toolbox

You're largely in control of this type of pain. Here are pain-relieving tips that work fast.

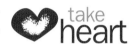
take heart

Indulge in a **postexercise massage**. An Australian study found that a 10-minute sports massage on a well-exercised arm 3 hours after exercise **reduced muscle soreness** by 20 to 40 per cent and **reduced swelling** as well.

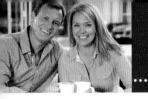

Nonprescription anti-inflammatories. 'Most people take only enough to relieve pain but not inflammation', says Mehul J Desai, MD, director of pain medicine at the George Washington University Hospital. 'Two hundred milligrams of ibuprofen may make you feel better but it won't address the inflammation.' If the dosage on the label instructions isn't enough to ease the pain, talk to your doctor. He may advise that you can take up to 800 milligrams of ibuprofen three times per day or 600 milligrams four times per day or 500 milligrams of naproxen twice daily. If you take either of these for 10 days and it doesn't help your pain, stop taking it and let your doctor know.

Active rest. Now's no time for a permanent return to the couch. 'Inactivity will lead to stiffness and a lack of flexibility, but if you go back to your activity too quickly, your pain will come back, too', says Desai. 'Take 3 days to 2 weeks off and then return gradually.'

Massage. Go ahead and get one from a pro. Several studies have shown that massage reduces soreness and swelling. Ohio State University researchers found that Swedish massage (which includes lots of kneading, long strokes and joint movement) done on rabbits after exercise speeded recovery and lessened swelling and inflammation. (Rabbit muscles have some parallels to ours.) The muscles recovered 60 per cent of their strength compared with a 15 per cent recovery rate in the control group.

Yoga. Researchers at the Medical College of Georgia found that women who did yoga several times a week had half the muscle soreness after a scream-inducing stint on a bench stepper than women who didn't. Yoga works because it stretches and loosens tight muscles. The key is to get a bit of yoga instruction a month before you take on a rigorous new exercise routine, or you'll be piling yoga muscle soreness onto your other troubles.

A peanut butter sandwich or a milk drink. Eating a mix of carbohydrates and protein 15 minutes to an hour after you exercise will help your muscles recover more quickly. During exercise, your body uses insulin more effectively to drive repairing nutrients into the cells, but that window only lasts an hour.

Variety. Instead of returning to the same activities that caused your soreness in the first place, try alternating activities. So, for instance, if you're a cyclist, alternate that with a day or two of swimming, which uses different sets of muscles.

Strengthening exercises. If your problem is tendon or ligament pain, work with a physiotherapist to learn range-of-motion and strengthening exercises that can help reduce soreness and increase the amount of stress the muscles, tendons and ligaments can absorb.

Water exercise. Stay active by taking up swimming or a water aerobics class, especially in a heated pool. Because of your buoyancy in water, you can exercise sore muscles, tendons and ligaments without stressing them as you would with weight-bearing exercises, such as walking and jogging.

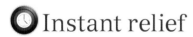

Instant relief

Here are a few suggestions to help your soreness subside.

Stretching. Although a number of studies indicate that stretching before exercise won't help muscle soreness, gently stretching out sore muscles *after* exercise can relieve the pain for 15 to 20 minutes. Stretching can also relieve ligament tightness that leads to soreness.

Heat wraps. Although cold's the best bet initially, after several days and after the inflammation subsides, heat can relax the muscles and help block pain. Therapeutic heat wraps, heating pads or sinking into a hot bath may make you forget that anything ever hurt.

Painkilling cream or ointment. Nonsteroidal anti-inflammatory drugs can also be applied topically, sidestepping some of the potentially dangerous side effects of taking them orally, such as gastrointestinal upset. Rub these creams or a sports cream over sore spots, and you should feel some relief.

Cherry juice. When researchers at the University of Vermont gave a 355-millilitre mix of apple and cherry juice, which is the equivalent of 50 fresh cherries, to men twice per day for 3 days before and 4 days after a bout of intense biceps curls, they ranked their worst pain at 2.4 on a 10-point scale in the days following the exercise, compared with a 3.2 rating by the non-cherry juice drinkers. Their pain peaked after 24 hours instead of 48. Cherries are rich in anthocyanins, anti-oxidants that have a natural pain-relieving effect. Berries and grapes are also good sources.

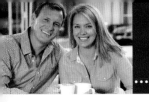

Repetitive stress injury

Carpal tunnel syndrome (see page 251) is just one of a number of types of repetitive stress injuries (RSIs). You've probably heard of tennis or golfer's elbow. And then there's Achilles tendinopathy, the runner's nightmare (see page 214). And rotator cuff injury, which is irritation to the muscles and tendons in the shoulder that can come from fun activities such as swimming or throwing a ball, or from those that are less so, such as painting the garage or stocking overhead shelves.

Repetitive stress injury is just what it sounds like: the irritation and injury to muscles and tendons that come from overuse, in other words, from repetitive stress. Initially, you may not suspect a thing. However, if you keep up that raking, say, hour after hour, day after day, then the irritation to the muscle accumulates until you are saying 'Ow!' with each stroke.

Who's most likely to get an RSI? The weekend warrior who exercises more in 2 days than she has since high school. Other prime candidates are those whose work requires repetitive movements: 'Athletes and factory workers, or someone at a computer straining neck muscles', says Mara Vucich, DO, an osteopathic physician at the Maryland Spine Center at Mercy Medical Center in Baltimore. 'And if you continue to put demand on the muscles involved, they will become fatigued and break down.'

To begin with, the area feels sore and stiff. It just seems to get worse until you may feel pain, tingling, numbness or weakness—and coordination loss—in that area.

With the combination of rest, anti-inflammatories, ice and other simple self-care measures, you can get yourself on the mend before the RSI becomes severe.

✅ Best first steps

To put yourself on a healing path, take the following steps, pronto.

1. Stop.
There's a reason our bodies yell at us: they're trying to tell us to stop. Give your muscles and tendons a rest when they ask you to do so.

2. Put your pain on ice.
Wrap an ice pack in a clean cloth—a bag of frozen peas will do—and place it on the painful spot for 20 minutes at a stretch to stop both pain and inflammation.

3. Take some nonprescription anti-inflammatories.
If the dosage on the label instructions isn't enough to ease the pain, talk to your doctor. He may advise that you can take up to 800 milligrams of ibuprofen three times per day or 600 milligrams four times per day or 500 milligrams of naproxen twice daily. If you take either of these for 10 days and it doesn't help your pain, stop taking it and let your doctor know. Don't take this much on your own.

4. See your doctor before the pain gets worse.
If the pain doesn't subside after a few days, let your doctor check it out. He can offer both medications and tips that can keep an RSI from getting worse and rule out other treatable conditions that may be causing your pain.

🩺 Doctor's bag

Your doctor will examine you, asking you about activities and patterns of pain. He may suggest tests of nerve function or imaging such as ultrasound, X-ray or MRI. Caution is needed interpreting results: it is easy to wrongly ascribe the cause of your pain to non-specific minor abnormalities that are often found. He may suggest one or several of the following.

Prescription anti-inflammatories. If you find that nonprescription anti-inflammatories aren't enough to tamp down your pain, your doctor may prescribe stronger ones.

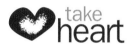
take heart

Researchers at Temple University have found that our bodies produce certain chemicals that signal the beginnings of inflammation in repetitive stress injuries, a finding that may eventually **help doctors detect and treat such injuries** before they become debilitating.

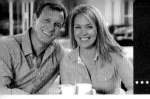

Dry needling. Sometimes dry needling can be performed by a doctor or therapist: this uses acupuncture-like needles to resolve irritable points in muscles.

Your pain toolbox

Trying one or several of the following may help reduce your pain and speed your healing.

Rest. Working a muscle more than 200 times in a row is overuse. So, if you're typing, painting, bowling, sweeping or whatever, stop every 20 minutes and do something else.

Better form. Ask a physiotherapist or athletic trainer to review your moves with you, particularly those that got you into trouble in the first place. She can suggest stretches and a shift in postures and techniques that can relieve stress on your muscles. She can also assess and show you how to balance the strength in opposing sets of muscles, such as triceps and biceps. Having one set of muscles stronger than the other can strain your joints.

Gentle exercise. Now's no time to try out for the Olympics, but remaining somewhat active is essential. Otherwise you'll grow stiff, losing range of motion. Gently stretch out the sore area. Continue doing some light exercise such as walking or swimming without using the stressed muscle. This will lower pain and increase blood circulation, speeding healing.

Serious help

Most RSIs will heal with rest, but an injured muscle or tendon occasionally requires more serious attention.

Steroid injection. If you're really hurting, your doctor might recommend a steroid injection to relieve the pain and inflammation. In recent times there have been studies looking at injections of your own blood, which contains factors that promote healing.

Endometriosis

Endometriosis is a puzzling condition that affects females in their reproductive years. The word is derived from the name for the lining of the inside of the uterus, or other pelvic organs—the bladder, bowel and rectum. The resulting pain can be severe. Infertility can also occur.

The endometrial tissue that grows outside the uterus responds to a woman's hormones just like the uterine lining does. Every 28 to 30 days, the lining thickens, preparing for a pregnancy. When that doesn't happen, the body sheds the lining by bleeding and a woman has her period. But with endometriosis, the uterine lining and blood are believed to go to the cavity outside the uterus and get trapped there, causing irritation and pain. Sometimes a blood cyst called an endometrioma can form. Trapped blood and ruptured cysts can result in scar tissue, or adhesions, that can bind pelvic organs together. When your cycle ceases during pregnancy, many of your symptoms may vanish, only to return after the baby is born and you've finished breastfeeding.

The symptoms can wax and wane and even disappear when a woman is not ovulating. Some women experience no symptoms. Most have pelvic pain, often during sex, during their periods, or when they urinate or have a bowel movement. You may have more severe cramping, and pelvic, back and stomach pain before and during your period than you used to. You may have heavier periods and bleed between your periods as well.

'Endometriosis is considered to have genetic, auto-immune and environmental components', says Dr Susan Evans, laparoscopic gynaecologist in Adelaide, South Australia, who has extensive experience in this condition.

Without treatment, the condition tends to get worse. Although it can't be cured, hormone treatments, pain medications and some lifestyle measures can help make you more comfortable.

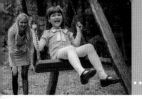

✅ Best first steps

You don't have to feel defeated by the pain of endometriosis. Here are some immediate steps you can take on the path to feeling better.

1. Take nonprescription pain relievers.
Pain-relieving NSAIDs, such as ibuprofen and naproxen, can help relieve pain and inflammation. There is no clear evidence to show that one of these agents is superior to any other. Start the medication immediately before or at the start of your period, following the dosage instructions on the label.

2. Get checked out.
Make an appointment with your gynaecologist if you're having symptoms such as chronic pelvic pain, more severe periods or intermittent bleeding. The sooner you get treated, the less risk of complications and more pain.

Doctor's bag

Your family doctor may need extra help to treat your endometriosis. You need a doctor who knows and understands endometriosis and can perform the right tests and offer the most effective treatments, including surgery, to ward off years of pain and to protect your fertility. Your specialist will begin by taking your medical history and performing a pelvic examination, looking for abnormalities such as pelvic tenderness or cysts. She may also do a vaginal ultrasound, inserting a scanner into your vagina, a test that can also detect cysts. To find out definitively if you have endometriosis and how widespread the disease is, she may perform a laparoscopy. In this surgical procedure done under general anaesthesia the doctor makes a small incision in your abdomen through which she inserts a laparoscope, a lighted instrument that allows her to view your pelvic area. Once she confirms a diagnosis, she may suggest one or several of the following.

Pain relievers. Your doctor will probably suggest that you continue taking nonprescription anti-inflammatories, but if she feels that those aren't strong enough, she may bump you up to more potent prescription doses.

Hormonal finetuning. Taking hormones can help ease pain and slow the growth of the displaced endometrial tissue. The options include birth control pills, patches or intra-uterine contraceptive devices (IUCDs), which shorten the menstruation period and thereby reduce your pain.

GnRH agonists and antagonists. GnRH is an acronym for 'Gonadotropin-Releasing Hormone', which is a naturally occurring chemical that helps regulate the menstrual cycle in a woman's body by stimulating ovarian hormones. Drugs that block GnRH create an artificial menopause that sends endometriosis into dormancy because your ovaries are no longer producing oestrogen. These drugs can be given as an injection, implant or nasal spray, and may have some side effects including hot flushes, headaches, vaginal dryness and bone loss. Your doctor may also suggest you take small doses of the hormones oestrogen or progestin in conjunction with GnRH drugs to diminish those effects. The aim of the 3-to-6-month treatment is to suppress the condition, putting the endometriosis into remission.

Progestin. Offered as a pill or injection, progestin is a synthetic form of progesterone, a female hormone that normally prepares the uterine lining for an egg. Taking it for endometriosis will usually shorten or even eliminate your period. More important, it helps shrink the tissue that's growing where it shouldn't. Side effects can include mood and weight changes, bloating, sore breasts, headache, nausea and dizziness.

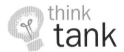

think
tank
'You may need acupuncture once or twice a week or more to treat period pain.'

—Professor Zhen Zheng, BMed, PhD,
Chinese Medical School of Health
Sciences, RMIT, Melbourne

Your pain toolbox

This condition may madden you, but there are things you can do to lower your pain and brighten your outlook.

Evening primrose oil. This oil, derived from the evening primrose plant, is high in linolenic acid, which promotes the production of good prostaglandins (hormone-like chemicals that act as anti-inflammatories) and interferes with the production of bad prostaglandins (hormone-like chemicals that cause inflammation and pain). Be sure to buy supplements from a reputable company and follow the directions on the bottle. The recommended dose is 1000 milligrams three times per day.

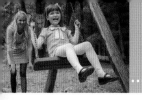

Acupuncture. 'The great part about acupuncture is its effects are not limited to pain relief', says Professor Zhen Zheng. 'Often there is an enhanced sense of wellbeing, reduced nausea and vomiting and reduced headache. So it is the overall effect of acupuncture that impresses the patient.'

Low-fat diet. Stick to a diet of vegetables, fruit, whole grains and lean meats. These types of food will make you feel a whole lot better than eating fatty foods. Diets that are rich in animal fat, dairy products and spicy foods should be avoided because they stimulate bad prostaglandins that boost the pain of endometriosis, says Barbara Soltes, associate professor of gynaecologic endocrinology, Rush University, Medical Center, Chicago. Linseed, soy and fish stimulate good prostaglandins that counteract inflammation. Fatty dairy products are also associated with the inflammation. In people with endometriosis, fatty foods may also cause gastrointestinal symptoms such as bloating, nausea and diarrhoea.

Fish oil. The oil in fatty fish is full of omega-3 fatty acids, which produce anti-inflammatory prostaglandins as well as fight inflammation. A typical dose is 1000 milligrams a day, but check with your doctor about a dose that's right for you.

⏱ Instant relief

You may feel like curling up into a ball of pain, but instead, take these small steps that can help you feel better fast.

Heat. Soaking in a warm bath is pampering, but it's also utilitarian, relaxing tight abdominal muscles and increasing blood flow. A heating pad or hot-water bottle can do much the same.

Movement. Muscles contract and tighten in response to pain; moving keeps those muscles loose, which can help reduce pain. Take yourself on a walk to get things moving.

Self-massage. Rubbing your abdomen in a circular motion gets the blood flowing and relaxes your stressed-out abdominal muscles.

Castor oil pack. Don't worry; you don't have to swallow anything. Put castor oil on a soft, clean cloth. Place it in a casserole dish and heat it in an oven at 175°C for about 20 minutes to a comfortable, not too hot temperature. Put it on your stomach and let it sit for 30 to 60 minutes covered with a towel or hot-water bottle.

Deep breathing. Sitting quietly, breathe in slowly through your nose to the count of five, then release your breath through pursed lips. This can help relax tense pelvic muscles and also get blood flowing in the reproductive system and elsewhere.

🐄 Serious help

If medication and changes in diet and exercise aren't enough, your doctor may recommend surgery. The options include the following.

Laparoscopy. In this procedure the doctor inserts a laparoscope, a thin, lighted instrument, through a small incision in your abdomen. She'll likely use a diathermy or perhaps a laser to remove or burn away endometrial nodules, scar tissue and adhesions without having to remove reproductive organs. If the endometriosis isn't too advanced, this procedure can improve the chances of fertility.

Laparotomy. If you have already had a laparoscopy or if your endometriosis is more advanced, your doctor may recommend laparotomy, or abdominal surgery, which requires an incision. The advantage is that the doctor can see and address more areas that may be damaged.

Hysterectomy. If your endometriosis is severe, your doctor may suggest a complete hysterectomy—the removal of uterus and cervix. Removing the ovaries is essential to putting an end to endometriosis. The menstrual cycle will end, and the pelvic pain will substantially decrease. This surgery is usually considered a last resort because it throws you into menopause, ending your chances of pregnancy forever.

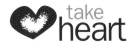
take
heart

An Australian study found that **laparoscopic treatment** of endometriosis reduced pain and improved quality of life.

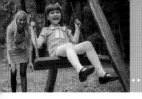

Interstitial cystitis

Having to visit every toilet en route to somewhere is no one's idea of fun. Add to that a range of pain from mild to intense, and you have a fair description of interstitial cystitis (IC), also called painful bladder syndrome. The condition, which primarily affects women, is perplexing: its symptoms, which can come and go, vary widely from person to person. It ebbs and flows as your bladder empties and fills. It can be worse during menstruation. Even sex can bring it on. And with the pain often comes urgency, including the need to urinate as many as 60 times a day and during the night—and still feeling the urgency to urinate.

Because IC can seem so varied, most researchers suspect different forms of the disease exist. In one form, nonulcerative IC, the bladder may become scarred and stiffen, its walls covered with glomerulations, or pinpoint bleeding. About 5 to 10 per cent of cases are ulcerative IC, in which patients develop a condition called Hunner's ulcers on the lining of the bladder.

IC can mimic a bacterial infection, but the condition seems unrelated to bacteria and doesn't respond to antibiotics. Scientists have found a substance called antiproliferative factor, or APF, in people with IC, which appears to block the growth of normal cells on bladder walls. People with IC often have other conditions such as irritable bowel syndrome, endometriosis and fibromyalgia, making researchers suspect that IC may be linked to a more general inflammatory condition. Bladder or pelvic surgery, bacterial infection or a dysfunction of the pelvic floor muscles may also trigger IC.

Fortunately, there is a combination of treatments that can help reduce your pain.

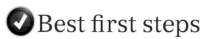 Best first steps

Your best bet for relief is to address IC's painful symptoms—the discomfort, urgency and frequency of urination—as soon as possible. Here are the best early steps to take.

1. See your doctor.
The sooner you get a diagnosis, the sooner you can take steps to minimise your pain and discomfort.

2. Pay attention to your foods.
Many people report that specific foods can cause a flare-up of symptoms. These include carbonated soft drinks, caffeine, alcohol and some fruit juices.

3. Take a nonprescription anti-inflammatory.
Ibuprofen and naproxen can help relieve pain and inflammation.

Doctor's bag

No definitive test exists for IC, so the first thing your doctor will do is rule out other conditions such as a urinary tract infection, bladder cancer, or, in men, prostatitis or chronic pelvic pain syndrome. The doctor may want do a urinalysis and urine culture to check for infection. He may also perform a cystoscopy, in which he inserts a tube with a camera and a light to see the bladder and urethra (the tube that drains urine from the bladder) and the entrance of the ureters (openings that drain urine from the kidney to the bladder). At the same time, he may perform bladder distension, filling the bladder to capacity with water or saline solution to get a better view. He may also take a biopsy, or tissue sample, to rule out bladder cancer. Once he rules out other conditions, he may suggest several of the following treatments.

Bladder distention. Your doctor performs this, as described above, to aid in diagnosis but also because it sometimes helps the pain for 3 to 6 months. It may work by increasing bladder capacity and by stretching bladder muscle. If it does stop the pain, your doctor may recommend repeating the procedure when the effect wears off. It requires general or regional anaesthesia. Your symptoms may worsen for several days after the procedure, but you should improve within 2 to 4 weeks.

Bladder instillation. This procedure entails filling your bladder with a therapeutic solution that you hold in for 15 minutes. The choice of solution depends on what each person needs, but may include dimethyl sulfoxide (DMSO); heparin, an anticoagulant;

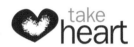

take
heart

Up to 62 per cent of people with IC find that **eliminating certain foods** helps relieve painful symptoms.

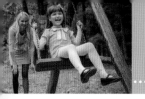

or Cystistat, a drug whose main ingredient is hyaluronic acid, an arthritis treatment approved by the FDA for IC. The medications all help reduce inflammation and block pain and reduce the muscle contractions that make you feel you have to urinate constantly. You have to repeat the treatment every 6 to 8 weeks (some doctors allow patients to do the treatment themselves), and it may take 3 to 4 weeks before you feel better.

Pentosan polysulfate (Elmiron). This is the only medication that is specifically approved by the Therapeutic Goods Administration in Australia. It may work by repairing damage to the bladder lining, but it can take up to 4 months to relieve pain, up to 6 for you to feel less urgency. It can be tough on the liver and can also make you lose at least some hair (although it grows back once you stop taking the medication).

Antidepressants. Antidepressants, such as amitriptyline (Endep), can help reduce urination frequency and block some pain signals, but they can also make you feel fatigued. Selective serotonin reuptake inhibitors (SSRIs), such as paroxetine, or serotonin-noradrenaline reuptake inhibitors (SNRIs), such as duloxetine (Cymbalta), may also help.

Antihistamines. Chlorpheniramine (Phenergan) is a nonprescription antihistamine that affects mast cells, large cells involved in allergic and other hypersensitive reactions. It helps decrease the frequency of urination as well as pain and pressure, especially in patients who have allergies. But it can make you sleepy and increase depression in already depressed people.

Muscle relaxants. Muscle relaxants such as baclofen (Lioresal) don't act directly on the muscles but on the central nervous system. They're especially helpful in relieving muscle spasms that make you feel the need to urinate.

Opioids. If pain is severe, your doctor may prescribe a short-term course of an opioid drug. If you need prolonged treatment with opioids, your doctor will refer you to a pain clinic.

Electrical nerve stimulation. Transcutaneous electrical nerve stimulation (TENS), the delivery of mild electrical impulses to the skin of the lower abdomen or back, helps relieve pain. Stimulation of the underlying nerves helps block pain signalling at the spinal cord. The impulses have to be delivered several times a day for several months before there is any effect, so a doctor or physiotherapist has to train the patient to operate a portable TENS unit at home.

Your pain toolbox

'If pain cannot be cured, you should learn how to manage it your-self', says Dr Angela Chia, Head of the Chronic Pelvic Pain Clinic at the Royal Women's Hospital, Melbourne. Since you're running the show, here are some self-care techniques you can try.

Diet consciousness. People with IC commonly find that particu-lar foods cause flare-ups, but it seems to be very individual, with many reporting a slow process of discovery over 6 months or longer of trial-and-error. Common triggers include alcohol, fruit juices, caffeine and processed foods. It is worth consulting a dietitian specialising in food allergy and intolerance if you are really stuck.

A tobacco-free life. Some patients find that smoking exacerbates their symptoms. Since smoking is a risk factor for bladder cancer, quitting is a great idea whether or not it quells IC symptoms.

Physiotherapy. 'Physiotherapy generally gives good results', says Angela Chia, 'but it has to be done by a physiotherapist trained in pelvic floor muscle dysfunction'. The treatment can involve inter-nal and external massage, in which the therapist manipulates your pain's trigger points—taut and painful bands of muscle—working to release and stretch tightened muscles. An experienced therapist will also teach you exercises you can do at home to strengthen and stretch the pelvic floor muscles.

Bladder training. Essentially, this is urinating by the clock. Begin by urinating every half an hour (or whatever beginning interval seems appropriate) whether you have to or not. Then gradually increase the time between urinations by 15 to 30 minutes every 3 to 4 weeks. In one study, gradual increase resulted in less frequency of urination, day or night, and less urgency in 71 per cent of patients. In another study that combined the training with weekly pelvic floor muscle exercises, which your physiotherapist will teach you, and use of relaxation tapes, 98 per cent of the patients had to urinate less frequently.

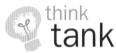

think
tank

'People with IC are more sensitive to acidic and spicy foods and chocolate as these foods may irritate the bladder and cause more inflammation.'

—Anne-Florence Plante, BA, PT, physiotherapist at the Royal Women's Hospital, Melbourne

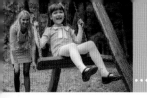

Stress-reducing therapies. Therapies such as yoga, meditation and progressive muscle relaxation can help lower stress levels. A study published by the Interstitial Cystitis Network found that 90 per cent of women who took an 8-week course in yoga said it reduced their symptoms, aided sleep and reduced stress.

Serious help

Surgery is a dicey proposition for IC because it can often make things worse. Your doctor will recommend it only when all other avenues have failed.

Sacral neuromodulation. If TENS does help address your pain (see 'Electrical nerve stimulation', page 268), your doctor may suggest trying sacral nerve stimulation, in which the electrical unit is implanted surgically. The electrical stimulation of the sacral nerves—the nerves at the lower end of your spine—helps inhibit the bladder so that you feel less pain and less frequent need to urinate. A wire is placed near the tailbone, and the stimulator is inserted under the skin near your upper buttocks or in the abdomen. The patient has an external device that allows her to adjust the level of stimulation. 'This can be useful in selected patients', says Dr Peter Courtney, interventional pain specialist, Royal Melbourne Hospital.

Instant relief

Here are more things you can do to relieve your pain by reducing muscle-tensing stress.

Heat therapy. Holding a hot-water bottle to your abdomen temporarily deactivates pain receptors, according to a British study. Hold it on the painful spot for 15 to 20 minutes at a time. Dr Angela Chia also suggests trying a heat wrap, worn up to 12 hours at a time, which allows you to go about your usual activities instead of lying in bed.

Deep breathing. Lie down, allowing your body to relax as much as possible. Close your eyes, then imagine scanning your body, releasing tension in each muscle group from scalp to toe. Breathe in deeply through your nose, letting your stomach rise as you do. Breathe out through your mouth. Continue for several minutes until you feel completely relaxed.

A tennis ball. If you have a trigger point in your buttocks (or back), sit or lie on a tennis ball, placing the ball directly under the trigger point, keeping a constant pressure there for at least 60 to 90 seconds.

Menstrual cramps

This may be the reason a woman's period is often called the curse, that cramping and aching in your lower abdomen that can even reach around to your back and down to your thighs. About 50 per cent of women suffer the dull or throbbing pain just before and during their periods, and for about 15 per cent, the pain can be bad enough to send them to bed for a day or two. The cramps that occur around your period may arrive with other unfriendly symptoms: nausea, diarrhoea, sweating, headache and dizziness.

Cramps usually result from the contractions of the uterus as it rids itself of the endometrial lining every month. The contractions are triggered by prostaglandins, hormone-like substances that can cause pain and inflammation. Other inflammatory compounds within the pelvis, called leukotrienes, also increase cramps. The cramps get worse as clots of the shed lining pass through the cervix.

Cramps can also stem from other causes such as endometriosis (the growth of uterine lining tissue outside the uterus, see page 261), adenomyosis (the growth of uterine lining in the muscle walls of the uterus), pelvic inflammatory disease (an infection of the fallopian tubes and ovaries as the result of a sexually transmitted disease), fibroids (benign growths on the inside and outside of the uterus) or an intra-uterine contraceptive device (IUCD), a birth control device placed in the uterus that can cause cramps, especially in the first months after placement.

The women at highest risk include those younger than 20 (about 90 per cent report cramps), women whose periods began at age 11 or younger, women with heavy periods, women who suffer from anxiety or depression, women who have never had children and women who smoke. Fortunately, for many women who experience cramps without secondary causes such as those listed here, cramps tend to lessen after age 30 or childbirth.

Cramps don't have to stalk you. There are lots of ways for you to lessen their ache.

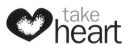
take
heart

Seventy per cent of women who take **low-dose contraceptives** find their cramps abate.

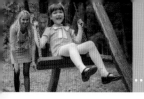

✔ Best first steps

Forget losing one or two days per month because of cramps. Here are steps you can take at the outset to quell your misery.

1. Take pain relievers before the pain begins.
Start taking nonprescription pain medications one or two days before your period begins and continue for one to two days into your period. If your doctor gives you the okay, try 400 milligrams of ibuprofen every 4 hours or 500 milligrams of naproxen.

2. Get severe pain checked out.
If you turn into a couch potato every time you get your period or if your period suddenly arrives with painful cramps you haven't had before, see your doctor so that he can check for a more serious cause.

🩺 Doctor's bag

Your doctor will begin by asking you about your menstrual cycle and reproductive history, and by doing a pelvic examination. She may also order imaging tests such as a pelvic ultrasound, computerised tomography (CT) scan or magnetic resonance imaging (MRI), which allow her to look inside your pelvis. She may do a laparoscopy, in which she inserts a tiny lighted camera through a small incision in your stomach to look at your abdominal and pelvic cavity. Or she may do a hysteroscopy, in which she inserts a tiny lighted instrument with a camera through your vagina and into the uterus to examine it. Then your recourse may include the following.

Low-dose oral contraceptives. 'There are now many other options of pills for women with heavy menstrual bleeding, some of which treat both pain and bleeding', says Dr Catarina Ang, Head of Gynaecology Unit 1, Royal Women's Hospital, Melbourne.

Prescription pain relievers. If nonprescription anti-inflammatories don't work, your doctor may prescribe a stronger version.

Treatment for the underlying cause. If your cramps stem from another condition, your doctor will treat that condition first. For instance, if cramping stems from an infection, she'll prescribe antibiotics. If it stems from fibroids, she may recommend surgery.

think tank

'The perfect homemade recipe for relief is a low-carbohydrate diet, anti-inflammatories, exercise, plenty of sunshine and 1200 milligrams of calcium every day. Those are the steps that women can do at home without having to rely on hormones or stronger medications.'

—Jamal Mourad, DO, SACOG, assistant clinical professor at Midwestern University in Glendale, Arizona

Your pain toolbox

You can push back the pain of menstrual cramps by persisting in a combination of new habits.

Exercise. True, you don't even feel like sitting up, but exercising 30 minutes per day at least three times a week relieves stress and releases endorphins, the body's natural painkillers.

Evening primrose oil. Its gamma-linoleic acid blocks the production of bad inflammatory prostaglandins and other substances involved in stoking your cramps. Take a standard extract containing 500 milligrams or more of fatty acids up to three times per day.

 # Instant relief

Knowing measures that can quickly take the edge off your pain can help you feel in control. Here are some shortcuts to relief.

The sock cure. Fill a large cotton sock or a small pillowcase with rice, knot the top, heat it in the microwave and you have an instant heating pad to hold to your cramping stomach.

Luxury bathing. Add a few drops of relaxing lavender oil and soak in a warm bath for 15 to 20 minutes. The heat increases blood flow and relaxes tight muscles, and the quiet soak washes away tension.

Rest and relaxation. 'The more stressed out you are, the more likely you are to have physical pain', says Dr Jamal Mourad, assistant clinical professor at Midwestern University, Glendale, Arizona. 'When your body says you're not doing well, take it easy.' Lie down for 5 minutes and listen to soothing music. Make sure you get 8 hours of sleep every night. Lack of sleep can lower your pain threshold.

Lip press. Pressing on the centre of your top lip just under the nose for 1 minute every 15 minutes several times a day is said to slow down a heavy menstrual flow, reducing pain. The only way to know if it works is to try it.

Pelvic tilts. Stretching out your pelvic muscles can help cramps skedaddle. Stand with your feet hip-width apart, your knees bent, your hands on your hips. Rock your pelvis back and forth 15 times. This should help loosen you up.

The foetal position. You probably do this instinctively when you have cramps. Lie on your side with your legs drawn up into your abdomen. This shifts the position of the uterus so that it doesn't press on the bundle of nerves at the front of the pelvis known as the solar plexus.

Self-massage. Try massaging your lower stomach and back. The massage increases blood flow and reduces muscle tension. A Korean study of 42 women found that just 5 minutes per day of abdominal massage for 5 days before menstruation through the first day significantly reduced cramping.

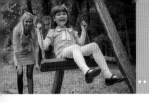

Calcium. Several studies have found that calcium helps alleviate symptoms of premenstrual syndrome, including menstrual cramps. In one study, researchers at Columbia University found that women who took 1200 milligrams of calcium per day for 2 months had a 54 per cent drop in pain and PMS symptoms compared with the placebo group, whose pain increased 15 per cent. Calcium protects bones as well. Take 600 milligrams twice per day.

Vitamin E. In a 4-month Iranian study of teenage girls, the ones who took 200 milligrams of vitamin E twice a day beginning 2 days before their periods and continuing for 3 days into their periods reported cramps for an average of 2 hours compared with 17 hours in the control group. Don't exceed 400 milligrams per day. Check with your doctor before taking vitamin E; it can increase the effect of blood thinners, and, in one large study, vitamin E users had a slightly elevated risk of heart failure. Natural vitamin E might be safer than synthetic; look for 'd-alpha' on the label.

Acupuncture. In a recent German study, women who had 15 acupuncture treatments over 3 months had up to a 33 per cent reduction in cramping.

The anticramp diet

We all want a fast fix for pain, but making a few dietary changes that are good for you, anyway, could help you experience fewer cramps and need less pain-relief medication.

More fibre. Make room in your diet for more high-fibre foods such as bran, brown rice and wholemeal bread by kicking out the simple carbohydrates, including sugary foods and drinks, white rice and white bread. Complex carbs make tryptophan, an amino acid, more available. Tryptophan is a precursor of serotonin, which not only boosts mood but also eases cramping and pain.

Less meat and dairy. Animal fat produces bad prostaglandins that rev up muscle cramps. Cut out the saturated fats and eat more fish, whole grains and vegetables. While calcium may help with PMS pain, dairy products have been associated with increased inflammation. It may help to forgo milk, cheese and yogurt on the days that you're cramping.

A kettle o' fish. Oily fish, such as salmon and tuna, contain omega-3 fatty acids, which reduce the production of cramp-producing prostaglandins. 'They're the same as taking NSAIDs but in a form more available to the body', says Mourad. If you find you can't eat fish at least twice a week, ask your doctor about taking 1000 to 3000 milligrams of fish oil per day.

Premenstrual syndrome

You're depressed, tired and cranky and if your husband shouts at the umpire one more time, you're breaking the television. Your breasts hurt, you're bloated and you know what's coming: in a week or so you'll get your period and you'll turn into your own worst nightmare, if you're not there already.

Premenstrual syndrome (PMS) is no picnic for anyone, but for some women it's debilitating. About 85 per cent of women from their late twenties to early forties have at least one symptom every month, including acne, insomnia, cramping, constipation or diarrhoea, headache or backache, food cravings, joint or muscle pain, trouble concentrating or remembering, irritability, mood swings and crying fits.

Fluctuating levels of hormones and neurotransmitters (brain chemicals) such as serotonin may be at the root of PMS; add stress and anxiety, and your symptoms bloat just like your stomach.

You don't have to suffer endlessly. There are a number of ways your doctor can help, from antidepressants to birth control pills to diuretics. You can make relatively small changes in your diet, vitamin intake and exercise habits that make a big difference.

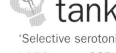

think tank

'Selective serotonin reuptake inhibitors, or SSRIs, are antidepressants that work quite well for severe PMS. Some women state that taking SSRIs changed their lives.'

—Dr Catarina Ang, MBBS. FRANZCOG, DSHR (UK), DUE AFSA (France), MBS, Head of Gynaecology Unit 1, Royal Women's Hospital, Melbourne

✔ Best first steps

If you suspect you have PMS, you can take several steps both to confirm your suspicions and to feel better.

1. Keep track of your symptoms.
Create a chart, numbering days 1 through 31 across the top, listing your five worst symptoms down the side. Each day, give each symptom a severity score from 0 to 3 (3 being the worst). Circle the days

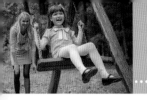

when you are bleeding. Complete this chart for one to two complete cycles. This will help you see whether your symptoms continue after your period, a sign that your difficulties may be more than PMS.

2. Try nonprescription PMS treatments.
Medicines containing ibuprofen or naproxen can address a range of symptoms, including bloating and pain. Also, make sure you are getting 1000 milligrams of calcium per day by taking nonprescription supplements twice daily, especially if you don't eat a lot of dairy products.

Doctor's bag

If you haven't already kept a diary of your symptoms, your doctor may ask you to track them for at least 2 months to help confirm a diagnosis of PMS. She'll ask you about your medical history and offer a physical and pelvic examination. If she suspects you have PMS, she may suggest several of the following treatments.

Antidepressants. Selective serotonin reuptake inhibitors (SSRIs) such as sertraline, fluoxetine and paroxetine taken daily or during the last 14 days of the menstrual cycle can lessen severe irritability, mood swings and depression and can even help food cravings, bloating and breast tenderness.

Low-dose oral contraceptives. These can reduce cramps, bloating, breast tenderness and, depending on the type of oral contraceptive, also help with irritability, mood swings, sleep problems and food cravings. Angelique, Yasmin and Yaz are birth control pills that contain drospirenone, a different kind of progestin from other contraceptives that is more effective at relieving both physical and emotional symptoms of PMS. Progestin is a synthetic form of progesterone, a hormone that helps prepare the uterus for pregnancy. Drospirenone also acts like the diuretic spironolactone.

Diuretics. Your doctor may suggest that you take the mild diuretic spironolactone (Aldactone, Spiractin) before your symptoms begin each month to help deal with water retention and bloating. It works by helping your kidneys flush out sodium and water. It can also reduce symptoms such as fatigue and depression. It's best taken during the day so that the need to urinate doesn't keep you up at night.

Your pain toolbox

You have more pain-relieving tools at your disposal than you may think, from changes in your diet to better sleep habits. Here are a few.

Nonprescription pain relievers. They can tamp down the discomfort of cramps, backaches, headaches and breast tenderness. If your doctor gives you the okay, try 400 to 600 milligrams of ibuprofen every 4 hours; 500 milligrams of naproxen to start, then 250 milligrams every 6 hours. Don't take these in addition to other nonprescription drugs marketed for PMS symptoms.

Calcium. Studies show that calcium helps reduce symptoms of PMS, including menstrual cramps. Researchers at Columbia University found that women who took 1200 milligrams of calcium a day for 2 months had a 48 per cent decrease in premenstrual symptoms compared with 30 per cent in the control group; a 45 per cent decrease in emotional symptoms, including depression; and a 54 per cent drop in pain compared with the placebo group, whose pain increased by 15 per cent. Mourad recommends 1200 milligrams per day (in two divided doses) for all women over age 20 to protect bones as well.

Instant relief

PMS can mire you in misery. Here's what you can do to feel better fast.

A cup of tea. The ritual of tea is psychologically comforting, but that's not all. Brew a cup using ginger, dandelion and juniper, and you have a natural diuretic that will help you lose some of the bloat. Fill a teapot with boiling water, add three slices of ginger and a teaspoon each of dried dandelion and juniper (available in health and natural foods stores) and brew for 5 to 15 minutes. Drink several times per day. Green tea is also a natural diuretic. If caffeine in black and green tea seems to make you more irritable, try the caffeine-free versions.

A bounce in your step. Putting your sneakers on is the hardest step. But walking (or swimming, biking or any other form of aerobic exercise) 30 minutes most days will lift your mood and give you more energy.

Sunlight. 'Increasing your exposure to natural bright light for at least 30 minutes a day is very effective at decreasing mood-related symptoms such as depression and irritability', says Mourad. 'Lying in bed wrapped in a quilt may make things a little bit worse.'

Progressive muscle relaxation. Lie down with your eyes closed. Inhale, and tense your feet as hard as you can for 8 seconds. Then release as you exhale, imagining pain and stress floating away, paying attention to how different tension and relaxation are. Rest for 15 seconds. Then repeat with your calves, proceeding body part by body part (thighs, buttocks, stomach, arms, hands, etc.) until you reach your head.

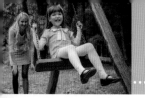

Less salt, more water. Cutting back on table salt and salty foods such as chips, pickles, soy sauce, canned soups and other packaged foods and deli meats, especially a few days before your period, may prevent bloating. And, as odd as it sounds, drink lots of water, which will help you flush out the sodium that holds on to fluids.

Vitamin B_6. International studies using vitamin B_6 in PMS have used high doses. In Australia and New Zealand, the recommended upper limit is 50 milligrams: amounts greater than 50 milligrams per day are not recommended.

Massage. In a study at the Touch Research Institute in Miami, women with PDD who had half-hour massages that included stomach massage twice a week for 5 weeks found their moods improved and their pain levels diminished. They also had less water retention.

Psychological strategies. A British study found that cognitive behavioural therapy, which is a form of counselling that focuses on examining the link among thoughts, behaviour and even physical symptoms, was as effective in treating PMS as the antidepressant fluoxetine. Relaxation techniques such as progressive muscle relaxation (see 'Instant relief', page 277), yoga and meditation can also be helpful. One study found that women with PMS who regularly used relaxation techniques showed a 58 per cent improvement in their symptoms.

Smaller meals. Eating smaller, more frequent meals instead of three big ones could help reduce bloating and that beached-whale feeling. It keeps your blood glucose stable, which can help with both cravings and mood swings. Make the meals high in fibre with plenty of fruit, vegetables and whole grains. Those complex carbs make tryptophan, an amino acid, more available. Tryptophan is a precursor of serotonin, which not only boosts mood but also eases cramping and pain.

Vulvodynia

This condition involves an intense burning or knifelike pain in the vulva, the fleshy area around the opening of the vagina, in response to touch or pressure. Up to 16 per cent of women are said to experience it during sex, whenever they insert a tampon, have a gynaecological examination or just sit down for any length of time. The actual number may be higher, since vulvodynia has no outward signs (though occasionally the area can look red and swollen) and many women are reluctant to discuss the problem with their doctors. Any woman can develop the condition at any age, though the largest group of sufferers is between ages 18 and 25.

The condition is tough to diagnose and the causes remain unknown but are probably complex. You may develop vulvodynia as the result of a yeast infection; allergies; nerve damage; structural problems in the pelvic floor, back, and/or buttocks; or even hormonal changes such as those that occur at menopause. According to recent studies, women with vulvodynia may have as much as a tenfold increase in the number of nerve endings in the vulva, which would intensify even minor problems that can cause pain. Not surprisingly, the condition can also lead to depression.

Once your doctor determines the pain's cause, she can prescribe helpful treatments. There's plenty you can do to lessen the discomfort, from changes in your hygiene routine to a switch in underwear.

✅ Best first steps

Vulvodynia means pain in the vulva, which tells you nothing you don't already know. One key to treatment is to find out the root cause, which means discussing the problem with your gynaecologist.

1. Go to a specialist.
'If you think that you have not been helped by your GP, go to a gynaecologist for evaluation', says Dr Ross Pagano, Head of the

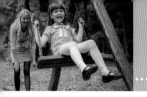

Vulvar Disorders Clinic at the Royal Women's Hospital, Melbourne. 'A thorough clinical assessment, recognition of the emotional and sexual implications and knowledge of the treatment options available can lead to effective management.'

2. Stop soaping.
Until you can see your doctor, stop putting soap, bath oil, cream or feminine deodorant sprays on your genital area, and avoid using harsh detergents and fabric softener on your underwear. Wash with plain water only. This may help ease symptoms.

3. Take a night-time antihistamine.
This may ease the itching so that you can get a good night's sleep, always important in fighting pain.

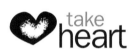

Doctor's bag

Your gynaecologist will examine you to determine the cause of your pain, checking for a bacterial or yeast infection. She may perform a colposcopy, an examination of the genitals using a magnifying instrument. She may do a biopsy, taking a small piece of numbed tissue from the genital area. Depending on what she finds, she'll recommend one or several of the following treatments. (Some doctors may also try prescription anti-inflammatory drugs to combat inflammation, or anticonvulsant drugs or muscle relaxants to combat muscle spasms that may contribute to pain.)

Tricyclic antidepressants. Antidepressants such as amitriptyline and nortriptyline can block pain signals and also improve your mood.

Oestrogen. Vaginal creams containing oestrogen can reduce the pain in some women, possibly because they calm inflammation beneath the skin. Oestrogen tablets inserted into the vagina once or twice weekly can cut back on itchy dryness as well as discomfort.

Anaesthetic ointments. Your doctor may prescribe a lignocaine (Xylocaine) ointment to use intermittently, say, 30 minutes before sex to make it less painful. (Warn your partner that he may be a bit numb afterwards too.) But using it nonstop can further irritate your skin.

Researchers at Cornell University have found two genetic variations that predispose women to vulvodynia. One results in a propensity for producing low levels of inflammation blockers; the other, a predisposition to produce low levels of a substance that normally protects against yeast or bacterial infections.

Your pain toolbox

Your doctor may prescribe medications, but there are more options.

Physiotherapy. If the pain is related to your pelvic floor muscles, a physiotherapist may use massage and biofeedback, teaching you exercises to help loosen tight and spastic pelvic muscles.

Transcutaneous electrical nerve stimulation (TENS). In TENS, electrodes are placed on an area of skin that shares neural pathways with the painful area. The gentle electric current stimulates the underlying nerves, which results in lessening of pain transmission at the spinal cord. The effect is transient so the stimulation has to be repeated frequently. Once you are trained by a therapist, you can manage this treatment.

Exercise. Aerobic activity, such as walking 30 minutes per day on most days, jump-starts the production of endorphins, the body's natural painkillers. However, for obvious reasons, don't choose cycling.

Lots of water. More urinating doesn't sound pleasant, but drinking more water dilutes your urine so it won't burn as much when you go.

Looser clothes. You need airflow and dryness. If you have to wear stockings, skip the panty version and wear a garter belt instead. Or buy only those with a cotton crotch, then slit the crotch to keep it loose. Wear only cotton underwear during the day and nothing when you sleep.

A foam doughnut cushion. If sitting hurts, one of these cushions, sold at pharmacies and medical supply companies, may help.

Instant relief

For those moments when you can't stand the pain and itching one second longer, try these.

Cold compresses. Wet a soft cloth with cold water and place it on your genitals to ease pain and itching, or after sex. Or use a cold pack wrapped in a face washer.

Ointments. If it burns when you urinate, try rubbing an ointment such as Desitin Nappy Rash Ointment, or similar ointment using zinc oxide or Vaseline on the area, which can keep the urine from burning.

A cup of water. After you urinate, immediately pour a cup of water over the area. This will both dilute and wash away the burning urine.

Leaning forwards when you urinate. This helps direct your urine straight down, so that not as much of it touches your skin.

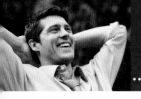

Burns

For most of us, the only time we experience the pain of a burn is when we accidentally grab a hot pan without a mitt or fall asleep on the beach. But burns also include skin damage caused by scalding water, flames, chemicals such as bleach and electric burns. And burns range broadly in severity, categorised as first, second or third degree.

First-degree burns are the ones you get from a slight brush with a hot baking pan: they affect only the top layer of skin, which turns red, swollen and painful. These usually resolve in 2 or 3 days, although you may lose a little skin. A second-degree burn involves both the first and second layers of skin. The skin turns red and painful, blisters form and healing takes longer. A third-degree burn damages all layers of skin and the deeper tissues as well—fat, muscle and possibly bone. Healing time depends on how deep and severe the burns are, but it can take months.

Chemical and electrical burns may not show up on the skin, but that doesn't mean they aren't painful and serious, possibly damaging internal organs. All chemical and electrical burns should be reviewed in the emergency department. So if you think you've had a chemical or electrical burn you should go to your local emergency department.

Minor burns, including first-degree burns or second-degree burns that are no more than 8 to 10 centimetres in diameter can be handled at home. Larger first-degree burns or those involving the face, hands, feet or genitals, and second- and third-degree burns need the immediate care of a doctor. So do burns to a child.

✅ Best first steps

Taking action fast can lessen pain, swelling and damage.

For minor burns

1. Run cold water over minor burns.
Keep the cold water coming for at least 5 minutes or until the pain lets up. Don't apply ice because it may cause more skin damage.

2. Cover.
Loosely cover minor burns with a sterile gauze bandage to protect the skin from infection.

3. Take a nonprescription pain reliever.
For the pain, take aspirin, ibuprofen or paracetamol as directed on the package.

4. Don't pop blisters.
If they pop on their own, don't snip or peel off the skin; it's nature's best bandage. If the top of the blister comes off on its own, apply petroleum jelly followed by a nonadhesive dressing to keep the area moist. This promotes healing in the first week. Avoid putting any kind of bandage on the affected skin; that skin is fragile, and pulling off the bandage can shear it off.

For severe burns

Call your local emergency number or go to the emergency department.
While awaiting an ambulance, run cool water over the affected area. Do not attempt to remove any materials that are stuck to the skin, but remove or cut away any loose material near the burn. Cover the area with a clean cloth. Keep the burnt area above heart level to lessen swelling.

⏱ Instant relief

Even minor burns can be extremely painful. When the pain's too much, try these measures.

Aloe vera gel. The inside of each leaf on an aloe vera plant contains a gel that works as an anti-inflammatory and also kills bacteria, relieving pain, itching and swelling. Apply one tablespoon of gel three times per day to first- and second-degree burns only. A review of four studies involving 371 patients found that people with burn wounds who were treated with aloe vera healed an average of 9 days earlier than those who were not.

An oatmeal bath. For minor burns or for windburn or sunburn, add one to two cups of oatmeal (you can grind oats in a blender to make oatmeal) to a warm bath and soak for 15 minutes. The oatmeal's vitamin E, and compounds called avenanthramides, work as anti-inflammatories, and the oatmeal also helps soothe the itching and reduce skin dryness.

Lemon and water. Don't use this if your burn is still open. However, in its aftermath, rinsing with lemon or vinegar and water can help to ease the itch.

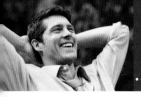

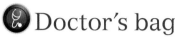 Doctor's bag

For more serious burns, including any burn to a child, deep burn or burns from chemical or electrical causes you should see a doctor immediately, even if the burn is not painful. He'll examine the wound, assessing the degree of damage. He'll also check you for other conditions that often accompany burns, such as smoke inhalation or carbon monoxide poisoning. He may then treat you with several of the following.

Pain relievers. The doctor will likely offer oral or intravenous opioids, such as morphine, for severe pain.

Tetanus injection. If you haven't had a tetanus injection in 5 years, your doctor may give you a booster. (Normally, adults need a booster only every 10 years, but within 5 years of a serious injury.)

Antibiotics. Your doctor may prescribe topical (skin cream or ointment), oral or intravenous antibiotics to prevent or treat infection.

Local anaesthesia. The doctor may numb the area so that he can clean the wound of any debris.

Your pain toolbox

For minor burns and even more serious burns, here are some options for diminishing pain.

Water. A bad sunburn can leave you dehydrated, which can make you feel sick. Be sure to drink plenty of fluids.

Calendula or chamomile. Both herbs reduce inflammation and act as a mild antiseptic for minor burns or sunburns. Calendula is available as a gel, or make a tea of either herb by steeping several teaspoons of the dried herb in one cup of hot water for 10 minutes. Soak a clean white cloth in the tea and apply to the sunburn.

Pawpaw ointment. This soothing ointment has antimicrobial properties.

St John's wort. Most of us associate this herb with boosting mood, but used topically in oil or cream, it can ease inflammation and pain, and help spur healing of minor burns. Don't forget to let your doctor know if you are taking this herb as it can interact with other medications.

Salmon for dinner. Fatty fish, such as salmon, contain omega-3 fatty acids that combat inflammation and also protect healing skin by keeping cell membranes fluid, allowing easy transport of healing nutrients and oxygen. Eat a 110-to-170-gram serving of fish twice per week or take up to four 1-gram fish oil capsules a day (check with your doctor first).

Antihistamines. As your burn heals, it will also begin to itch. Scratching opens the door to infection. An antihistamine may help.

Massage therapy. In the recovery stage, people with serious burns may get pain relief from massage. In one study, burn patients who were massaged weekly for 20 minutes had less anxiety, depression and anger, experienced a drop in their pulse rate and decreased levels of the stress hormone cortisol and reported less pain.

Serious help

For serious burns that cover a large area of your body, your doctor may have to turn to more involved measures, which may include the following.

Intravenous fluids. If your body has lost significant amounts of fluid from the burnt area, he may supply fluids intravenously.

Breathing tube. If your lungs have been damaged or if you are having difficulty breathing, the doctor may provide you with oxygen through a face mask. It may be necessary for your safety to insert a breathing tube into your throat (you'll be sedated before the tube is inserted).

Skin grafting. The surgeon will begin the procedure by removing the dead tissue. He will then take skin from a healthy part of your body and place it on the burnt area. In some cases, artificial skin is used to replace dead skin.

Surgery. Healed burns can leave large, tight scars that can make it difficult for the spot (for instance, at a joint) to move as it once did. The doctor may recommend surgery that can both improve the appearance of the scar and return the spot to more normal function.

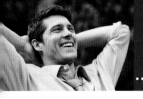

Psoriasis

Your elbow feels like you've run it across a cheese grater, its raised red patches painful, itchy, even bleeding, blistered or covered with pus. This scaly skin condition, psoriasis, stems from a dysfunction in your immune system. Specialised white blood cells, called T-cells, which normally protect you from viruses and other invaders, go awry, attacking your skin cells, which respond by swelling and multiplying. Normally, skin cells turn over once a month, but if you have psoriasis, the process takes only days. As a result, skin cells build up, creating thick, scaly patches that can appear anywhere on your body. The condition, which is not contagious, is often genetic.

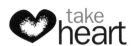

According to a 10-week study at Baylor University Medical Center in Dallas, **infliximab** (Remicade) **reduced symptoms** of psoriasis in every body area by **at least three-quarters** in 80 per cent of 1500 patients.

Stress, smoking, a current cold or infection, trauma, surgery or cold weather can also trigger a flare-up, as can conditions that weaken the immune system, such as alcoholism and HIV.

Around 10 per cent of patients with psoriasis will develop psoriatic arthritis in which the joints are affected as well as the skin. It causes irreversible erosive damage to the joints. If you have persistent joint pain, especially in the small joints such as the hands, wrists, elbows, ankles or knees, it is important to see your dermatologist or a rheumatologist to prevent the progression of psoriatic arthritis.

Psoriasis is not an easy one, both because of its cosmetic effects and its discomfort. It can lead to infection and also to complicated emotions of anxiety, low self-esteem and depression. Patients with psoriasis also have a greater incidence of high blood pressure, elevated blood fats including cholesterol and triglycerides, diabetes and obesity. This puts them at higher risk of heart disease, heart attack and stroke. Make sure your doctor regularly monitors you for the development and/or treatment of these conditions.

✅ Best first steps

You can act quickly to start yourself on a path to more comfort.

1. Head to a doctor.
If you develop red, itchy patches on your skin, visit your doctor as soon as possible.

2. Moisturise.
This is key to minimising flare-ups. Use nondetergent soaps, such as Dove or Oil of Olay Wash, for bathing: they clean the skin and add necessary moisturisers. Immediately after bathing, while the skin is damp, apply a thick moisturising cream (no lotion) to prevent further loss of moisture from the skin. Petroleum jelly (Vaseline) works best and is inexpensive. Other less greasy but still effective creams are made by MooGoo, Cetaphil and Eucerin. Reapply several times per day. When the skin is well moisturised, any topical prescription creams that you apply afterwards will penetrate and work better.

Doctor's bag

The doctor will examine you, perhaps taking a skin sample to rule out other disorders. Once he confirms that you have psoriasis, he may suggest one or more of the following treatments. He may also recommend involvement of a dermatologist.

Steroid creams. Your doctor may prescribe topical corticosteroids, which help relieve inflammation and itching. It's important that you don't use steroids on your skin for extended periods without medical approval. In particular, don't use steroid preparations on your face or neck for even a short time without your doctor's approval.

Vitamin D cream. Calcipotriene (Dovonex) lowers inflammation and slows skin cell production. It's often used in conjunction with a steroid cream and other treatments, such as light therapy.

Light therapy. Judicious doses of ultraviolet light help slow skin cell production and decrease inflammation. Depending on the kind of light therapy, this may involve treatments three or more times per week for weeks. After light therapy your skin may be red, dry and itchy.

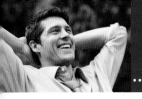

Oral medications. Three traditional options include methotrexate, cyclosporin (Neoral) and oral retinoids. Methotrexate decreases inflammation and skin cell production and is often effective when other methods fail. Cyclosporin works by suppressing the immune system but isn't used for more than 1 to 2 years because it's linked to toxic side effects, such as kidney and blood pressure problems. Retinoids, derivatives of vitamin A, such as acitretin (Neotigason), also reduce the production of skin cells and, like cyclosporin, can have serious side effects, including birth defects, high cholesterol and diminished liver function.

Biologics. Usually prescribed only for people with severe psoriasis, these drugs, given by injection or infusion, block the overactive immune response involved in psoriasis, which helps to lower inflammation. These drugs include etanercept (Enbrel), infliximab (Remicade), adalimumab (Humira) and ustekinumab (Stelara). These drugs are less likely to harm the kidney or liver than some other medicines, but, because they suppress the immune system, they may increase the risk of serious infection or cancer.

Your pain toolbox

Moisturising your skin regularly is your first line of defence. Beyond that, try these options to help make your skin look and feel better.

Stop smoking. Psoriasis is yet another reason to stop smoking. Ask your doctor for assistance and look on the web, for example http://www.quitnow.gov.au.

Nightly plastic wrap. Before bed, after you've smoothed on a thick moisturiser, wrap the area with plastic wrap. You may feel a bit like a leftover, but the wrap will make the moisturiser more effective. Remove the wrap in the morning and wash away any accumulated scales.

Instant relief

When you need relief straightaway, try this soother.

A warm bath. Warm (not hot) baths help loosen and soothe the irritated skin. Add bath oil, Epsom or Dead Sea salts or one cup of ground oatmeal to the bath and soak for at least 15 minutes.

Some sunlight. Getting out in the sun for short periods at least three times per week can help clear up patches. However, too much sun can make them worse. Start with 15-minute sessions, protecting unaffected parts of your body with sunscreen. Keep a record of the sessions and your skin's reaction after each one until you have a good idea how much sun helps and how much is too much.

A trigger diary. Keep a diary tracking what seems to set off flares, such as a cut or scrape, an infection somewhere in your body, emotional stress, smoking too many cigarettes, drinking too much alcohol or getting too much sunlight. The next step, of course, is to avoid those triggers whenever possible.

Weight loss. Excess body fat triggers the production of inflammatory chemicals in the body, which may raise the risk of psoriasis. Some researchers suggest that weight loss may help active psoriasis die down.

Relaxation. Stress and anxiety make psoriasis worse. Put aside at least 15 minutes a day to unwind by listening to music or meditating.

Salmon. Add fatty fish to your menu two or three times per week for its inflammation-fighting omega-3 fatty acids. A British study found that people with psoriasis who ate 170 grams of fatty fish, such as salmon, mackerel or herring, every day for 6 weeks improved by 15 per cent; those who ate nonfatty white fish had no improvement.

Orange-red vegetables. Pile on the carrots, tomatoes and other brightly coloured vegetables high in beta-carotene. One Italian study found that eating a diet high in these orange-red vegetables lowered the risk of psoriasis.

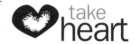

A promising treatment is **indigo ointment**, which contains emollients, as well as *Indigo naturalis*, a dark-blue powder derived from **dried Chinese herbs** that decreases inflammation. Taiwanese researchers found that after **12 weeks of treatment** with indigo ointment, psoriasis patients showed an **81 per cent improvement**. It stains the skin, but the colour washes off. **More research is needed**.

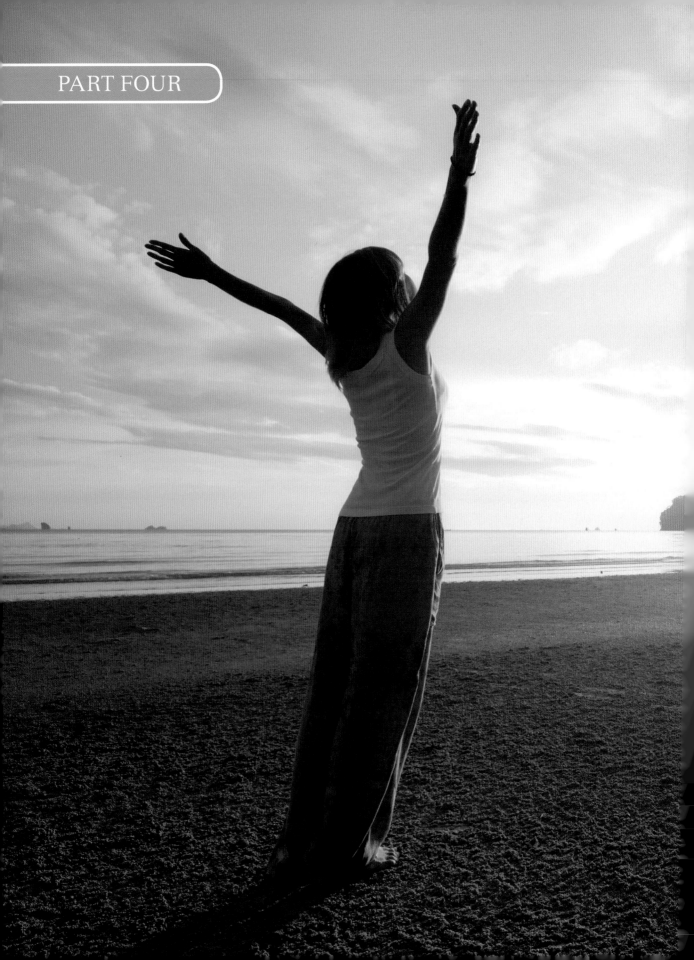

PART FOUR

Exercises
for pain relief

Ease your pain with exercise

For many people, the word 'exercise' has a negative connotation that has nothing to do with its actual definition. Mention the word, and they immediately think of hard work, pain, gyms and expensive gym fees, weights, sweat, lycra, high-tech sneakers and big muscles. We understand. But exercise can also be very enjoyable so it's now time to explode that definition.

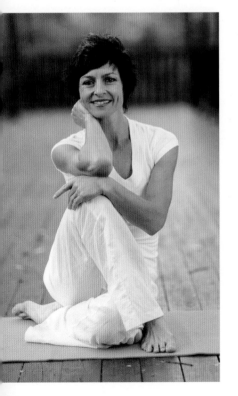

Exercise, in its broadest definition, is *any* exertion done for the sake of training or improvement. It can be mental or physical, short or long, simple or complex, done in bed, in the kitchen or even in line at the shop. Nowhere in the dictionary definition of exercise does it say you need to change your clothes, sweat, join a class, leave your home or spend hours doing it.

Why are we telling you this? Because for many people, intimidating stereotypes and preconceived notions cause them to *not* exercise. And as we've said so many times, for pain management to be truly effective, exercise needs to be part of the program.

The exercises in the pages ahead are a perfect place to start. These are gentle, therapeutic movements, developed by experts in pain management and rehabilitation, not by fitness trainers. They won't make you sweat, and in some cases, they won't challenge your muscles all that much. But that is their beauty. Each is highly targeted and proven effective at relieving the joints and muscles that are causing you pain, in an easy-to-live-with way.

Getting started

Like a restaurant menu, we offer a wide selection of exercise choices, leaving it to you to read the descriptions and decide which ones best suit your unique needs. Start by browsing the exercises targeted to your specific type of pain, then select a few moves you feel are most suited to your particular situation. If you're not certain, get your doctor or physiotherapist involved. Bring this book to your next appointment, and get his recommendations.

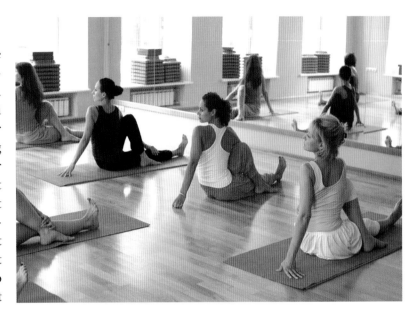

Before you even start to do any of the moves, read and make sure you thoroughly understand the instructions. Then carefully test them out. What exactly is the movement? Does it look right? Does it feel right? That way, when you start doing the exercise regularly, you can be confident your technique is correct.

Once you have that down, the next step is to develop a routine: a regular time and place to do the moves. First thing in the morning? During commercials while watching the news? After taking your evening walk? By committing to a specific time, you'll be more likely to make doing the exercises a habit.

Then do them! Move slowly and carefully, without any jerky motions. While you do the exercise, breathe deeply; don't hold your breath, as is often the natural inclination. If the move causes you to hurt beyond what seems appropriate or natural, stop.

Finally, keep your ultimate goal in mind as you exercise. For a small investment in time and energy, you are doing precisely what you need to do to greatly reduce pain, improve mobility and live the life you want. Let's get started!

Pelvic tilt

Strengthens and stabilises back muscles affected by spinal osteoarthritis, disc problems and general lower back pain

LIE on your back with your knees bent, feet flat on the floor, knees about shoulder-width apart. You should be able to fit your fist between your knees. Push the small of your back into the floor by pulling your lower abdominal muscles up and in. Inhale and exhale normally. This is a subtle, not dramatic, movement. Hold position for 5 seconds, then slowly relax. Start with 3 sets of 3, build up to 3 sets of 5, then 7, then 10.

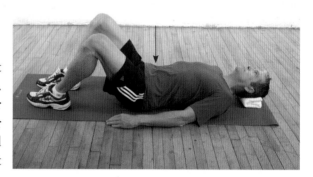

A

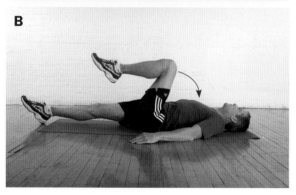

B

Single knee to chest

Increases flexibility and range of motion for those affected by spinal osteoarthritis and general lower back pain

A. Lie face up. You may bend your knees, keeping your feet flat on the floor.
B. Bring one knee towards your chest, so that you feel a stretch but no pain. If you wish, you can place your hands behind your knee and gently pull your knee towards your chest. Start with 3 repetitions on each side, build up to 5, then 7, then 10.

Static crunches

Gently strengthens abdominal muscles that support your lower back; stronger ab muscles take pressure off your lower back, reducing pain

LIE on your back with your knees bent, feet flat on the floor. Tighten your stomach muscles and press your lower back into the floor. Raise your left knee, so that your leg forms a 90-degree angle. Place your left hand on the top of your left thigh and, exhaling, press forwards, while resisting the force, so that your knee doesn't move. Hold for 5 seconds. Relax for 5 seconds. Perform 10 repetitions. Repeat on the other side. Start with 3 sets of 3, build up to 3 sets of 5, then 7, then 10.

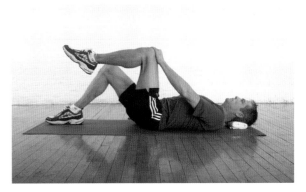

A

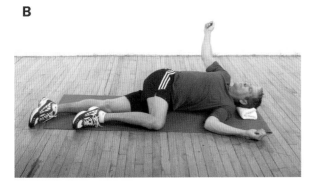

B

Trunk rotation

Increases flexibility in the lower back for those affected by spinal osteoarthritis, disc problems and general lower back pain

A. Lie on the floor on your left side with your knees bent, right knee brought towards your chest. Place your hands by your head.
B. Rotate your shoulders and head as though you are trying to look over your right shoulder, letting your right arm follow. You should feel a slight stretch in your lower back. Hold this position for 10 seconds. Repeat 3 times. Turn onto your right side and repeat. Build up to 5, then 7, then 10.

Clamshell ●

Strengthens hip and lower back for those affected by spinal osteoarthritis and general lower back pain

A. Lie on your left side with your knees bent.
B. Tightening your abdominal muscles, lift your right knee while keeping your ankles together. Keep your hips aligned vertically. Slowly lower leg to starting position. Do 3 sets of 3 repetitions, then switch sides. Build up to 3 sets of 5, then 7, then 10 repetitions.

A

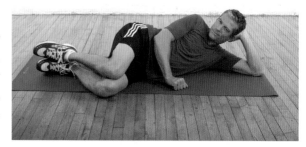

B

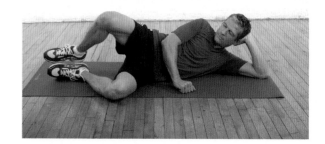

● Heel taps

Gently strengthens your hips and lower back; for greater effect, lift your heel further from the ground

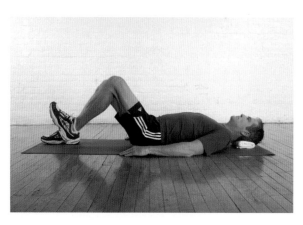

LIE on your back with your knees bent, feet flat on the floor. Tighten your stomach muscles and press your lower back into the floor. Hold this position while tapping your right heel 5 centimetres up from and down to the floor 3 times. Repeat on the other side. Do 3 sets. Build up to 3 sets of 5, then 7, then 10 repetitions.

Press-ups on elbows

Increases flexibility and range of motion, alleviating disc problems and sciatica

A. Lie facedown on the floor, your hands by your head.
B. Keeping your back relaxed and your hips on the floor, slowly press up on to your elbows. Hold for 10 seconds. Repeat 3 times. Build up to 3 sets of 5, then 7, then 10 repetitions.

A

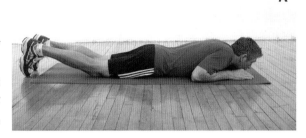

B

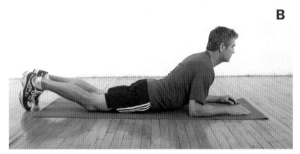

Alternate arm and leg extensions

Strengthens and stabilises supporting muscles, alleviating disc problems and general lower back pain

A. Lie on the floor facedown, arms extended in front of you. If desired, rest your forehead on a small pillow or rolled towel.
B. Lift your right arm and left leg about 5 to 7.5 centimetres off the floor. Hold for 3 seconds, relax and do the same with the left arm and right leg. Do 3 sets (both sides) of 3 repetitions. Build up to 3 sets of 5, then 7, then 10 repetitions.

A

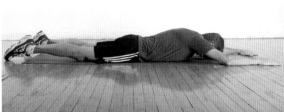

B

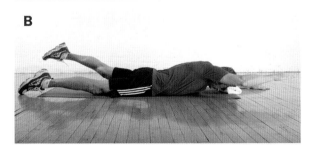

- Do exercises with a green dot when your pain is active.
- Do exercises with a red dot when you're feeling better, to keep future flares at bay.

  Remember to start slowly and gradually build up your repertoire and your repetitions.

Piriformis stretch ●

Increases flexibility for those affected by spinal arthritis, general lower back pain, sciatica and hip pain

LIE on your back, knees bent and lower legs parallel to the ground. Cross your right leg over the left, just above the left knee. Grip your left knee with both hands and slowly pull towards your chest. Hold for 15 to 30 seconds, then repeat on the right leg. Do 3 sets of 3 repetitions per leg. Build up to 3 sets of 5, then 7, then 10 repetitions.

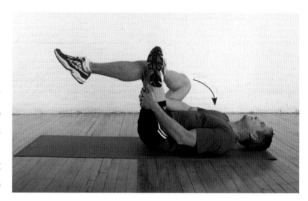

● ## Pelvic bridge

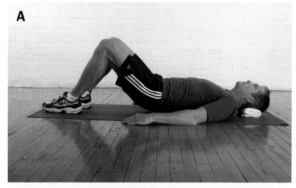

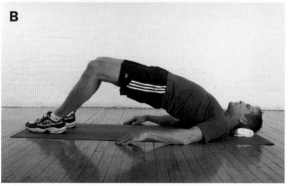

Strengthens abs, glutes and thigh muscles to stabilise hip joints

A. Lie on your back with your knees bent. Tighten your abdominal muscles to flatten your lower back against the floor.
B. Lift your buttocks off the floor so that your body forms a straight line. (Don't sag in the middle or arch your back.) Squeeze your buttocks. Return to start. Do 3 sets of 3 repetitions. Build up to 3 sets of 5, then 7, then 10 repetitions.

Double knees to chest •

Increases flexibility and range of motion for those affected by spinal osteoarthritis and general lower back pain

LIE face up, knees bent. Gently pull your knees towards your chest so that you feel a stretch but no pain. If you wish, place your hands behind your knees and use them to pull your legs forwards. Hold for 10 seconds. Repeat 3 times. Build up to 3 sets of 5, then 7, then 10 repetitions.

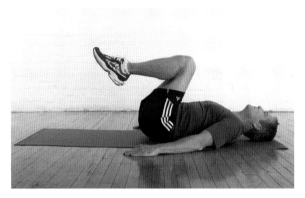

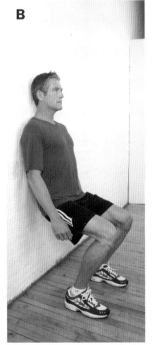

A   B

• Wall squat

Strengthens supporting muscles (quadriceps and glutes) affected by spinal arthritis, general lower back pain, hip pain and knee pain

A. Stand with your back against a wall, heels about two steps (45 centimetres) from the wall, shoulder-width apart.
B. Pulling in your abdominal muscles, slide slowly down the wall until your knees are bent at about 90 degrees, as though you're seated. If that's too difficult, bend your knees to a 45-degree angle and gradually build up from there. Count to 5 and slide slowly back up the wall. Do 3 sets of 3 repetitions. Build up to 3 sets of 5, then 7, then 10 repetitions.

- ● Do exercises with a green dot when your pain is active.
- ● Do exercises with a red dot when you're feeling better, to keep future flares at bay.
  Remember to start slowly and gradually build up your repertoire and your repetitions.

Heel slides ●

Strengthens hip, hamstring and back muscles affected by general lower back pain

LYING on your back, press your lower back into the floor and hold while you slide one heel away from you along the floor until your leg is straight. Return to start. Repeat 3 times with each leg. Do 3 sets. Build up to 3 sets of 5, then 7, then 10 repetitions.

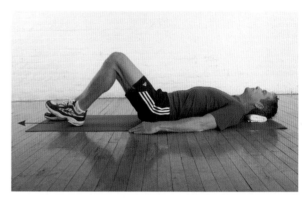

A

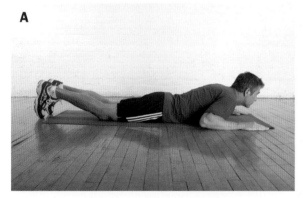

B

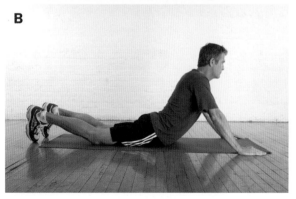

● Press-ups on hands

Increases flexibility and range of motion for those affected by disc problems and sciatica

A. Lie facedown with your palms flat on the floor about level with your head. Toes can be pointed straight back or straight down onto the floor, whichever is more comfortable.
B. Pushing down on your hands, straighten your arms, keeping your hips on the floor. Relax your lower back and buttocks. Hold for 10 seconds. Repeat 3 times. Build up to 3 sets of 5, then 7, then 10 repetitions.

Kneeling arm and leg extensions

Strengthens and stabilises muscles affected by general lower back pain, hip pain and disc problems

A. Get on all fours, hands directly below your shoulders, fingers pointing forwards, knees directly below your hips. Keep your back straight during this exercise. Pretend you're balancing a bowl of water on your back and trying to avoid spilling it, or place a broomstick along your spine lengthways to keep your back in place.

B. Tightening your abdominal muscles, raise your right arm and extend it in front of you. At the same time, raise your left leg and extend it behind you. Hold for 5 seconds, relax and switch sides. Do 3 sets (both sides) 3 times. Build up to 3 sets of 5, then 7, then 10 repetitions.

A

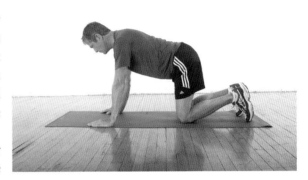

B

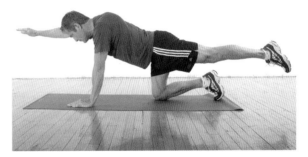

● ● ● All these exercises can be performed when your pain is acute,
as well as when it's calmed down, in order to keep future flares at bay.
Remember to start slowly and gradually build up your repertoire and your repetitions.

Carpal tunnel stretch ● ●

Increases flexibility

Do each of these exercises 5 times. Hold each position to a count of 15. Repeat up to 3 times.

Position 1 Hold your hand up, wrist relaxed and close your fingers and thumb into a relaxed fist.

Position 2 Extend your fingers and thumb so that they're pointing towards the ceiling.

Position 3 Keeping your fingers extended, bend your wrist back as if trying to make your palm face the ceiling.

Position 4 Repeat position 3, but move your thumb away from your fingers.

Position 5 Repeat position 4 with your forearm facing the ceiling, as though you're carrying something.

Position 6 Repeat position 5, but use the other hand to gently stretch thumb.

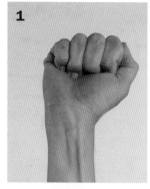
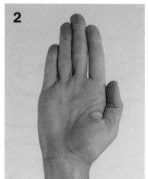
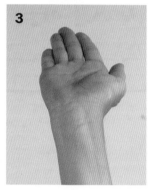
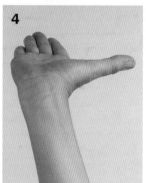
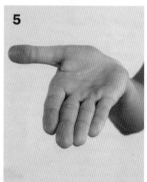
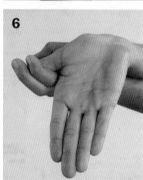

Interior forearm stretch ● ●

Increases flexibility

SIT with your left arm extended, palm facing up. Use your right hand to stretch the palm back by gently applying pressure until you feel a stretch in your forearm. Hold for 30 seconds and repeat up to 3 times. Switch arms.

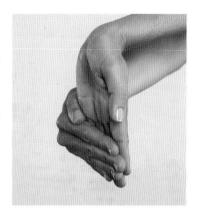

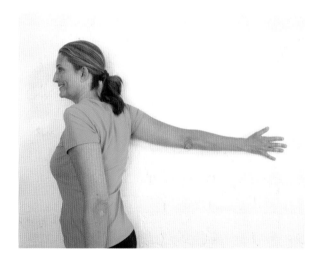

● ● Wall stretch

Stretches your fingers, wrist, arm and chest muscles

STAND facing directly towards a wall. Place your open palm on the wall with your fingers facing backwards. Keep your shoulder relaxed and down. Turn your body away from the wall, moving your feet as needed. You should feel a stretch across your chest and down into your hand.

● Do exercises with a green dot when your pain is active.
● Do exercises with a red dot when you're feeling better, to keep future flares at bay.
Remember to start slowly and gradually build up your repertoire and your repetitions.

Interior forearm stretch ● ●

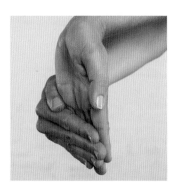

Increases flexibility

SIT with your left arm extended, palm facing up. Use your right hand to stretch the palm back by gently applying pressure until you feel a stretch in your forearm. Hold for 30 seconds and repeat up to 3 times. Switch arms.

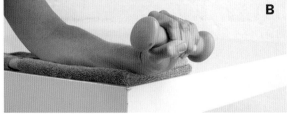

A

B

● Wrist extension

Strengthens muscles

A. While seated, rest your forearm on a pillow or towel on a table, with your palm facing the floor holding a 500-gram dumbbell.
B. Without moving your forearm, lift the weight towards the ceiling. Do 3 sets of 3 repetitions with each wrist. Build up to 3 sets of 5, then 7, then 10 repetitions. Increase weight in small increments when 10 reps become too easy.

Exterior forearm stretch ● ●

Increases flexibility

SIT with your left arm extended, palm down, wrist relaxed. Use your right hand to stretch the wrist so that your fingers point to the floor, or until you feel a stretch in the top of your forearm. Hold for 30 seconds. Repeat 3 times, then switch arms.

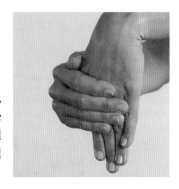

Wrist flexion •

Strengthens muscles

A. While seated, rest your forearm on a pillow or towel on a table, with your palm facing the ceiling holding a 500-gram dumbbell.
B. Without moving your forearm, bend your wrist up. Return to start. Do 3 sets of 3 repetitions with each wrist. Build up to 3 sets of 5, then 7, then 10 repetitions.

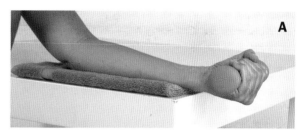

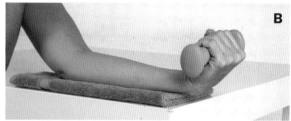

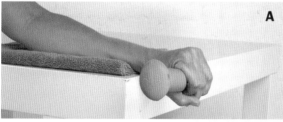

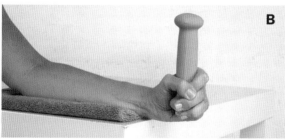

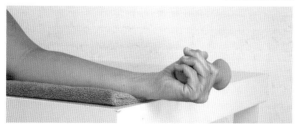

• Pronation/supination

Strengthens muscles

A. While seated, rest your forearm on a pillow or towel on a table, with your palm facing the floor, grasping the end of a 500-gram dumbbell.
B. Without moving your elbow, slowly turn your palm up. Return to start. Do 3 sets of 3 repetitions. Build up to 3 sets of 5, then 7, then 10 repetitions.

- Do exercises with a green dot when your pain is active.
- Do exercises with a red dot when you're feeling better, to keep future flares at bay.

Remember to start slowly and gradually build up your repertoire and your repetitions.

Simple ankle and foot stretch ●

Increases flexibility and restores range of motion

WHILE seated, place your right ankle on your left knee. Rotate your foot clockwise 10 times, then anticlockwise. Do 3 sets of 3 repetitions and then switch feet. Build up to 3 sets of 5, then 7, then 10 repetitions.

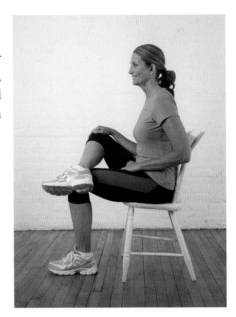

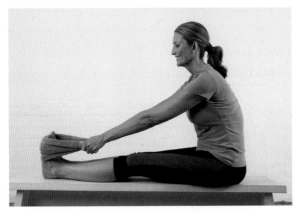

● Seated calf stretch

Increases flexibility in toes, feet and ankles

SIT on the floor or a bench with your feet extended in front of you. Wrap a hand towel or bath towel around the ball of one foot. Pull the towel towards you, keeping your leg straight until you feel a comfortable stretch in your calf. Hold for 30 seconds. Repeat 3 times with each foot.

Towel curls

Stretches and improves range of motion in toes, feet and ankles

WITH your foot resting on a towel on the floor, curl your toes under and grasp the towel with them and pull it towards you. Then relax your toes. Do 3 sets of 3 repetitions, then switch feet. Build up to 3 sets of 5, then 7, then 10 repetitions.

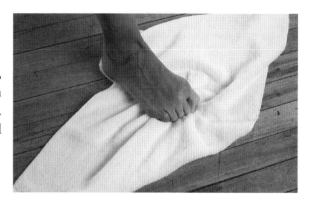

A

Seated calf raises

Strengthens and increases range of motion in toes, feet and ankles

A. Sit in a chair with feet flat on the floor.
B. Raise feet up onto toes. Return feet to the ground slowly. Do 3 sets of 3 repetitions and then switch feet. Build up to 3 sets of 5, then 7, then 10 repetitions.

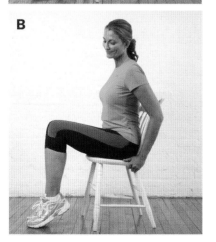

B

• Do exercises with a green dot when your pain is active.
● Do exercises with a red dot when you're feeling better, to keep future flares at bay.
Remember to start slowly and gradually build up your repertoire and your repetitions.

Plantarflexion •

Strengthens calf muscles affected by tendinopathy, ankle pain and foot pain

A. Make a loop in a plastic resistance band (such as a Thera-Band) or use a band that comes with a loop. Sitting on the floor with your legs extended, place the loop around the ball of your painful foot, holding the other end of the band at your waist.
B. Starting with your toes pointed upwards, push your foot down against the resistance of the band. Slowly return to start position. Do 3 sets of 3 repetitions, then switch feet. Build up to 3 sets of 5, then 7, then 10 repetitions.

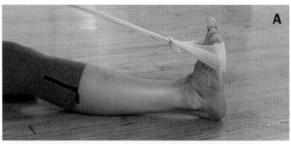

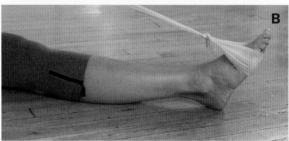

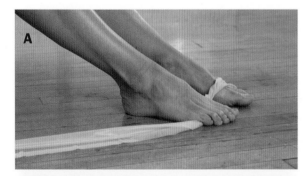

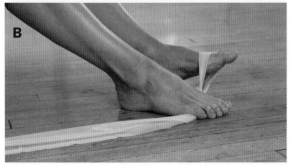

• Dorsiflexion

Strengthens ankles and feet to alleviate various types of pain

A. Sit on the floor with your legs extended, feet close together. Place the loop of a resistance band around your left foot and run the band under the front of the right foot. Hold the end of the band in your hand.
B. Pull your left foot upwards against the resistance band, while your right foot remains stationary. Return to start position slowly. Do 3 sets of 3 repetitions, then switch feet. Build up to 3 sets of 5, then 7, then 10 repetitions.

Eversion

Strengthens ankles and feet affected by Achilles tendinopathy, osteoarthritis and other conditions

A. Sit on the floor with your legs extended, feet close together. Place the loop of a resistance band around your left foot. Run the band under the front of your right foot and hold the end of the band by your waist. Keep your right leg stiff.

B. Keeping your foot relaxed and your leg stationary, pull the left foot outwards. Don't allow the knee to twist. Slowly return to start position. Do 3 sets of 3 repetitions, then switch feet. Build up to 3 sets of 5, then 7, then 10 repetitions.

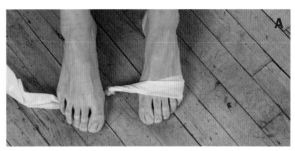

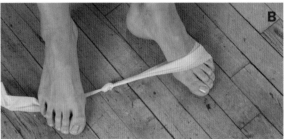

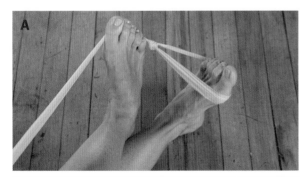

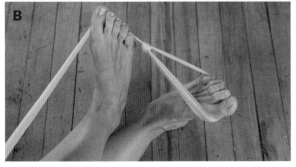

Inversion

Strengthens ankles and feet affected by Achilles tendinopathy, osteoarthritis and other conditions

A. Sit on the floor with your legs extended, your right leg crossed over the top of your left leg. Place the loop of a resistance band around the ball of your left foot and bring the band under the front of your right foot. Hold the end of the band by your waist.

B. Keeping both legs stationary, pull your left foot inwards against the band's resistance. Slowly return to start position. Do 3 sets of 3 repetitions, then switch feet. Build up to 3 sets of 5, then 7, then 10 repetitions.

● Do exercises with a green dot when your pain is active.
● Do exercises with a red dot when you're feeling better, to keep future flares at bay.
   Remember to start slowly and gradually build up your repertoire and your repetitions.

Calf raise ● ●

Strengthens calf muscles affected by tendinopathy

A. Stand on the edge of an aerobic step placed against a wall or a step in your home that will allow you to hold on to a rail or wall for balance.

B. With your hand on the wall or rail, slowly lower both heels. Adjust the pressure on the injured leg by putting most of your weight on your good leg. Now rise up on tiptoe. Start with just a few repetitions when you're in the acute phase of your injury, gradually working up to 3 sets of 10 to 15 repetitions.

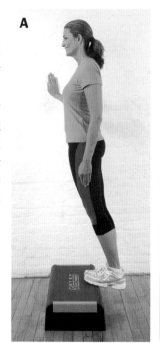

A

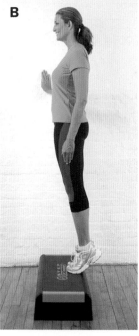

B

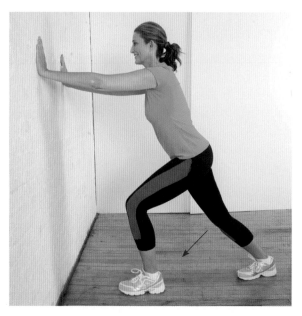

● Standing calf stretch

Increases flexibility in muscles affected by tendinopathy, ankle pain and foot pain

STANDING about 45 centimetres from a wall, place both hands on the wall. Bring your left leg forwards and your right leg back. Bend your left knee towards the wall, keeping your right foot flat on the floor. Point your right foot slightly inwards. You should feel a stretch in your right calf. Hold for 30 seconds, then switch legs.

Plantar fasciitis stretch •

Promotes flexibility

IN a seated position, cross your right leg over your left. Grasp the toes of the affected foot with the corresponding hand, and pull your toes and foot upwards towards your shin, bending until you feel a stretch on the sole of your foot. Hold for 30 seconds. Repeat 3 times. Switch to the other foot if it's also affected.

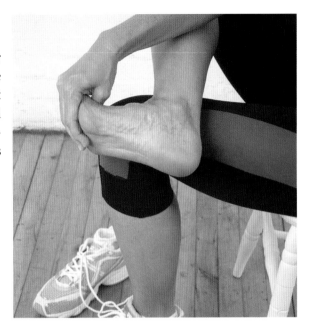

• ## Soft tissue release with ice

Decreases muscle tension in painful heel area

FILL and freeze a small plastic water bottle. Place the bottle on the floor and place your foot on top. With gentle pressure, roll the bottle under your foot back and forth. Perform for about 7 minutes or until the bottom of the foot is chilled.

● Do exercises with a green dot when your pain is active.
● Do exercises with a red dot when you're feeling better, to keep future flares at bay.
Remember to start slowly and gradually build up your repertoire and your repetitions.

Finger bends ●

Increases flexibility

A. Hold your hand upright, fingers close together and pointing to the ceiling.

B. Bend the top two joints of your fingers, keeping your wrist and knuckles straight. Move slowly and smoothly to return your hand to the starting position. Repeat with other hand. Start with 3 sets of 3 repetitions with each hand. Build up to 3 sets of 5, then 7, then 10 repetitions.

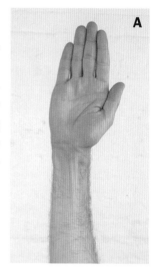
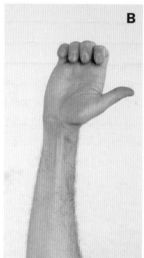

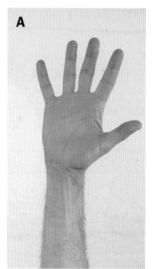
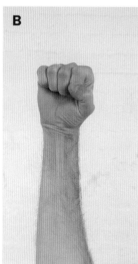

● **Fist**

Increases flexibility

A. Hold your hand upright, fingers pointing to the ceiling, and spread apart.

B. Make a loose fist, wrapping your thumb around the outside of your fingers. Don't clasp your fingers tightly. Return to the starting position. Do this 10 times, then switch hands.

Wide hands

Increases flexibility

A. Spread your fingers as far apart as you can and hold for a count of 10.

B. Slowly relax your fingers and bring them together. Return to the wide-open position. Repeat with the other hand, gradually increasing the number of repetitions.

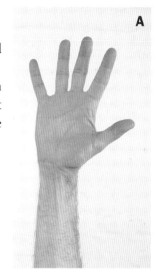
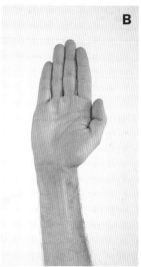

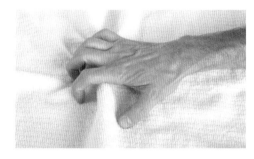

Towel curls

Increases flexibility

WITH your hand resting on a towel on a table, curl your fingers under so that you pull towel towards you, then relax your fingers. Start with 3 sets of 3. Build up to 3 sets of 5, then 7, then 10 repetitions.

Ball squeeze

Strengthens muscles

GRAB a rubber ball or a folded sponge in the palm of your hand and squeeze lightly. Hold for a count of 10. Start with 3 sets of 3. Build up to 3 sets of 5, then 7, then 10 repetitions.

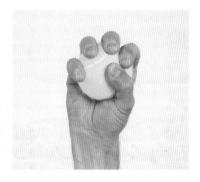

• Do exercises with a green dot when your pain is active.
• Do exercises with a red dot when you're feeling better, to keep future flares at bay.
  Remember to start slowly and gradually build up your repertoire and your repetitions.

Finger extension •

Strengthens muscles

A. Place a rubber band around all 5 fingertips.
B. Spread your fingers, then relax them. Start with 3 sets of 3 repetitions with each hand. Build up to 3 sets of 5, then 7, then 10 repetitions. If the exercise feels too easy, add a second rubber band or a thicker band to provide more resistance.

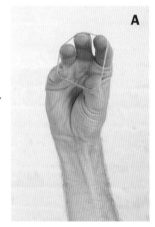
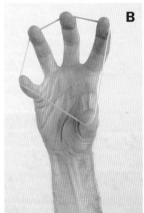

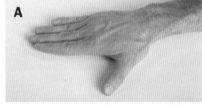
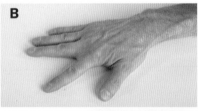
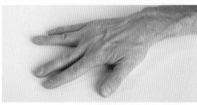
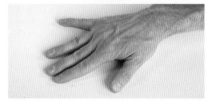

• Finger walk

Increases flexibility

A. Rest your hand on a flat surface, such as a table, with your palm down and your fingers relaxed and slightly apart.
B. Moving one finger at a time, slowly walk your fingers towards your thumb, starting by lifting and moving your index finger, followed by your middle finger, ring finger and pinkie. Keep your wrist and hand stationary. Do 10 repetitions. Repeat with your other hand.

Fingertip touch •

Increases flexibility

A. Hold your hand upright, fingers and thumb straight.

B. Bend your thumb across your palm, touching it to the pad of your palm just under your pinkie or as far as you can comfortably reach. Return to start position.

C. Slowly and smoothly form the letter 'O' by touching your thumb to each fingertip, straightening thumb and fingers after each motion. Repeat with your other hand. Do 10 repetitions.

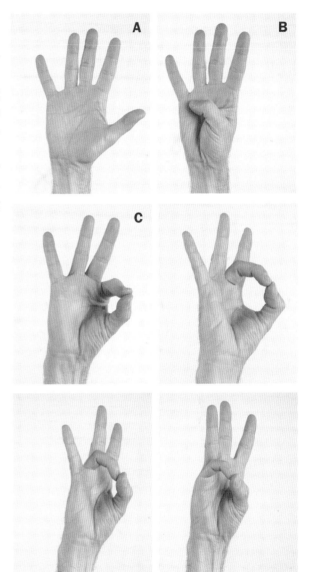

- Do exercises with a green dot when your pain is active.
- Do exercises with a red dot when you're feeling better, to keep future flares at bay.
  Remember to start slowly and gradually build up your repertoire and your repetitions.

Hip hula

Improves range of motion in those affected by hip arthritis or other hip pain

PRETEND you're twirling a hula hoop and slowly rotate your hips in a circle one way, then the other. Your motion should be controlled and pain-free.

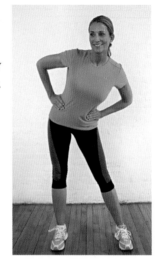 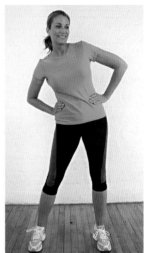

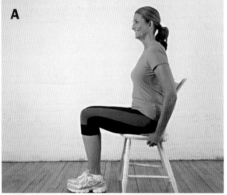

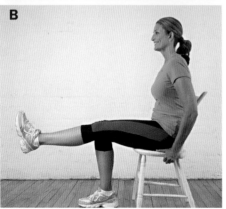

Seated knee extension

Warms up joints before exercise and improves flexibility

A. Sit with your feet flat on the ground and your back and neck straight up. For stability, grab the sides of your chair.
B. Slowly straighten your left leg without moving your body. Pause, then return. Repeat this movement for 30 to 60 seconds. Then repeat with your other leg.

Supine clamshell ●

Strengthens supporting muscles of the hip, knee and back

A. Lie on your back with your knees bent. Tie a resistance band around your thighs just tightly enough to just keep them together.

B. Slowly, pull your knees apart. Hold for 5 seconds, then slowly return to the starting position. Start with 3 sets of 3 repetitions. Build up to 3 sets of 5, then 7, then 10 repetitions.

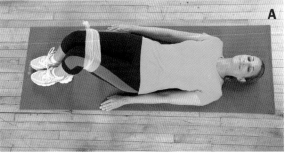

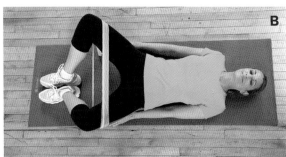

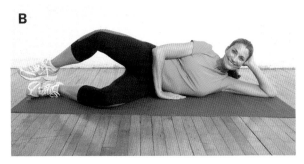

● Clamshell

Strengthens hip and lower back

A. Lie on your left side with your knees bent.

B. Pulling in your abdominal muscles, lift your right leg while keeping your ankles together. Keep your hips vertically aligned. Slowly lower leg to starting position. Start with 3 sets of 3 repetitions then switch sides. Build up to 3 sets of 5, then 7, then 10 repetitions.

- Do exercises with a green dot when your pain is active.
- Do exercises with a red dot when you're feeling better, to keep future flares at bay.
  Remember to start slowly and gradually build up your repertoire and your repetitions.

Towel squeeze

Strengthens hip and knee to stabilise and support knee and hip joints

LIE on your back with your knees bent. Place a rolled towel between your knees. Squeeze the towel and hold for 5 seconds. Start with 3 sets of 3 repetitions. Build up to 3 sets of 5, then 7, then 10 repetitions.

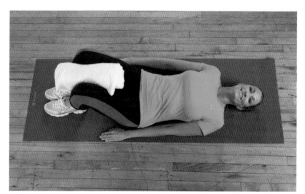

A

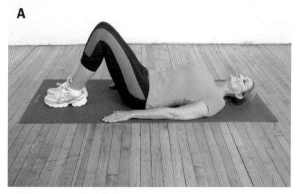

B

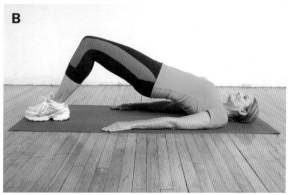

Pelvic bridge

Strengthens abs, glutes and thigh muscles to stabilise hip joints

A. Lie on your back with your knees bent. Tighten your abdominal muscles to flatten your lower back against the floor.
B. Lift your buttocks off the floor so that your body forms a straight line. (Don't sag in the middle or arch your back.) Squeeze your buttocks. Return to start. Start with 3 sets of 3 repetitions. Build up to 3 sets of 5, then 7, then 10 repetitions.

Piriformis stretch

Increases flexibility for those affected by spinal arthritis, general lower back pain, sciatica and hip pain

LIE on your back, knees bent, lower legs parallel to the ground. Cross your left leg over the right, just above the right knee. Grab your right knee with both hands and slowly pull your knee towards your chest. Hold for 15 to 30 seconds, then repeat with the right leg. Do 1 set of 2 repetitions per leg.

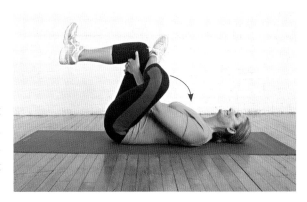

Hamstring stretch

Improves flexibility in hips and knees

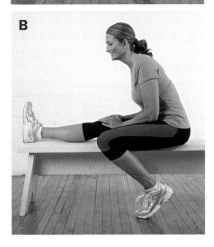

A. Sit on a bench or the edge of a bed. Extend one leg in front of you while resting the other foot on the floor (or on a step beside the bed if the bed is high). Straighten your back.

B. Bend forwards at the waist, without curving your back, as you feel a stretch in the back of the extended leg. Hold the position for 30 seconds. Do this exercise 3 times, then repeat with other leg.

● Do exercises with a green dot when your pain is active.
● Do exercises with a red dot when you're feeling better, to keep future flares at bay.
Remember to start slowly and gradually build up your repertoire and your repetitions.

Quad squeezes ●

Strengthens quadriceps muscles, which support the knee

LIE on your back with a rolled towel under the affected knee. Bend the other knee. Tightening your abdominal muscles, push your knee down into the towel, straightening the leg. Hold for 5 to 10 seconds, then relax. Do 3 sets of 5 repetitions. Switch legs if both are affected. Build up to 3 sets of 10, then 15, then 20 repetitions.

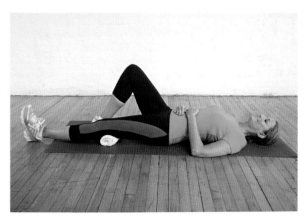

● ● Quadriceps stretch

Improves flexibility in hips and knees

STAND with one hand on a chair or bench for balance. Keeping your stomach and buttocks tight, bend one knee to raise your foot at the back of you, using your free hand to grab the foot until you can feel a stretch in the front of your thigh. Keep your knees next to each other. Hold for 30 seconds. Do this exercise 3 times, then switch legs.

Short arc quadriceps

Strengthens and stabilises knee and hip joints

A. Lie on your back, your right knee bent, your left knee resting on a rolled towel.
B. Tighten your abdominal muscles, then raise your left leg, Hold for 5 to 10 seconds, then relax slowly. Switch legs if both are affected. Do 3 sets of 5 repetitions. Build up to 3 sets of 10, then 15, then 20 repetitions.

A

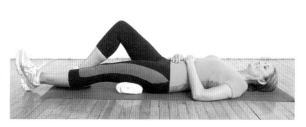

B

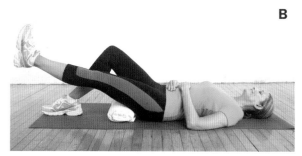

A

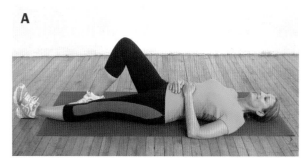

B

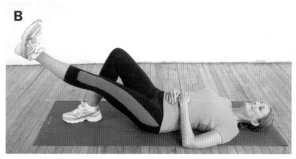

Straight leg raise

Strengthens muscles that support the knee

A. Lie on your back on the floor with one knee bent and the other straight.
B. Slowly raise the straight leg and lower slowly. Keep your stomach muscles tight so your lower back lies flat on the floor. Keep your knee locked during the motion and your foot perpendicular to the floor. Do 3 sets of 3 repetitions. Build up to 3 sets of 5, then 7, then 10 repetitions.

● Do exercises with a green dot when your pain is active.
● Do exercises with a red dot when you're feeling better, to keep future flares at bay.
Remember to start slowly and gradually build up your repertoire and your repetitions.

Prone hip extension ●

Strengthens hips and knees

A. Lie on your stomach with a pillow under your hips (and a small pillow or rolled towel under your forehead if it's more comfortable).

B. Slowly raise one leg off the floor, with your toes facing down. Make sure to not arch your back, and keep your knee locked. Return to start. Do 3 sets of 3 repetitions on each side. Build up to 3 sets of 5, then 7, then 10 repetitions.

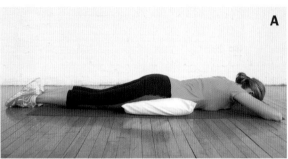

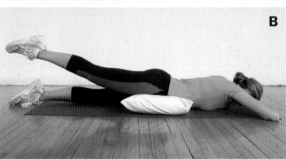

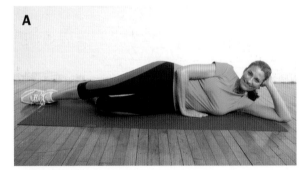

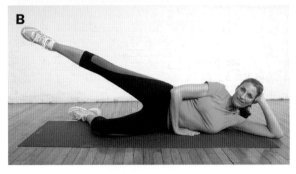

● Hip abduction

Strengthens muscles that support the hip and knee

A. Lie on your side with your bottom leg bent slightly and the top leg straight. Make sure your hips are vertically aligned.

B. Lift your top leg up, then lower slowly. Make sure your knee is locked and your foot is pointing in front of you, not downwards. Do 3 sets of 3 repetitions on each side. Build up to 3 sets of 5, then 7, then 10 repetitions.

Hip adduction •

Strengthens hip and knee muscles

A. Lie on your side with your bottom leg straight and your top leg bent at the knee, the foot in front of the bottom knee.

B. Tighten your abdominal muscles and slowly raise your bottom leg, then lower slowly. Keep your knee locked and your foot bent. Do 3 sets of 3 repetitions on each side. Build up to 3 sets of 5, then 7, then 10 repetitions. If you feel pain in your groin, stop.

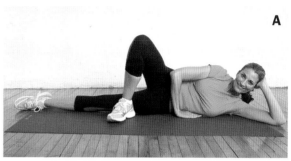

A

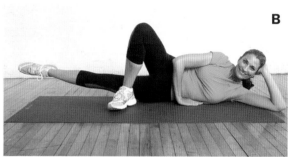

B

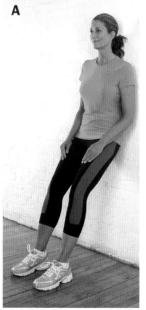

A

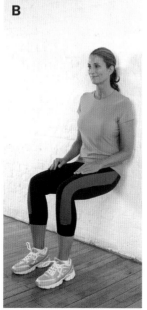

B

• Wall squat

Strengthens supporting muscles (quadriceps and glutes) to alleviate hip and knee pain

A. Stand with your back against a wall, heels about two steps (45 centimetres) from the wall, feet shoulder-width apart.

B. Pulling in your abdominal muscles, slide slowly down the wall until your knees are bent at about 90 degrees, as though you're seated. If that's too difficult, bend your knees to a 45 degree angle and gradually build up from there. Count to 5 and slide slowly back up the wall. Repeat 3 times. Build up to 5, then 7, then 10 repetitions.

● Do exercises with a green dot when your pain is active.
  Do exercises with a red dot when you're feeling better, to keep future flares at bay.
  Remember to start slowly and gradually build up your repertoire and your repetitions.

Neck stretch 1 ●

Increases flexibility

STANDING or sitting, drop your chin towards your chest. Hold for 10 seconds and repeat 2 to 3 times.

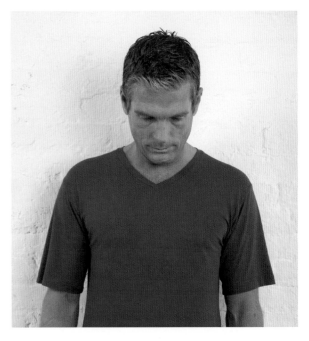

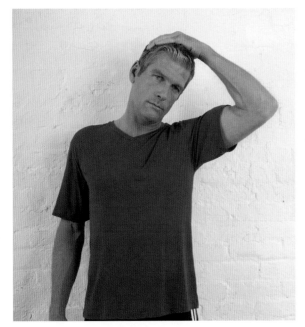

● Neck stretch 2

Increases flexibility, releases muscle tension

BRING your chin slightly towards your chest. Drop your left ear to your left shoulder. Support your head with your left hand but do not pull your head. Hold for 10 seconds. Repeat 2 to 3 times, then switch sides.

For an added stretch, grasp a chair with your right hand and lean your body to the left.

Neck stretch 3 •

Increases flexibility, releases muscle tension

BRING your chin towards your chest. Drop your left ear towards your left shoulder, and look down towards your left side. Support your head with your left hand but don't pull your head. Hold for 10 seconds. Repeat 2 to 3 times, then switch sides.

For an added stretch, grasp a chair with your right hand and lean your body to the left.

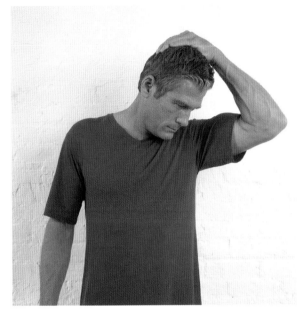

• Neck stretch 4

Strengthens neck muscles and the muscles affected by TMD

LIE on your back with a rolled towel or small pillow under your head, knees bent. Tuck your chin towards your chest and hold for 10 seconds. Relax. Repeat 2 to 3 times.

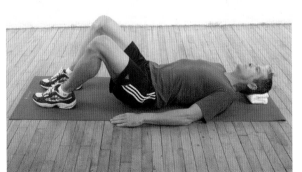

● Do exercises with a green dot when your pain is active.

Do exercises with a red dot when you're feeling better, to keep future flares at bay.

Remember to start slowly and gradually build up your repertoire and your repetitions.

Jaw stabilisation ● ●

For TMD pain

KEEPING your tongue relaxed, grasp your chin and gently apply pressure sideways to the right as you slowly open and close your mouth. Repeat 3 times, then switch to the left side. Build to 5, then 7, then 10 repetitions.

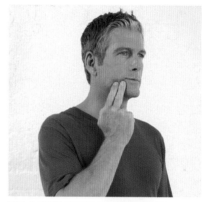

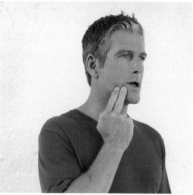

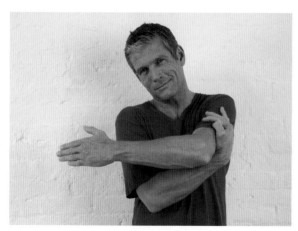

● ● Cross arm stretch

Stretches and increases flexibility in neck muscles and the muscles affected by TMD

STANDING up straight, bring your right arm across your chest, using your left arm to cradle and hug it towards your chest. Lean your head towards your left shoulder. Hold for 30 seconds. Return to start. Repeat 3 times on each side.

Standing pec stretch

Stretches and increases flexibility in neck muscles and the muscles affected by TMD

STANDING beside a wall, place your elbow on the wall at shoulder height, your forearm resting on the wall. Take a step forwards with the leg away from the wall. Lean your body forwards, but do not twist towards the wall. You should feel a gentle stretch in the front of your shoulder and chest. Hold for 30 seconds. Repeat 3 times on each side.

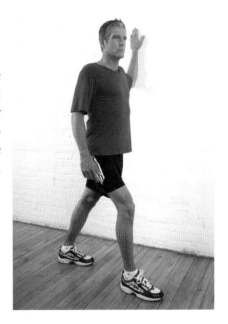

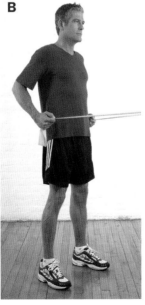

A   B

Scapular retraction

Strengthens shoulder and neck muscles to relieve and prevent general shoulder, neck and TMD pain

A. Anchor the middle of a resistance band (such as a Thera-Band) to a door and, holding an end in each hand, stand facing the door about 60 centimetres away. With your shoulders back, slowly pull the band towards you with your elbows bent at 90 degrees. Focus on squeezing your shoulder blades together.

B. Slowly return to the starting position with your shoulders relaxed. Complete 3 sets of 3 repetitions each. Build up to 3 sets of 5, then 7, then 10 repetitions.

● Do exercises with a green dot when your pain is active.
  Do exercises with a red dot when you're feeling better, to keep future flares at bay.
  Remember to start slowly and gradually build up your repertoire and your repetitions.

Cervical spine isometrics ●

Strengthens neck muscles and those muscles affected by TMD

This series of motions, which should be done together, may be done seated or standing

A. Place one hand on the side of your head. Press the front of your head into your hand and try to push the hand to the side, but don't let your head or hand move. Hold that position for 10 seconds. Do this 3 times, then repeat with the opposite side. Build up to 5, then 7, then 10 repetitions.

B. Place both of your palms on your forehead. Push your head into your hands but don't let it move. Hold for 10 seconds. Do this 3 times, then switch to the back of your head. Build up to 5, then 7, then 10 repetitions.

C. Place one hand on one side of your head and hold it there. Turn your head onto your hand as if you were going to look over your shoulder, but don't let your head move. Hold this position for 10 seconds. Repeat 3 times, then switch sides. Build up to 3 sets of 5, then 7, then 10 repetitions.

See also Corner stretch, External rotation, Internal rotation, Scapular retraction, Shoulder extension, T stretch and Posterior and Anterior shoulder stretches, all of which are preventive exercises for neck pain covered in the following pages.

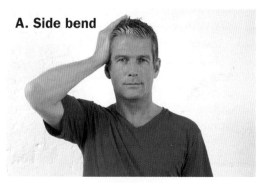

A. Side bend

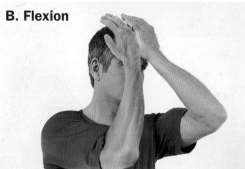

B. Flexion

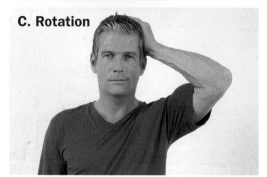

C. Rotation

Pendulum swing

Stretches rotator cuff muscles

STAND straight, then lean forwards slightly from the hips. Keep your painful shoulder and arm relaxed and hanging straight down. Gently and slowly swing the arm back and forth, then in a circle. Continue for 30 to 60 seconds.

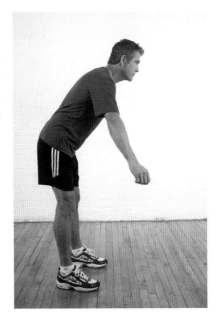

Corner stretch

Stretches and increases flexibility to relieve and prevent neck, shoulder and TMD pain

STAND facing a corner and place both hands on the wall with elbows roughly at shoulder level. Lean forwards until you can feel a gentle stretch across your chest. Hold for 20 seconds, then return to starting position. Repeat 2 times, twice a day.

- Do exercises with a green dot when your pain is active.
- Do exercises with a red dot when you're feeling better, to keep future flares at bay.
   Remember to start slowly and gradually build up your repertoire and your repetitions.

External rotation

Strengthens rotator cuff muscles, relieves and prevents neck, shoulder and TMD pain

A. Tie one end of a resistance band (such as a Thera-Band) around a door handle, or tie a knot in the end of the band and close it in a door so that the knot is on the other side of the door to you. Stand about a metre from the door, with the affected shoulder away from the door. Place a rolled towel between your body and the arm on the affected side. Hold the band in your hand, resting near your stomach. Keep your elbow bent at 90 degrees.
B. Slowly move your hand away from your body, keeping the towel in place. Slowly return to start. Do 3 sets of 3 repetitions. Build up to 5, then 7, then 10 repetitions.

Create more resistance by moving further from the door.

Note that your range of movement may differ from that demonstrated on this page.

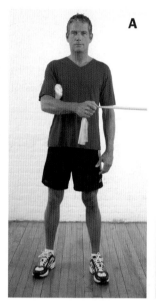
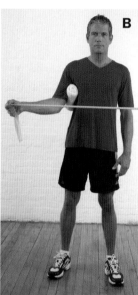

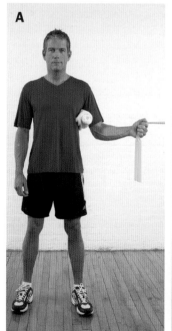
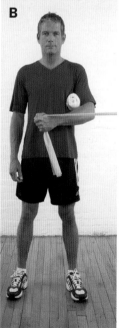

Internal rotation

Strengthens rotator cuff muscles, relieves and prevents neck, shoulder and TMD pain

A. Tie one end of a resistance band around a door handle and stand about 45 centimetres from the door, with the affected shoulder towards the door and that hand holding the band. Place a rolled towel between your body and the arm on the affected side. Hold your forearm in at an angle away from your body, keeping your elbow bent at 90 degrees. (For an easier stretch, start with your arm straight in front of you.)
B. Slowly bring your arm towards your stomach, keeping the towel in place, then return to start position. Complete 3 sets of 3 repetitions. Build up to 3 sets of 5, then 7, then 10 repetitions.

Scapular retraction

Strengthens shoulder and neck muscles to relieve and prevent general shoulder, neck and TMD pain

A. Anchor the middle of a resistance band to a door. Holding an end in each hand, stand facing the door several feet away with your shoulders pulled back.

B. Slowly pull the band towards you by squeezing your shoulder blades together. Slowly return to the starting position. Complete 3 sets of 3 repetitions. Build up to 3 sets of 5, then 7, then 10 repetitions.

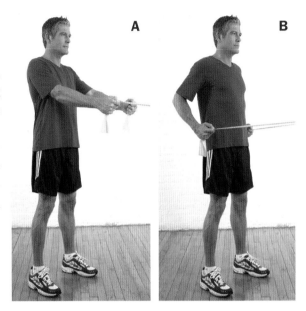

Shoulder extension

Strengthens neck and shoulder to relieve and prevent general neck, shoulder and TMD pain

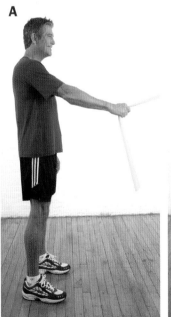
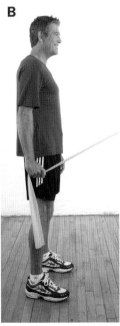

A. Tie a knot in a resistance band and close it in a door near the top of the door so that the knot is on the other side of the door to you. Stand facing the door, several feet away. Hold the band in the hand of the affected shoulder with your arm outstretched in front of you.

B. Slowly pull the band down to your side. Return to the start position with your shoulder relaxed. Complete 3 sets of 3 repetitions. Build up to 3 sets of 5, then 7, then 10 repetitions.

- Do exercises with a green dot when your pain is active.
- Do exercises with a red dot when you're feeling better, to keep future flares at bay.

  Remember to start slowly and gradually build up your repertoire and your repetitions.

The T stretch •

Strengthens upper back to relieve and prevent neck, shoulder and TMD pain

IF you can safely and comfortably get into and out of this position, lie facedown with your arms straight out to your sides at shoulder level. Lift your arms towards the ceiling, squeezing your shoulder blades together. (You can also do this exercise with your thumbs up towards the ceiling or with your elbows bent.) Lower your arms. Do 2 sets of 5 repetitions. Build up to 2 sets of 10 then 15 repetitions.

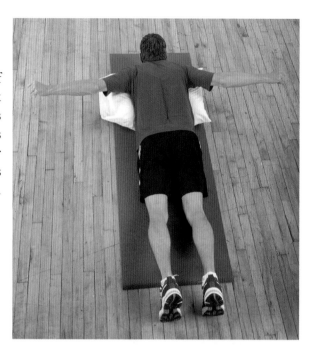

• • Simple posterior shoulder stretch

Stretches and increases flexibility in shoulder muscles

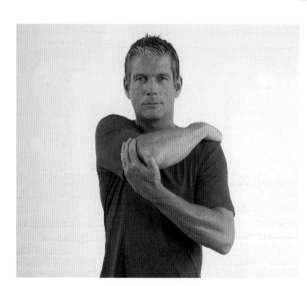

STAND straight with your shoulders relaxed and back. Reach your right arm across your chest and over your shoulder. Grab your right elbow with your left hand. Pull the right elbow in as far as you can, so that your right fingertips reach your shoulder blades. Hold for 5 to 10 seconds. Switch sides. Do 2 sets of 5 repetitions. Build up to 2 sets of 10 then 15 repetitions.

Simple anterior shoulder stretch •

Stretches and increases flexibility

A. Standing, hold about 30 centimetres' worth of towel or resistance band behind your back in both hands at waist level, with your arms straight and the band pulled tight.

B. Stick out your chest and raise the band up and away from your body until you feel a stretch. Do 2 sets of 5 repetitions. Build up to 2 sets of 10 then 15 repetitions.

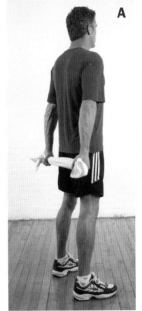
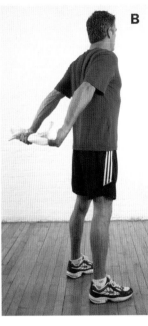

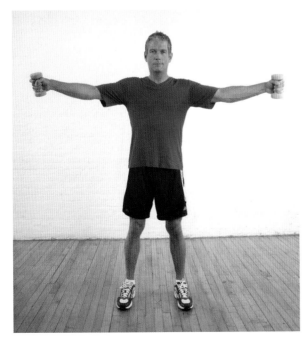

• Shoulder abduction

Strengthens the neck and shoulder muscles

STAND up straight with 250–500-gram hand weights in your hands at your sides. In one controlled motion, lift the weights outwards and upwards until your arms are horizontal at shoulder level, thumbs up. Keep your elbows slightly bent. Do not lift your arms above horizontal. Return to start. Do 5 repetitions. Build up to 10 then 15 repetitions. Gradually increase the weight when it feels easy to do so.

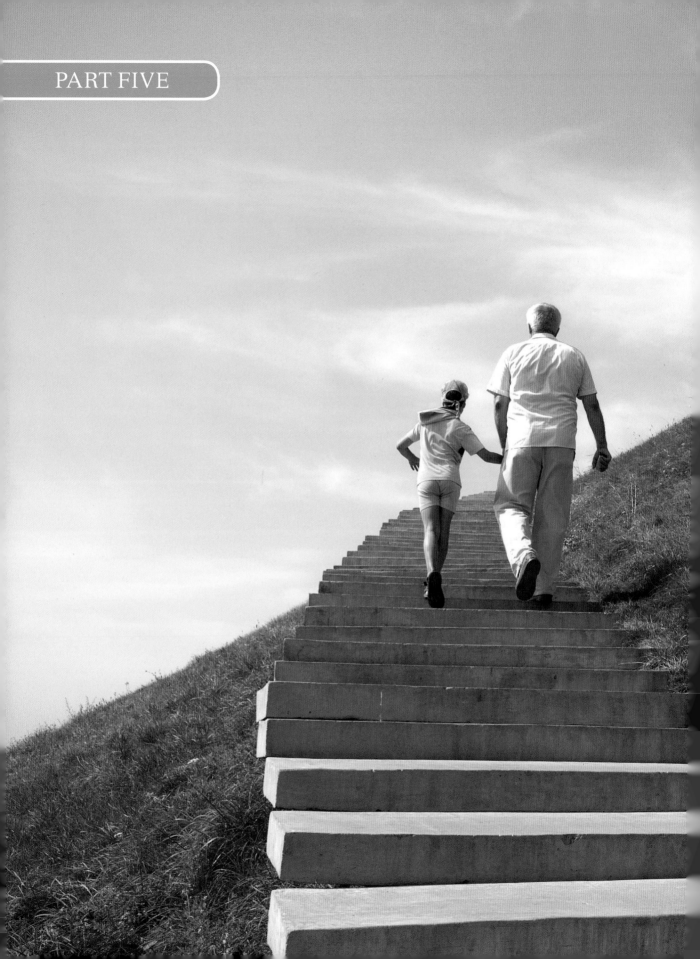

PART FIVE

Useful resources

Help yourself to manage your pain

You are not alone in managing your pain. Help is available from countless sources, including doctors, other health care experts and even family and friends. This section of the book will help you tap into useful resources and keep track of what you and your doctors and therapists—your pain management team—are doing to alleviate your pain. You'll find logs to help you remember how things have gone.

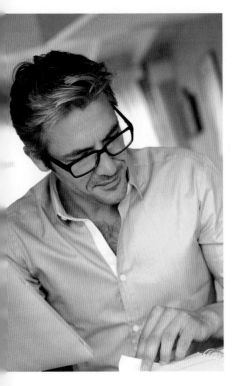

Keeping tabs on your pain, the medications you take, the treatments you undertake and how well they work for you, provides helpful information for your doctor and can even help you deal with the challenge of living with chronic pain. On days when you're discouraged you can flip through your pain diary to remind yourself that there are times when things have gone well. You'll see that even though you've had setbacks, you've got through them.

The following pages suggest ways for you to keep track of your efforts. Use them all or pick and choose, but you'll be glad you tried at least a few. Photocopy the logs you want to use or make copies on your laptop or tablet; adapt them for your use.

Are you ready to start managing your pain? Signing a self-care contract is a way for you to reinforce your resolution to manage your pain, to work with your doctor, to treat yourself like someone who deserves the best care. Photocopy and post the signed contract where you'll see it every day, to remind yourself of your commitment.

My self-care contract

I acknowledge that I need and deserve a good quality of life.
I hereby vow to take steps to manage my _____ pain so that I can:

1) _____

2) _____

3) _____

I expect my doctors and other health care providers to work with me to help manage my pain. I promise to be an active partner and help them help me. With my doctor's help and on my own, I will educate myself about pain management. I will prepare for doctor visits by making a list of questions and writing down details about my pain, including when I experience it and what seems to trigger it. I acknowledge that if my doctor's approach isn't working for me, I will talk to her and see whether there is something we could be doing better as a team.

I know that treating pain often requires more than one approach, often at the same time, and that those approaches include many steps that I can take at home.

I'm willing to take active steps to

Get more, better quality sleep
Get more exercise appropriate for my condition
Limit my pain triggers
Keep a good attitude, even on difficult pain days

I agree to seek the help of other experts besides my doctor to help me accomplish my goal of achieving pain relief, such as a psychologist, a psychotherapist or other therapists.

I acknowledge that pain can affect me emotionally, adding tension and lowering my spirits. I resolve to lower stress by practising deep breathing, visualisation or simply making time to listen to music I love or taking hot baths. If I am depressed, I will tell my pain management team so that they can assist me.

I vow to build a support network for myself. I will alert my family and friends to my pain and explain the important things I do to manage it, and the ways in which I am making shifts in my life. I will ask them to respect and support those changes.

I commit to managing my pain and improving the quality of my life.

Signature _____

Date _____

Pain diary

Keeping track of your pain is one of the most useful strategies for managing it. Knowing when your pain is worst and what seems to trigger it can help you and your pain management team begin to see patterns and devise strategies for helping you manage.   Date_____

Time	Pain intensity from 0 to 10	Pain description (sharp, stabbing, throbbing, etc.)	Activity when pain started	Pain relievers you tried (drug and nondrug)	Comments (mood, other symptoms, sleep quality, etc.)
Midnight					
1 am					
2 am					
3 am					
4 am					
5 am					
6 am					
7 am					
8 am					
9 am					
10 am					
11 am					
Noon					
1 pm					
2 pm					
3 pm					
4 pm					
5 pm					
6 pm					
7 pm					
8 pm					
9 pm					
10 pm					
11 pm					

Pain-trigger log

Understanding what triggers your pain is a key part of managing that pain. This log will help you shine a light on which aspects of your life may be worsening your pain. The possibilities are broad, from your emotions, physical activities and foods to weather conditions. Once you identify your triggers, you can take steps to reduce them or create a plan for dealing with the ones you can't avoid.

Date and time	Pain description	Foods and drinks within last 12 hours	Weather	Emotions (stressed, depressed, anxious, etc.)	Activities (exercise, lifting, climbing, etc.)	Sleep the night before (hours, quality)

Exercise record

Movement helps the body feel better. Your doctor or physiotherapist can help you set specific exercise goals appropriate for you. Most people should aim for at least 30 minutes of physical activity on most days. Keeping a record of your exercise will help you articulate reasonable goals and stick with them. It will also help you to see and appreciate how far you've come from day 1, when walking to the letterbox seemed like a feat.

Exercise log for week of _____

Weekly goals			Goals accomplished				
			Yes No				
Date and time	Type of exercise	Duration/ distance (if applicable)	Pain before exercise (from 0 to 10)	Pain after exercise (from 0 to 10)	Satisfaction level (from 0 to 10)	What can I do differently?	

Medication log

If you are in pain, you are likely to be taking medication. Keeping track of what you're taking, who prescribed them, when you started them and what effect they have, can help you understand what's helping your pain. Tracking medications can also keep you better prepared for every doctor visit.

Medication/ prescribing doctor	Start date/ end date	Dosage per day	Effect on pain	Side effects	Comments

Management log

The best approach to treating pain is one that combines a variety of strategies and therapies. Keeping track of management strategies and how they affect you can help you finetune pain approaches so that you're not putting energy into an intervention that's not effective for you. Remember that interventions are not expected to cure pain, but to allow you to do the things that give you meaning in your life!

Intervention strategy	Intervention date	Response (excellent, good, fair, poor, none so far)	Pain before treatment (from 0 to 10)	Pain after treatment (from 0 to 10)	Comments

Stress diary

Stress and pain are like siblings who live in the same house: one inevitably stirs up the other. Pain itself can be stressful, but many other factors contribute to stress as well: work, family, bills, major events and so on. Stress tightens muscles, speeds breathing, increases heart rate and blood pressure and makes pain worse. Tracking stressors and your body's responses can help you learn to get a handle on them, which translates to better pain control.

Date and time	Stressor	Physical reaction	Emotional reaction	Your solution	My satisfaction with my effort (from 0 to 10)	What can I do differently?

index

abscesses, 143, 145
accrediting agencies, 52
ACE inhibitors, 224, 241
Acetyl-L-carnitine, 242
Achilles tendon, 211, 227, 228
Achilles tendon pain, 67, 212, 213, 214–16, 258, 309
aciclovir, 245
acid backup, 160
acid blockers, 161–2, 175
acitretin, 288
acknowledging pain, 16, 25, 41–2
active lifestyle, 14, 18, 25, 26, 42
active rest, 256
acupuncture, 52, 55
    back pain &, 111
    diabetic retinopathy &, 242
    fibromyalgia &, 130
    introduction to, 56
    neck pain &, 116
    pelvic pain &, 263, 264, 274
acute and chronic pain, 12, 53
adalimumab, 166, 198, 209, 288
adenomyosis, 271
adhesive capsulitis, 119
adrenaline, 79, 90, 94
Advil, 34, 174
aerobic exercise, 36, 60, 61, 62, 63–5, 74, 233, 281 see also water aerobics
alcohol
    face and mouth pain &, 142, 149
    gastrointestinal pain &, 156, 169, 170, 173
    head pain &, 177, 180, 186
    joint pain &, 192, 194, 203
    nerve pain &, 243
    pain trigger, 91, 92, 93, 269
    pelvic pain &, 269
    psoriasis &, 286, 289
    sleep &, 85
Aldactone, 276
aldose reductase inhibitors, 242
alendronate, 236
all-or-nothing thinking, 22
Allegron, 32, 138, 231, 235, 240, 246
allergy medications, 148, 149
allopurinol, 194
aloe vera, 144, 283
alpha-linolenic acid, 242

alternative pain fighters, 32
    see also complementary and alternative medicine
aluminium hydroxide, 161
aminosalicylates, 165
amitriptyline, 85, 109, 138, 142, 152, 184, 231, 235, 240, 246, 268, 280
anaesthetic local, 284
anaesthetic ointment, 280
anaesthetists, 48, 52–3
Anamorph, 35, 202, 231
anchovies, 98, 204, 209
Angelique, 276
anger, 18, 22, 23, 85–6, 90
anger versus depression, 84–5
angina, 161
ankle pain
    arthritis, 220–2
    exercise for, 72, 306–9, 310
antacids, 161, 174, 175
anterior shoulder stretch (exercise), 333
anthocyanins, 98, 257
antibiotics, 145, 148, 154, 155, 166, 174, 190, 191, 284
anticipating pain, 89
anticonvulsants, 33, 35, 137, 138, 142, 179, 184, 236, 241, 246, 249, 280
antidepressants, 14, 16
    back pain &, 109
    body pain &, 33, 123–4, 128–9
    cancer pain &, 137, 138
    depression &, 84, 85
    face and mouth pain &, 142, 152
    gastrointestinal pain &, 160, 170
    introduction to, 31–3
    migraine &, 33, 184
    mystery pain &, 231
    nerve pain &, 31–3, 235–6, 240–2, 244, 245–6, 248–9
    pain killing, 31–3, 84, 85
    pelvic pain &, 33, 262–3, 267–9, 272, 275, 276, 277, 280
antihistamines, 149, 160, 246, 268, 280, 285
anti-inflammatory foods, 98, 99, 100

anti-inflammatories see under name e.g. naproxen
antinausea medications, 183
anti-oxidants, 94, 98, 100, 104, 210, 257
anti-Parkinson's disease drugs, 129
antiproliferative factor, 266
antiviral drugs, 245
anxiety, 13, 27, 42, 45, 49, 53, 140, 142, 169, 186, 230, 232, 233, 275
apples, 98, 103, 146, 158, 176
Arava, 206
arch supports, 218
arm-strengthening exercise, 69, 70, 297, 301
Aropax, 33
arteriosclerosis, 223
Arthrexin, 193
arthritis, 220–2
    aids, 205, 209
    exercise for, 72, 306–9, 310
Arthritis Australia, 203
Arthritis Foundation of South Africa, 127
Arthritis New Zealand, 127
arthritis pain
    diet &, 98, 99
    exercise &, 60, 65, 298, 299, 319
    foot and ankle, 220–2
    knee, 60, 99, 101, 198, 202
    medication for, 28, 30, 34
    shoulder, 119, 120
    stress &, 94
    thoughts &, 86
    triggers for, 89, 93, 94, 97
    see also osteoarthritis; psoriatic arthritis; rheumatoid arthritis
Arthritis Self-management Program, 203
arthrodesis, 222
arthroscopic surgery, 120, 199
artificial discs, 112
artificial skin, 285
asparagus, 98, 105
aspirin, 158, 173, 182, 186, 224, 283
Associated New Zealand ME Society, 123

associations and societies, 48, 123
Atacand, 183
atenolol, 183
atropine, 165
Atrovent spray, 148
attitude adoption, 41–5
attitude of gratitude, 43–5
Australian Health Practitioner Regulation Agency, 48, 52, 54, 55
Australian Medical Association, 122
Australian Pain Management Association, 48
Australian Pain Society, 48
Australian Physiotherapy Association, 48, 54
Australian Psychological Society, 54
autoimmune diseases, 170
autonomic nervous system, 177, 239
avenanthramides, 283
avocados, 98
avoidance, 83
azathioprine, 133, 166, 207

babies and lupus, 131
back pain
    acupuncture for, 111
    anger &, 90
    best first steps for, 108–9
    CBT for, 112
    depression &, 83
    diet &, 98
    doctors &, 53, 109, 112–13
    exercise for, 61, 65, 66, 71, 75, 110–11, 294–301
    heat/ice for, 109, 111
    instant relief for, 111
    learning about, 110
    leg pain &, 108
    lifting &, 19
    massage therapy for, 111
    medication for, 30, 34, 108–9, 110
    obesity &, 101
    physiotherapy for, 110
    recurrence of, 110
    rest &, 108, 111
    spinal manipulation for, 111
    surgery for, 112–13

thoughts &, 86
triggers for, 93
willow bark for, 32
back stretches, 71, 110, 111
baclofen, 268
bad pain/good pain, 74
ball squeeze (exercise), 313
bananas, 67
barbecued vegetables, 105
Barrett's oesophagus, 160
baths
  body pain &, 124, 129, 130, 133
  burns &, 283
  gastrointestinal pain &, 155, 157, 166, 171
  menstrual cramps &, 273
  mystery pain &, 233
  nerve pain &, 241, 246
  psoriasis &, 288
  PVD &, 225
beans, 99, 249
beer, 194
benzodiazepine hypnotics, 35, 142, 232
berries, 98, 159, 257
beta-blockers, 183, 224
beta-carotene, 289
Betaloc, 183
biceps curls, 69
biofeedback, 184, 187, 281
biofeedback therapists, 56, 95
biological response modifiers, 206, 208–9
biologics, 166, 198, 288
birth control pills, 183, 263, 271, 272, 275, 276
bite guards, 152
black tea, 99
blackberries, 159
bladder cancer, 269
bladder distention, 267
bladder instillation, 267–8
bladder training, 269
bleeding
  haemorrhoids &, 157
  IBD &, 164
  NSAIDs &, 30, 31
  ulcers &, 176
blood clotting risk, 31, 32, 34, 224, 225
blood fats, 243, 286
blood glucose, 97, 225, 239, 240, 243
blood thinners, 31, 32, 34, 162, 274
blueberries, 159
body clock, 35, 36, 177
body scan, 87
bok choy, 99
bone fusion, 205, 222
bone realignment, 205
bone spurs, 200, 222, 251
Botox injections, 115, 184

bowel cancer, 157
brain
  chronic fatigue syndrome &, 121, 124
  exercise &, 63, 84
  fibromyalgia &, 129
  laughter &, 79
  mystery pain &, 230, 231
  pain levels &, 13, 20, 29, 77, 81, 89, 230, 231, 243
  relaxation &, 81
  specialists in, 48, 53
brain chemicals, 63, 78, 79, 84, 85, 95, 124, 129, 169, 177, 185, 186
bran, 274
'breakthrough' pain, 136, 137
breast cancer, 61
breathing and breathing techniques, 70, 75, 82, 83
  see also deep breathing
breathing tubes, 285
Bridges & Pathways Institute Incorporated, 123
broccoli, 98, 104, 175, 195
bromelain, 32, 99, 195
brown rice, 98, 104, 194, 274
Brufen, 34
brussels sprouts, 175
bunionectomy, 219
bunions, 217–19
buprenorphine, 35, 202, 231, 241
burning mouth syndrome, 140–2
burns, 282–5
bursectomy, 191
bursitis, 34, 97, 118, 188–91, 196
Buscopan, 170
butorphanol, 29
butyrate, 167
bypass surgery, 226

cabbage, 98, 104, 175
Cafergot, 183
caffeine, 30, 36, 85, 91, 130, 134, 170, 184, 269, 277
calcipotriene, 287
calcitonin, 236
calcium, 274, 276, 277
calcium channel blockers, 179
calf raises (exercise), 307, 310
calf stretches (exercise), 72, 306, 310
cancer pain, 86
  best first steps, 135–6
  'breakthrough', 136, 137
  chemotherapy &, 139
  constipation &, 136
  doctors &, 53, 135, 136–8
  exercise &, 66, 139
  instant relief for, 138
  introduction to, 135
  medications for, 135–8

progressive muscle relaxation &, 138
  radiotherapy for, 139
  surgery for, 139
  visualisation &, 138
  wellness and supportive care &, 138–9
  see also under name e.g. bladder cancer
candersartan, 183
canola oil, 98, 195, 204, 209, 226, 242
capsaicin cream, 32, 128, 189, 198, 201, 210, 221, 242, 246, 249
capsicums, 195
Carafate, 175
caraway seeds, 171
carbamazepine, 138, 249
carbohydrates, 97, 256, 274
carbon monoxide poisoning, 284
cardamom seeds, 171
cardiovascular drugs, 183
carotenoids, 99
carpal tunnel syndrome, 97, 99
  best first steps, 252
  doctors &, 53, 252
  ergonomics &, 253
  exercise for, 302–3
  introduction to, 251
  medications for, 252
  splints for, 253
  surgery for, 252, 253
carrots, 102, 104, 146, 289
cartilage, 196, 199, 200, 220, 222
castor oil heat pack, 264
catastrophising, 21–2
cauliflower, 98, 175
causalgia see complex regional pain syndrome
celery, 102, 146
CellCept, 133
central nervous system, 12, 33, 53, 128
cereal grains, 91
  see also whole grains
cervical spine fusion, 117
cervical spine isometrics (exercise), 328
Cetaphil, 287
chair stretches, 111
chamomile, 171, 284
chard, 99
chemical burns, 282, 284
chemotherapy, 133, 139
cherries, 98, 159, 191, 195, 257
chewing gum, 91, 93, 141, 146, 162
chickenpox, 244
children
  burns &, 284
  lupus &, 131
  sinusitis &, 145

chilli, 91, 94, 100
Chinese medicine, 52, 55, 56, 187, 289
chiropractors, 55, 111, 115
chlorpheniramine, 268
cholesterol, 224, 243, 286
chondroitin, 204
chronic fatigue syndrome, 93, 121–5
Chronic Pain Australia, 48
chronic pain defined, 8, 12
cilostazol, 225
cimetidine, 175
cinnamon, 94
circulation, 71
clamshell (exercise), 296, 317
clonazepam, 138, 142
clopidogrel, 162, 224
cluster headaches, 177–80
Cochrane Collaboration database, 55
codeine, 35, 129, 182, 183, 231–2
coeliac disease, 170
coffee, 36, 93, 156, 163, 184, 186, 194
cognitive behavioural therapy, 14, 37, 48, 54, 90, 170
  back pain &, 112
  chronic fatigue syndrome &, 124
  fibromyalgia &, 130
  introduction to, 85, 86–7
  PMS &, 278
  tension headaches &, 187
  TMD &, 153
cognitive restructuring, 87
colchicine, 193, 194
cold packs see ice and cold treatments
colds and sore throats, 30, 34
collagen, 210
Colofac, 170
colon cancer, 170
colonoscopy, 158
comfort foods, 97
communication skills, 17
complementary and alternative medicine (CAM), 55–6, 124
complex regional pain syndrome, 234–8
concentration problems, 122
consistency, 17
constipation
  cancer pain &, 136
  diverticulitis &, 154, 155, 156
  haemorrhoids &, 157
  IBS &, 169, 171, 172
contour pillows, 117
coping plans, 129
coping skills, 33, 85–7
core body temperature, 36
core strength exercises, 70, 75
coriander seeds, 171

corner stretch (exercise), 329
corticosteroids
    gastrointestinal pain &, 165, 174
    joint pain &, 190, 197, 202, 208, 212
    lupus &, 132, 133, 134
    nerve pain &, 245
    overuse injuries &, 252, 255
    plantar fasciitis &, 228
    psoriasis &, 287
    sinusitis &, 148
cortisol, 79, 94, 121, 285
cortisone, 218, 222
Coumadin, 34
counselling, 27, 49, 51, 170
cramps, 100
    exercise for, 67
    IBD &, 164, 165, 167
    IBS &, 169, 171, 172
    menstrual, 30, 34, 67, 93, 171, 271–4
    PVD &, 223
cranberry juice, 98
cravings, food, 103–4
Crohn's disease, 164, 166, 167, 168
cross arm stretch (exercise), 326
curcumin, 100
curry powder/pastes, 100
cycling, 36, 65, 129, 203, 209
cyclosporin, 288
Cymbalta, 32, 109, 123, 128–9, 231, 235, 240, 268
Cystistat, 268
cystitis see interstitial cystitis
cytoprotective agents, 175
Cytotec, 175

dairy products, 91, 93, 99, 167, 169, 194, 212, 249, 264, 274
dandelion tea, 277
decompression surgery, 252, 253
deep breathing, 81, 237
    fibromyalgia &, 128, 130
    gastrointestinal pain &, 166, 171
    introduction to, 70, 83
    pelvic pain &, 264, 270
    shoulder pain &, 120
    TMD &, 151, 153
degenerative disc disease, 110
dehydration, 67, 91, 93, 105, 187, 284
dental abscesses, 143, 145
dental hygiene, 145
dental pain
    best first steps, 143–4
    causes of, 143
    diet &, 144, 145–6
    instant relief for, 144
    introduction to, 143
    medications for, 30, 34, 144, 145

prevention of, 144–6
referred sources of, 143
treatment for, 144–5, 146
triggers for, 89, 93
dental products, 145
dentists, 141, 143, 144–5, 146, 152, 153
depression
    anger and stress &, 84–5
    CRPS &, 237
    exercise &, 63, 84
    fibromyalgia &, 33, 83
    involvement &, 84
    mind and body solution for, 16, 83–5, 86
    music &, 86
    mystery pain &, 232, 233
    pelvic pain &, 276, 277, 279
    persistent pain &, 13, 14, 16
    rheumatoid arthritis &, 33
    sleep &, 84, 85, 231
    speaking up about, 16, 83–4
    specialist help for, 53, 85
    tension headaches &, 186
    treating pain &, 85
    see also antidepressants
desvenlafaxine, 32
devil's claw, 204
dexamethasone, 137
diabetes, 31, 32, 33, 192, 225, 286
diabetic neuropathy, 239–43
diabetic peripheral neuropathy, 53
diaphragmatic breathing, 70
diaries, 42
diarrhoea and gastric pain, 155, 157, 164, 165, 169, 172
diazepam, 109
diclofenac, 201
diet
    adding foods to, 97–9, 104–5
    body pain &, 125
    burns &, 285
    cramps &, 67
    cravings &, 103–4
    dental problems &, 144, 145–6
    gastrointestinal pain &, 154, 155, 156, 157, 158–9, 161, 163, 167–8, 169, 170, 172, 175–6
    joint pain &, 98, 99, 192, 194, 195, 203, 204, 209, 210
    migraines &, 98, 185
    mindfulness &, 102–3
    muscle and tendon soreness &, 256
    neck pain &, 98, 117
    nerve pain &, 19, 242, 248, 249
    pain-proofing, 97–105
    pain relief &, 19, 29
    pain triggers, 93

pelvic pain &, 264, 267, 269, 274, 278
psoriasis &, 289
PVD &, 226
soothing spices in, 100
vegan, 19
see also fruit; vegetables; water consumption
diet foods and drinks, 91
dihydroergotamine, 183
Dilaudid, 35, 202, 231, 241
diphenoxylate, 165
disc pain, 108, 112
discectomy, 112
discoid lupus erythematosus, 131
distraction, 13, 42, 45, 78, 79, 86, 138
diuretics, 275, 276
diverticulitis, 97, 154–6
DMARDs, 133, 198, 206, 207–8
DMSO, 236, 267
doctors
    CAM &, 55
    communication with, 48, 50
    discussing other therapists with, 51
    exercise plans &, 60
    favourite pain remedies of, 19
    finding the right, 48–9
    mystery pain &, 231–2
    partnership with, 50
    planning your visit to, 16–17
    reassurance from, 25
    red flags &, 51
    reporting of, 52
    second opinions &, 47
    sharing information with, 27
    see also specialists
dopamine, 63, 124, 129
dorsiflexion (exercise), 308
Dove soap, 287
Dovonex, 287
drospirenone, 276
drug-induced lupus, 131
drug interactions, 34, 52, 162, 174
drugs see medications
dry needling, 115, 260
duloxetine, 32, 109, 123, 128–9, 231, 235, 240, 268
duodenal ulcers, 173
Durogesic, 35, 109, 136, 202, 231, 235, 241
Dyhydergot, 183

eating habit pain triggers, 91
eating, mindful, 102–3
Effexor, 32, 85, 231, 235
eggplant, 105
elbow pain exercises, 304–5
electrical burns, 282, 284
Elmiron, 268
emergencies, 13, 283

emotions, 13, 17, 22, 23
    see also mind–body solutions; thinking patterns
Enbrel, 198, 209, 288
Endep, 32, 33, 85, 109, 138, 142, 152, 184, 231, 235, 240, 246, 268
endodontists, 146
endometriosis, 261–5, 266, 271
Endone, 35, 202, 231, 235
endorphins, 13, 63, 64, 78, 79, 84, 95, 185, 186, 233, 273, 281
endoscopy, 174, 176
energy diary, 125
energy levels, 81
environmental change pain trigger, 92
Epilim, 184
Epsom salts baths, 63, 159, 288
ergonomics, 116, 191, 213, 253
ergotamine medications, 183
essential oils, 198
etanercept, 198, 209, 288
eucalyptus oil, 147, 201, 221
Eucerin, 287
evening primrose oil, 263, 273
eversion (exercise), 309
exercise
    back pain &, 61, 65, 66, 75, 110, 111, 294–301
    bad days &, 61
    cancer pain &, 66, 139
    carpal tunnel syndrome &, 302–3
    chronic fatigue syndrome &, 124, 125
    cooling down after, 66–7
    cue up your, 75
    depression &, 63, 84
    doctors &, 60
    easing your pain with, 292–3
    elbow pain &, 304–5
    energy &, 59, 60, 62
    fears about, 62
    fibromyalgia &, 60, 61, 126, 128, 129, 130
    flexibility &, 59, 65, 71–2, 75
    foot, ankle and leg pain &, 216, 220, 225–6, 228, 229, 306–11
    gastrointestinal pain &, 156, 157, 159, 167, 171
    hand osteoarthritis &, 312–15
    head pain &, 67, 185, 187
    heart rate &, 62–3
    hip and knee pain &, 316–23
    joint pain &, 60, 65, 66, 75, 191, 198, 199, 203, 208, 209, 211, 212, 213, 298, 299, 319
    lupus &, 134

medical conditions
    benefitting from, 60, 61, 66–7, 71–2
    motivation to, 72–5
    muscle aches &, 61, 63
    muscle working &, 65, 68
    neck pain &, 115, 116, 117, 324–8
    nerve pain &, 243, 248
    overuse injuries &, 253, 256, 257, 260
    pain-free hints and tips, 66–7
    pain management &, 17, 19, 26
    pain triggers &, 91, 93
    pelvic pain &, 273, 281
    physiotherapists &, 54
    posture &, 69, 71
    rehabilitation program, 74
    shoulder pain &, 67, 71, 115, 118, 119, 120, 329–33
    sinusitis &, 148
    sleep &, 36, 59, 62, 84, 90
    starting, 68
    strengthening, 54, 59, 60, 61, 62, 63, 65, 68–70, 75, 115, 191, 213, 257
    stress relief, 62–3, 75, 95
    stretching, 59, 61, 63, 66, 67, 69, 70–2, 75, 110, 111, 128, 130, 152–3, 191, 198, 212, 213, 216, 228, 229, 253, 257, 260
    TMD &, 152–3, 324–8
    variety &, 73
    warming up before, 66–7, 68, 211, 229
    weight loss &, 59, 63
    where and how of, 74
    see also aerobic exercise; cycling; Pilates; swimming; tai chi; walking; yoga
exercise baseline, 68
exercise record, 340
exercise tracking, 72
exercises for pain relief, 291–333
expectations, 50, 82
expressed anger, 90
exterior forearm stretch (exercise), 304
external rotation (exercise), 330

face and mouth pain see burning mouth syndrome; dental pain; sinusitis; temporomandibular disorder
facet joint denervation, 117
Faculty of Pain Medicine (ANZCA), 48, 53
famciclovir, 245
family, 41, 125, 233
fantasising, 45

fast food, 93
fat (body), 100
fat (dietary), 91, 93–4, 97, 101, 103, 104, 134, 163, 167, 170, 264
fatigue see chronic fatigue syndrome
fatigue pain trigger, 93
fears, 16, 27, 49, 62, 137
Fellow of the Faculty of Pain Medicine (ANZCA), 53
fennel, 91, 171
fentanyl, 35, 136, 137, 202, 231, 235, 241
fibre (dietary), 98, 134, 136
    gastric pain &, 156, 157, 158, 163, 167, 176
    pelvic pain &, 274, 278
fibre supplements, 158, 165, 167
'fibrofog', 126
fibroids, 271, 272
fibromyalgia, 123, 266
    acupuncture &, 130
    best first steps, 127
    capsaicin &, 129
    CBT for, 130
    coping plan &, 129
    deep breathing &, 128, 130
    depression &, 83
    diagnosis of, 127
    doctors &, 127, 128–9
    educating yourself about, 127
    exercise &, 60, 61, 126, 129, 130
    flare-ups of, 127
    instant relief for, 128
    introduction to, 126
    medications for, 32–3, 127, 128–9
    pain triggers for, 93, 94, 97
    sleep disturbances &, 33, 126, 130
    stress &, 94, 126, 130
    warm baths for, 128, 130
    yoga for, 130
fight-or-flight response, 90
finger bends (exercise), 312
finger extension (exercise), 314
finger walk (exercise), 314
fingertip touch (exercise), 315
first-degree burns, 282, 283
fish and seafood, 91, 93, 97, 98, 99, 134, 194, 204, 209, 226, 249, 264, 274, 285, 289
fish oil, 32, 264, 274
fist (exercise), 312
flavonoids, 99, 159
flaxseed oil, 98
flexibility, 59, 65, 71–2, 75
fluid consumption see water consumption
fluoxetine, 33, 184, 276, 278
fluvoxamine, 33
focal neuropathy, 239

focus, 43, 44–5, 50, 81
food
    all-you-can eat, 102
    cravings for, 103–4
    early dinners, 163
    mindful eating of, 102–3
    pain-fighting shopping list, 97–9
    pain perception &, 103
    pain trigger, 91, 92–4, 97
    savouring of, 102
    soothing spices, 100
    spicy, 91
    see also diet; junk food; snacks
food additives, 91, 94
food allergies, 170, 269
food diary, 163
food elimination, 92–3
food intolerances, 125, 170, 269
food portions, 94, 101–2, 162, 175, 202, 278
foot cramps, 67
foot pain
    arthritis, 220–2
    bunions, 217–19
    exercise for, 67, 72, 306–9, 310
    plantar fasciitis, 227–9
foot pain triggers, 93
foot soaks, 187, 221
foot splints, 228
footwear, 199, 215, 216, 217–18, 219, 221, 222, 226, 227, 228, 229
forearm stretches (exercise), 303, 304
Fosamax, 236
friends, 41, 125, 233
fruit, 91
    body pain &, 125, 134
    face and mouth pain &, 145, 146
    gastrointestinal pain &, 156, 158, 159, 163, 167, 176
    joint pain &, 194, 195, 209, 210
    pain-fighting shopping list for, 98, 99
    pelvic pain &, 264, 278
    PVD &, 226
    weight loss &, 94, 101, 185

GABA see gamma-aminobutyric acid
gabapentin, 33, 123, 138, 142, 184, 236, 241, 246, 249
gabapentinoids, 33, 241, 246, 249
gamma-aminobutyric acid, 232
gamma-knife radiosurgery, 250
gamma-linoleic acid, 273
gangrene, 223, 243
Gantin, 33
gardening, 60
garlic, 94, 99, 100

gastrointestinal pain, 93, 100
    see also diverticulitis; haemorrhoids; heartburn and GORD; inflammatory bowel disease; irritable bowel syndrome
gastrointestinal ulcers, 173–6
Gastrostop, 165
Gaviscon, 161
general practitioners, 15, 16–18, 47
    see also doctors
genes, 42
ginger, 32, 91, 100, 210
ginger essential oil, 198
ginger tea, 277
gingivitis, 144–5
GKR see gamma-knife radiosurgery
glucosamine, 204
glutamine, 175
glutathione, 98
glycine, 171
GnRH drugs, 263
goal setting, 17, 26, 72
golfer's elbow, 258
good pain/bad pain, 74
GORD see heartburn and GORD
gout
    best first steps, 192–3
    co-conditions &, 188, 190, 196, 200, 201
    diet &, 92, 192, 194, 195
    doctors &, 193
    instant relief for, 193
    introduction to, 192
    medications for, 34, 192, 193, 194
    triggers for, 91, 92, 93
    weight loss &, 194–5
graded motor imagery, 235, 237
grapefruit, 98
grapes, 99, 257
gratitude, attitude of, 43–5
gratitude journal, 43–4
great toe arthritis, 220, 222
green tea, 99, 103, 277
guaifenesin, 149
guided imagery, 81–2
guilt, 85
gum disease, 143, 144–5, 146
gyms, 74
gynaecologists, 262, 279–80

H2-receptor blockers, 161–2, 175
haemorrhoidectomy, 159
haemorrhoids, 93, 157–9
halibut, 226
hamstring stretches (exercise), 72, 319
hand osteoarthritis, 202, 312–15

hatha yoga, 75, 130
hazelnuts, 99
headaches
    anger &, 90
    chronic fatigue syndrome &, 122
    cluster, 177–80
    depression &, 83
    exercise &, 67, 185, 187
    fibromyalgia &, 126
    medications for, 30, 33, 34, 178–9, 182–4, 186
    migraine, 28, 33, 61, 81, 91, 92, 94, 100, 181–5
    neurologists &, 53
    rebound, 30, 182, 183
    tension, 186–7
    triggers for, 94
health professionals
    CAM, 55–6
    combination approaches &, 51–2
    describing pain to, 50–1
    evaluation of, 57
    finding the right, 48–9
    red flags, 51
    reporting of, 52
    rundown on, 52–4
    second opinions &, 47
    teamwork &, 15–16, 336
    working with, 15, 17, 50
    see also dentists; doctors; general practitioners; physiotherapists; psychologists; specialists
Health Services Commissioner, 52
heart problems, 31, 143, 223, 286
heart rate, 62–5, 68, 81, 90, 94
heartburn and GORD, 91, 92, 93, 160–3
heat treatment
    back pain &, 111
    cancer pain &, 138
    diverticulitis &, 155
    fibromyalgia &, 127, 129
    joint pain &, 189, 201, 207, 208, 212
    muscle and tendon soreness &, 257
    mystery pain &, 232
    neck pain &, 114, 116
    pelvic pain &, 264, 270, 273
    plantar fasciitis &, 228
    sinusitis &, 148
    tension headaches &, 187
    TMD &, 151
heel raises, 216
heel slides (exercise), 300
heel stretches, 66
heel taps (exercise), 296
Helicobacter pylori, 173, 174, 175, 176

help
    acceptance of, 41–2
    CAM practitioner, 55–6
    getting the right, 47–57
    health professional, 47, 48–54, 57, 336
    see also self-education
heparin, 267
herbal teas, 105, 277, 284
herpes zoster, 244, 246
herring, 289
hiatal hernia, 160
high blood pressure, 31, 90, 93, 94, 286
hip and knee pain exercises, 72, 298, 316–23
histamine, 177
HMG-CoA reductase inhibitors, 242
holistic approach, 37
hormone treatments, 263
hormones, 140
    see also sex hormones; stress hormones
horseradish, 148
hospitals, 48, 52
humidifiers, 147
Humira, 166, 198, 209, 288
humour, 13, 78–80, 95
hunger, 103
Hunner's ulcers, 266
hyaluronic acid, 198, 202, 268
hydralazine, 131
hydrocodone, 183
hydromorphone, 35, 129, 136, 137, 202, 231, 241
hydrotherapy, 199
hydroxychloroquine, 133, 207
hypnosis, 25, 95, 130, 167, 169, 170
hypothalamus, 121, 177
hysterectomy, 265

ibuprofen, 29, 30, 34
    burns &, 283
    back, neck and shoulder pain &, 108, 114, 119
    body pain &, 123, 127, 132
    cancer pain &, 137
    face and mouth pain &, 144, 147, 151
    gastrointestinal pain &, 155, 158, 173
    head pain &, 182, 186
    joint pain &, 189, 192, 197, 198, 203, 207, 208, 212
    leg and foot pain &, 215, 218, 221, 228
    nerve pain &, 245, 248
    overuse injuries &, 252, 256, 259
    pelvic pain &, 262, 267, 272, 276, 277
ice and cold treatments

    back pain &, 109
    burning mouth syndrome &, 141
    cancer pain &, 138
    haemorrhoids &, 157, 159
    head pain &, 179, 184, 187
    joint pain &, 188, 193, 196, 201, 207, 208, 212
    leg and foot pain &, 215, 219, 228
    muscle pain &, 63
    neck pain &, 114
    overuse injuries &, 255, 258
    post exercise &, 66, 67
    shoulder pain &, 119
    soft tissue release exercise &, 311
    vulvodynia &, 281
idiopathic pain, 230
ileoanal anastomosis, 168
Imigran, 177, 179, 183
imipramine, 231
immune system, 78, 81, 93, 100, 121, 131, 206, 207, 244–5, 286, 288 see also lupus
immune-system suppressors, 166
Imodium, 165, 167
Imovane, 35, 232
Imrest, 35, 232
Imuran, 133, 166
independence, 42
Inderal, 183
Indocid, 193
indigo ointment, 289
indomethacin, 193
inflammatory bowel disease, 164–8
infliximab, 166, 209, 286, 288
information see self-education
infrared coagulation, 158
inner vacations, 86
insulin, 256
insulin growth factor, 130
interactive imagery, 79, 82
interior forearm stretch (exercise), 303, 304
intermittent claudication, 223
internal rotation (exercise), 330
Internet, 48, 49, 52, 55
interstitial cystitis, 266–70
intrathecal drug pump, 238
intravenous fluids, 285
inversion (exercise), 309
ipratropium spray, 148
irritable bowel syndrome, 91, 92, 97, 98, 169–72, 266
Isocover, 162
IUCDs, 263, 271
iyengar yoga, 75

jaw stabilisation (exercise), 326
joint pain
    anticipation &, 89

dehydration &, 105
depression &, 83
diet &, 98, 99, 192, 194, 195, 203, 204, 209, 210
exercise &, 65, 66, 75, 191, 198, 199, 203, 208, 209, 211, 212, 213, 298, 299, 319
psoriasis &, 286
see also bursitis; gout; knee pain; osteoarthritis; rheumatoid arthritis; tendon pain
joint replacement, 199, 204, 210, 222
juniper tea, 277
junk food, 93–4, 97
Jurnista, 35, 109, 136, 202, 231

kale, 99, 175
Kapanol, 35, 109, 136, 202, 231, 235, 241
kappa-opioids, 29
kefir, 176
kidney damage, 31
knee pain
    arthritis &, 60, 99, 101, 198, 202
    best first steps, 196–7
    causes of, 196
    compression and support for, 198
    doctors &, 197–8, 199
    exercise &, 60, 65, 66, 69, 198, 199, 299, 316–18, 319–21
    instant relief for, 198
    introduction to, 196
    medications for, 197–8, 202
    physiotherapy for, 197, 199
    surgery for, 199
knee replacement, 199, 204, 205

lactic acid, 254
lactose, 93, 167, 170
laparoscopic surgery, 168, 265
laparotomy, 265
laughter, 13, 78–80, 81, 95
laughter club, 78, 79
lavender baths, 133
lavender oil, 273
lavender-oil massage, 187
laxatives, 136, 167
Ledertrexate, 133
leflunomide, 206, 207
left-sided colitis, 164
leg pain
    Achilles tendinopathy &, 214–16
    back pain associated with, 108, 113
    diabetic neuropathy &, 239, 243
    exercise &, 67, 69, 72, 297, 301, 310–11, 321
    PVD &, 223–6

leg pain triggers, 93
lemons, 146, 283
lentils, 99
leukotrienes, 271
lidoderm, 241, 245–6
lifestyle, 14, 18, 25, 26, 42
lifting and carrying, 19, 92, 93, 116, 118, 205
light therapy, 287
lighting pain trigger, 92, 93
lignocaine, 236, 245–6, 280
limit setting, 17, 43
linolenic acid, 263, 273
linseeds, 98, 204, 209, 226, 242, 264
Lioresal, 268
lip press, 273
lipid-lowering drugs, 241–2
lisinopril, 183
lithium, 34, 179
liver damage, 30, 127, 203
Lofenoxal, 165
lollies, 103, 167
Lomotil, 165
loperamide, 165, 167
Losec, 162, 175
loss, sense of, 23
Lovan, 33
low-fat dairy products, 91
low-level laser therapy, 212
lupus, 131–4
lupus pain triggers, 93
Luvox, 33
Lyrica, 33, 123, 128, 138, 142, 236, 241, 246, 249

mackerel, 289
Magicul, 175
magnesium, 98, 180, 249
magnesium hydroxide, 161
magnifying problems, 24
malaria medication, 93, 133
Malaysian Association for the Study of Pain, 48
management log, 341
mannitol, 170
massage therapy, 52, 55, 95
    back pain &, 111
    burns &, 285
    knee pain &, 198
    muscle and tendon soreness &, 63, 255, 256
    neck pain &, 116
    pelvic pain &, 264, 273, 278, 281
    tension headaches &, 187
massaging showerheads, 208
mattresses, 90, 124, 130
Maxalt, 183
Maxolon, 183
meal size, 91, 94, 101–2
    see also food portions
meat, 91, 92, 93, 94, 101, 145, 167, 192, 194, 264, 274, 278

ME/CFS Australia (Victoria), 123
medication log, 341
medications, 33
    back pain, 30, 34, 108–9, 110
    blood pressure, 93, 224, 241
    burn, 283, 284, 285
    burning mouth syndrome, 140, 141
    cancer pain, 135–8
    cardiovascular, 183
    chronic fatigue syndrome, 123–4
    common pain reliever, 29–30
    conditions caused by, 30, 32, 34, 36, 93, 129, 131, 141, 173, 201, 235
    dental pain, 30, 34, 144, 145
    diverticulitis, 154, 155
    fever reducing, 34
    fibromyalgia, 32–3, 127, 128–9
    gender specific, 29
    habit forming, 16, 35, 37, 183, 202, 232, 235
    haemorrhoids, 158
    head pain, 30, 33, 34, 178–9, 182–4, 186
    heartburn, 160, 161–2
    IBD, 165–6
    IBS, 170
    joint pain, 34, 189, 192, 193–4, 197–8, 201–2, 203, 206, 207–9, 212, 221, 222, 236
    leg and foot pain, 215, 218, 221, 224–5, 228
    lupus, 132–3
    malaria, 93, 133
    mystery pain, 231–2
    neck pain, 30, 114, 115
    nerve pain, 235–6, 240–2, 244, 245–6, 248–9
    NSAID dangers, 30–1
    overuse injury, 251, 252, 255, 256, 259
    pelvic pain, 262–3, 267–9, 272, 275, 276, 277, 280
    psoriasis, 287, 288
    safety of, 28, 29, 30–1
    shoulder pain, 34, 119
    side effects of, 28, 30–1, 32, 34, 37, 93, 132, 133, 134, 136, 138, 160, 182, 193, 201, 202, 203, 208, 231, 235, 263, 288
    sinusitis, 147, 148, 149
    sleep, 35, 123, 232
    taking appropriate, 17
    TMD, 151, 152
    ulcer, 174–5
    see also chemotherapy; codeine; opioids
meditation, 14, 27, 78, 81, 82, 185, 235, 237, 248, 270, 278

memory loss, 122, 126, 131
men
    cluster headaches &, 177
    gout &, 192
    osteoarthritis &, 99
    pain medications &, 29
    pain tolerance &, 29
    soy protein &, 99
meningitis, 147
meniscus, 196
menopause, 263, 265
menstrual cramps
    acupuncture for, 274
    best first steps, 272
    calcium &, 274
    diet &, 274
    doctors &, 272
    evening primrose oil for, 273
    exercise &, 67, 273
    IBS &, 171
    instant relief for, 273
    introduction to, 271
    medications for, 30, 34, 272
    triggers for, 93
    vitamin E for, 274
menstrual cycle, 29
mental energy, 18
mental filters, 23
menthol, 100
Metamucil, 158, 165
methadone, 136, 137
Methoblastin, 133
methotrexate, 133, 198, 206, 207, 288
methylphenidate, 124
metoclopramide, 183
metoprolol, 183
Miacalcin, 236
microvascular decompression, 250
midfoot arthritis, 220, 222
migraine diary, 182
migraines
    auras &, 181, 182
    best first steps, 181–2
    biofeedback &, 184
    butterbur for, 185
    diet &, 98, 185
    doctors &, 182–4
    exercise &, 61, 185
    instant relief for, 184
    introduction to, 181
    medication for, 28, 33, 182–4
    obesity &, 100, 185
    prevention of, 182, 183–4
    treatment plans for, 182
    triggers to, 89, 91, 92, 94, 181
milnaciprin, 123
mind–body solutions
    dealing with depression, 83–5
    endorphins &, 78, 79
    humour &, 78–80, 81
    introduction to, 77–8

learning to cope, 85–7
    relaxation &, 80–2
mind control, 45
mindful eating, 102–3
mindfulness, 82, 130, 237
minerals, 104
mint, 100
misoprostol, 175
moment-to-moment nonjudgmental awareness, 82
mood
    depression &, 83, 84
    exercise &, 19, 26, 63, 84, 129
    fibromyalgia &, 129
    lupus &, 131, 133, 134
    stress &, 83, 95
    thinking patterns &, 23
MooGoo, 287
morphine, 29, 35, 37, 129, 136, 202, 231, 232, 235, 241, 284
morphine myths, 137
motivation to exercise, 72–5
mouthguards, 152
MS Contin, 35, 136, 202, 231, 235, 241
mulberries, 99
Murelax, 35
muscle aches and pains, 30, 34, 56
muscle and tendon soreness, 83
    best first steps, 254–5
    diet &, 256
    exercise &, 61, 257
    instant relief for, 257
    introduction to, 254
    massage for, 63, 255, 256
    medications for, 255, 256, 257
    rest for, 254, 256
    RICE for, 254–5
    yoga &, 256
muscle relaxant medications, 109, 268
muscle strains, 32
muscle strengthening, 65, 68, 70–1, 75
muscle tightness, 70
mushrooms, 105
music, 45, 86, 90, 124, 130, 139, 210, 232
myalgic encephalomyelitis see chronic fatigue syndrome
mycophenolate mofetil, 133
Mylanta, 161, 174
mystery pain, 230–3

nalbuphine, 29
Naprosyn, 34
naproxen, 29, 30
    back, neck and shoulder pain &, 108, 114, 119
    body pain &, 127, 132
    cancer pain &, 137

face and mouth pain &, 151
gastrointestinal pain &, 173
head pain &, 186
joint pain &, 189, 193, 197, 203, 207, 208, 212
leg and foot pain &, 218, 228
nerve pain &, 245, 248
overuse injuries &, 252, 256, 259
pelvic pain &, 262, 267, 272, 276, 277
naproxen guide, 34
naps, 36, 85, 130
Naramig, 183
naratriptan, 183
narcotics *see* opioids
nasal sprays
head pain, 178, 179
sinusitis, 147, 148
naturopaths, 52, 55
neck pain
best first steps, 114–15
diet &, 98, 117
doctors &, 53, 114–16, 117
ergonomics &, 116
exercise for, 115, 116, 117, 324–8
heat/ice for, 114
instant relief for, 116
medications for, 30, 114, 115
pinched nerves &, 53
posture &, 114, 116
rest for, 116
spinal manual therapy for, 115–16
surgery for, 117
TENS &, 115
triggers for, 89, 93
weightlessness &, 116
neck pillows, 117
neck stretches (exercise), 71, 116, 324–5
needle interventions, 250
Neoral, 288
Neotigason, 288
nerve blocks, 236
nerve damage, 31–2, 53
nerve pain
complex regional pain syndrome, 234–8
diabetic neuropathy, 239–43
shingles, 32, 33, 53, 244–6
trigeminal neuralgia, 247–50
nerve pain signals, 12, 20, 22, 30, 31–2
neural activity suppression, 33
neuralgia, 53
neurologists, 53
Neurontin, 33, 123
neuropathic pain, 33, 35, 138
neuropathy, 31–2
neurostimulation therapy, 113
neurosurgeons, 48, 53

neurotransmitters, 84, 85, 124, 129, 152, 169, 231, 232, 275
New Zealand Medical Association, 122
New Zealand Pain Society, 48
Nexium, 162, 175
nitrates, 91, 94
nitroglycerine, 177
noise pain triggers, 90, 93
non-benzodiazepine hypnotics, 35
nonprescription medications, 28, 29, 31, 34, 52
nonsteroidal anti-inflammatory drugs, 29, 30–1, 173, 174, 255, 257
noradrenaline, 31, 79, 85, 124, 129
Normison, 35
Norspan, 35, 109, 202, 231, 241
nortriptyline, 32, 138, 231, 235, 240, 246, 280
Noten, 183
NSAIDs, *see* nonsteroidal anti-inflammatory drugs; *see also under drug* e.g. naproxen
Nurofen, 34, 174
nuts, 98, 99, 103, 145, 167

1-minute zone out, 85
oatmeal, 176
oatmeal baths, 246, 283, 288
obesity pain link, 100–1, 154, 185, 192, 200, 286
occupational therapists, 235, 237
odour pain triggers, 93
oesophageal sphincter, 160, 161, 163
oestrogen, 183, 263, 280
Olay Wash, 287
oleocanthal, 99
olive oil, 91, 98, 99, 195, 204, 209, 210
omega-3 fatty acids, 32, 98, 117, 134, 204, 209, 226, 242, 264, 274, 285, 289
onions, 99, 104, 105
opioid-induced hyperalgesia, 129, 235
opioids, 48, 90
back pain &, 109
burns &, 284
cancer pain &, 136–7
fibromyalgia &, 129
heartburn &, 160
joint pain &, 202
migraine &, 183
mystery pain, 231–3
myth and reality, 37
nerve pain &, 235, 241, 245
overview of, 16–17, 35, 37
pelvic pain &, 268

oral contraceptives, 183, 263, 271, 272, 275, 276
orange essential oil, 198
orange juice, 99
oranges, 98, 134, 195
osteoarthritis
best first steps for, 200
diet &, 99, 203, 204
doctors &, 201–2, 204–5, 221–2
exercise &, 61, 110, 203, 294, 295, 296, 299, 309, 312–15
foot and ankle, 221
hand, 202, 312–13
instant relief for, 202, 221
introduction to, 200
knee, 99, 101, 196
medications for, 30, 31, 201–2, 203, 221
overweight &, 94, 101
shoulder, 118, 119
sunshine &, 204
supplements &, 204
surgery for, 204–5, 222
TMD &, 150
weight loss &, 203
osteopaths, 55, 111, 115
osteoporosis, 162, 167
otolaryngologists, 149
overeating, 161
overexercise, 93
overgeneralising, 23
overuse injuries
carpal tunnel syndrome, 97, 99, 251–3
muscle and tendon soreness, 83, 254–7
repetitive stress injury, 258–60
overweight, 93, 94, 97, 98, 100–1, 154, 160, 185, 192, 200, 286
see also obesity pain link; weight loss
oxazepam, 35, 232
oxcarbazepine, 249
oxycodone, 35, 129, 136, 137, 183, 202, 231, 235, 241
OxyContin, 35, 109, 136, 202, 231, 235, 241
oxygen, 178, 179
OxyNorm, 35, 109, 202, 231, 235
oxytocin, 95

pacing, 15, 17, 26, 129
Pain Australia, 48
pain clinics/centres, 14, 15, 17, 48, 85
pain control, 19, 42
pain diary, 50, 92, 138, 336, 338
pain-free exercise hints and tips, 66–7
pain interpretation, 43

pain levels, 12–13, 28, 30, 45, 50
pain-management attitudes, 41–5
pain management obstacles, 15–16
pain monitoring, 86
pain patterns, 42
pain perception, 103
pain rating, 18, 77, 135, 138
pain reactions, 20
Pain SA (South Africa), 48
The Pain Society of Singapore, 48
pain, talking to your, 80
pain threshold, 29, 42, 83
pain tolerance, 29, 78
pain trigger inventory, 90–2
pain trigger log, 339
pain triggers, 87, 89–95, 97
painful bladder syndrome *see* interstitial cystitis
painkiller guide, 34
painkillers, 28–37
see also medications
Panadeine, 109
Panadeine Forte, 35, 231–2
pancolitis, 164
paracetamol, 29
back and neck pain &, 108, 114
body pain &, 127, 129, 132
burns &, 283
cancer pain &, 136
face and mouth pain &, 144, 147
gastrointestinal pain &, 155, 158, 165
head pain &, 182, 186
joint pain &, 203, 212
leg and foot pain &, 221, 228
nerve pain &, 245, 248
overview of, 30, 31, 34
Pariet, 162, 175
paroxetine, 33, 268, 276
Parsol 1789, 133
pasta, 97
patella tendinosis, 213
pawpaw ointment, 284
Paxamation, 138
peaches, 98
peanuts, 99
peas, 249
pec stretch, standing (exercise), 327
pelvic bridge (exercise), 318
pelvic inflammatory disease, 271
pelvic pain, 33
endometriosis, 261–5, 266, 271
interstitial cystitis, 266–70
menstrual cramps, 30, 34, 67, 93, 171, 271–4

premenstrual syndrome, 275–8
vulvodynia, 279–81
pelvic tilts (exercise), 273, 294
pencil smile, 80
pendulum swing (exercise), 120, 329
pentosan polysulfate, 268
pepper, 94
peppermint-oil capsules, 171
peppermint-oil massages, 187
periodontal cleaning, 144–5
periodontists, 146
periodontitis, 144–5
peripheral neuropathy, 239
peripheral vascular disease, 223–6
persistence, 17
persistent pain, 13–14
personal background, 20–1
personalising, 24
perspective, 25
Petadolex, 185
pets, 95
PHARMAC, 123, 184, 236, 246, 249
Pharmaceutical Benefits Scheme, 123, 184, 236, 246, 249
pharmacists, 52
Phenergan, 268
Physeptone, 136
physiotherapists, 14, 15, 52, 54, 68
physiotherapy
    back pain &, 110
    cancer pain &, 139
    CRPS &, 235, 236
    joint pain &, 197, 198, 199, 203, 212
    leg and foot pain &, 216, 218, 221
    lupus &, 134
    mystery pain &, 231, 233
    neck pain &, 115
    pelvic pain &, 269, 281
Pilates, 74, 75
piles *see* haemorrhoids
pillows, contour, 117
pineapple, 99, 195
piriformis stretch (exercise), 298, 319
planning
    doctors visits, 17–18
    exercise, 60–2, 68
    successful pain management, 17
plantar fasciitis, 61, 66, 227–9, 311
plantarflexion (exercise), 308
Plaquenil, 133
Plavix, 162
Pletal, 225
pleurisy, 131, 133

podiatrists, 218, 221
polyphenols, 210
posterior shoulder stretch (exercise), 332
postherpetic neuralgia, 244, 245–6
posture, 69, 71, 93, 114, 116, 211
potassium, 67
potatoes, 97, 98
powerlessness, 24
pramipexolc, 129
prayer, 44–5
prebiotics, 166
prednisolone, 132, 137
prednisone, 165, 179, 193, 194, 208, 245
pregabalin, 33, 123, 128, 138, 142, 236, 241, 246, 249
pregnancy, 157, 160, 162, 261
premenstrual syndrome, 97, 274, 275–8
prescription medications, 28, 29, 31
press-ups (exercise), 297, 330
Pristiq, 32
probenecid, 194
probiotics, 164, 166
procainamide, 131
prochlorperazine, 183
progesterone, 263
progestin, 263, 276
progressive muscle relaxation, 81, 82, 138, 153, 185, 270, 277, 278
prolactin, 95
pronation/supination (exercise), 305
propranolol, 183
prostaglandins, 30, 34, 254, 263, 264, 271, 273, 274
proton-pump inhibitors, 162, 165
proximal neuropathy, 239
Prozac, 33
pseudoephedrine, 36
psoriasis, 286–9
psoriasis triggers, 93, 289
psoriatic arthritis, 198, 211, 286
psychiatrists, 48, 53, 170
psychological counselling, 49, 51
psychological strategies, 14
psychologists, 14, 15, 27, 49, 52, 54, 170, 231, 233, 235, 237
psychotherapy, 85
pumpkin seeds, 98, 204, 209, 249
purines, 192, 194
Puri-Nethol, 166
pushing through pain, 14–15

quad squeezes (exercise), 320
quadriceps stretch (exercise), 320

quality of life, 28, 37
Quick-Eze, 174
quinidine, 131
quizzes, 44, 73
radiation, 250
radiotherapy, 138, 139
ranitidine, 175
raspberries, 98, 159
realism, 25, 41, 42, 50
reassurance, 25
rebound headaches, 30, 182, 183
reflex sympathetic dystrophy
    see complex regional pain syndrome
reflux oesophagitis, 160
rehabilitation medicine physicians, 48, 53
rehabilitation programs (exercise), 74
relationships, 41
relaxation, 14, 29, 54, 233, 237
    fibromyalgia &, 128, 129
    leg and foot pain &, 221, 225
    migraine &, 185
    painkilling power of, 79
    pelvic pain &, 273, 277, 278
    psoriasis &, 289
    rheumatoid arthritis &, 208
    shoulder injuries &, 120
    sleep &, 36
    stress reduction &, 80–1, 94–5, 289
    see also deep breathing; progressive muscle relaxation
relaxation techniques, 36, 81–2
Remicade, 166, 209, 288
repetitive stress injury, 258–60
    see also Achilles tendon pain; carpal tunnel syndrome
research groups, 49
resources, 334–42
rest
    lupus &, 133, 134
    overuse injuries &, 254, 256, 260
    see also relaxation
resveratrol, 99
retinoids, 288
rewards (exercise), 73
rheumatoid arthritis
    aids for, 209
    ankle, 220
    best first steps, 207
    cause of, 206
    co-conditions, 150, 188, 190, 196, 198, 200, 201, 251
    diet &, 99, 100, 209, 210
    doctors &, 207–9, 210
    exercise &, 208, 209
    fish oil for, 32
    instant relief for, 208
    introduction to, 206

medications for, 33, 206, 207–9
music &, 210
overweight &, 94
surgery for, 210
rheumatoid factor, 207
rheumatologists, 127
rice, 98, 99, 104, 194, 274
RICE, 254–5
Ritalin, 124
Rivotril, 138, 142
rizatriptan, 183
root canal therapy, 146
rotator cuff injuries, 119, 120, 258, 329, 330
routine, 18
rubber band ligation, 158
rubber band sensory cue, 101

6-mercaptopurine, 166
sacral neuromodulation, 270
sadness, 23, 42
St John's wort, 284
salads, 104
Salazopyrin, 165
salicylates, 201, 221
salmon, 98, 134, 204, 209, 226, 274, 285, 289
salt, 97, 278
saltwater mouth rinses, 144
saltwater nasal flushes, 147, 149
sardines, 226
saturated fats, 91, 97, 274
Savella, 123
scapular retraction (exercise), 327, 331
sciatica, 33, 53, 297, 298, 300, 319
scleroderma, 160
sclerotherapy, 158
second-degree burns, 282, 283
second opinions, 47
seeds, 98, 99, 171
self-care contract, 336, 337
self-education, 27, 42, 52
    CAM &, 55
    chronic fatigue syndrome &, 122–3
    fibromyalgia &, 127
    overview of, 47–8, 49
sense of loss, 23
sensory signals, 12
Serepax, 35
serotonin, 63, 85, 95, 124, 129, 169, 177, 186, 274, 275, 278
sertraline, 33, 276
sesame seeds, 99
sex, 95
sex hormones, 29, 37
shame, 23
shingles, 32, 33, 53, 244–6
shock treatment
    Achilles tendinopathy &, 213, 216

patella tendinosis &, 213
plantar fasciitis &, 229
shopping list, pain-fighting, 97–9
short arc quadriceps (exercise), 321
shoulder pain
  best first steps for, 118–19
  deep breathing for, 120
  doctors &, 119, 120
  exercise &, 67, 71, 115, 118, 119, 120, 329–33
  ice for, 119
  injections for, 119
  instant relief for, 120
  introduction to, 118
  medications for, 34, 119
  pillow padding for, 120
  relaxation &, 120
  surgery for, 120
  triggers for, 89, 93
shoulder replacement, 120
showerheads, massaging, 208
Sifrol, 129
sigmoidoscopy, 158
silverbeet, 99
single knee to chest (exercise), 294
sinusitis, 32, 100, 143, 147–9
Sjögren's syndrome, 141
skin grafting, 285
skin pain
  burns &, 282–5
  psoriasis &, 286–9
skin rashes
  lupus &, 131, 132, 133
  nerve pain &, 236, 244–6
  sleep habits, 29, 35, 36
sleep, hours of, 91
sleep medications, 35, 123, 232
sleep practices, 54
sleep routine, 85, 91
'sleep wave', 36
sleep problems
  alcohol &, 91
  chronic fatigue syndrome &, 122, 123, 124
  depression &, 84, 85, 231
  exercise &, 36, 59, 62, 84, 90
  fibromyalgia &, 33, 126, 130
  head pain &, 177, 180, 181, 185
  heartburn &, 163
  lupus &, 134
  music &, 86, 90, 210
  mystery pain &, 231, 232, 233
  pain triggers &, 90, 91, 93
  thought change &, 86
  trigeminal neuralgia &, 249
slippery elm tea, 175
smoke inhalation, 284
smoking
  diabetic neuropathy &, 243

gastrointestinal pain &, 93, 162, 167, 173, 174
head pain &, 93, 177, 180, 186
joint pain &, 206
lupus &, 93, 134
pelvic pain &, 269
psoriasis &, 93, 286, 288, 289
PVD &, 223, 225
sleep &, 36, 85
snacks, 94, 101, 102, 103, 104
snow peas, 104
SNRIs, 32, 128–9, 231, 268
societies and associations, 48, 123
sodium hyaluronate injections, 119
soluble fibre, 176
Somac, 162, 175
somatomedin-C, 130
soy products, 99, 192, 226, 242, 264
specialists
  bunions &, 218
  CAM, 55–6
  combination approach &, 51–2
  describing your pain to, 50–1
  evaluation of, 57
  expectations &, 50
  fibromyalgia &, 126
  finding the right, 48–54
  interviewing of, 48
  partnership with, 50
  qualifications of, 55
  questions for, 50
  red flags, 51
  reporting, 52
  rundown of, 52–3
  second opinions &, 48
  vulvodynia &, 279–80
  see also dentists
spices, soothing, 100
spicy food, 93, 94
spinach, 99, 158, 249
spinal cord
  mystery pain &, 231
  neck pain &, 115
  pain levels &, 13, 20
  peripheral nerve damage &, 33
  specialists &, 53
spinal cord stimulators, 237–8, 243
spinal decompression, 117
spinal fusion, 112
spinal manipulation, 111
spinal manual therapy, 115–16
spinal stenosis, 110
Spiractin, 276
spironolactone, 276
splints, 228, 253
sports clinics, 15
sports creams, 128
squats (exercise), 111, 299, 323

SSRIs, 33, 268, 275, 276
stair climbs, 69
static crunches (exercise), 295
statins, 224, 242
stationary bikes, 65, 110, 199, 209
steam inhalation, 147
Stelara, 288
Stemetil, 183
stents, 226
steroids, 119, 137, 193, 222, 260, 287
Stilnox, 35
stoicism, 22, 25
stomach bleeds, 30, 31
stomach pain, 83
strawberries, 98, 159, 210
strength moves, 68–70
strength-training exercise, 59, 60, 61, 62, 63, 65, 70, 115, 191, 213
stress
  biofeedback therapists &, 56
  depression &, 84–5
  exercise for, 62–3, 75, 95
  fibromyalgia &, 94, 126, 130
  head pain &, 185, 186
  IBS &, 169
  instant busters for, 83
  laughter &, 81
  lupus &, 134
  neck pain &, 114
  pain triggered by, 93, 94–5
  pelvic pain &, 269, 270, 273, 275, 277
  persistent pain &, 13, 27
  psoriasis &, 286, 289
  relaxation &, 81
  signs of, 80
  timeouts for, 85
  TMD &, 151, 152, 153
stress diary, 342
stress hormones, 78, 81, 94, 121
stress ulcers, 173
stretching basics, 71–2
stretching exercise, 59, 61, 63, 66, 67, 69, 70–2, 75, 110, 111, 116, 129, 130, 152–3
  see also exercises for pain relief
strictureplasty, 168
stroke and stroke risk, 33, 34, 53, 116, 132, 223, 286
'strong stoics', 22
substance P, 249
sucralfate, 175
sugar, 93, 94, 97, 101, 103, 104, 134, 146, 167, 185, 203, 274
sulfasalazine, 165, 206, 207
sulforaphane, 175
sumatriptan, 177, 179, 183
sunburn, 283, 284
sunflower seeds, 99
sunlight

importance of, 19
lupus &, 131, 133
osteoarthritis &, 204
pain trigger, 93
PMS &, 277
psoriasis &, 289
stress reduction &, 95
sunscreen, 133, 289
surgery
  back pain &, 112–13
  burns &, 285
  cancer pain &, 139
  carpal tunnel syndrome &, 252, 253
  dental pain &, 146
  diverticulitis &, 156
  endometriosis &, 265
  GORD &, 163
  haemorrhoids &, 158, 159
  IBD &, 168
  interstitial cystitis &, 270
  joint pain &, 191, 199, 204–5, 210, 213
  leg and foot pain &, 216, 219, 226, 229
  neck pain &, 117
  nerve pain &, 238, 243, 249
  shoulder pain &, 120
  sinusitis &, 149
  TMD &, 153, 250
  ulcers &, 176
Swedish massage, 256
sweeteners, artificial, 170
swimmer's shoulder, 211
swimming, 60, 187
  back pain &, 110
  fibromyalgia &, 129
  joint pain &, 64, 199, 203, 209
  leg and foot pain &, 221
  muscle and tendon soreness &, 257
  nerve pain &, 243
swimming strategies, 64
symbiotics, 166
sympathectomy, 238
synovectomy, 210
systemic lupus erythematosus, 131, 132–4

T-cells, 286
T stretch (exercise), 332
Tagamet, 161, 175
tai chi, 75, 209
Targin, 202, 235
tea, 93, 99, 103, 156, 277
Tegretol, 138, 249
telephoning
  CTS &, 253
  neck pain &, 117
Temaze, 35
temazepam, 35, 232
temporomandibular disorder, 150–3, 324–8
tendinopathy, 34, 118, 211–13

tendinosis, 211
tendon injections, 119
tendon pain
    best first steps, 211–12
    compression for, 213
    doctors &, 212–13
    exercise for, 213
    instant relief for, 212
    introduction to, 211
    medications for, 212
    physiotherapy for, 212
    rest for, 211, 213
    surgery for, 210, 213
    see also muscle and tendon
        soreness
tennis elbow, 211, 212, 258
TENS, 115, 242, 268–9, 281
tension headaches, 186–7
Teril, 249
tetanus injections, 284
tetracycline, 174
thankfulness, 43
Therapeutic Goods
        Administration (TGA), 268
thinking patterns
    all-or-nothing, 22
    catastrophising, 21–2
    changing, 20–7
    magnifying, 24
    mental filter, 23
    mind–body solutions &, 77
    other helpful, 25–7
    outsmarting, 23
    overgeneralising, 23
    personalising, 24
    'shoulds', 22
third-degree burns, 282
thoughts
    changing of, 16, 41, 54, 86
    chronic fatigue syndrome &,
        124
    management of, 17
    pain &, 13, 14, 80, 86, 87
    replacement of, 45
    writing down, 24
    see also cognitive behavioural
        therapy
thyme, 100
tic douloureux *see* trigeminal
        neuralgia
timeouts, 85
TNF-alpha inhibitors, 208–9
toe separators, 219
Tofranil, 231
tofu, 99
Tolerade, 231
tomatoes, 98, 195, 289
toothache *see* dental pain
toothpaste, 145
Topamax, 179
topiramate, 179, 184
towel curls (exercise), 307, 313
towel squeeze (exercise), 318
toxin removal, 62

tramadol, 123, 129, 245
Tramal, 123, 129
trans fats, 91, 97
transcutaneous electrical
        stimulation, 115, 242,
        268–9, 281
tricyclic antidepressants, 32, 33,
        85, 142, 152, 184, 231, 235,
        240, 246, 280
trigeminal nerve, 53, 93, 181,
        186
trigeminal neuralgia, 53, 93,
        153, 247–50
triggers *see* pain triggers
triglycerides, 239, 241, 243, 286
Trileptal, 249
triptans, 178, 183
trout, 98, 204, 209
trunk rotation (exercise), 295
tryptophan, 99, 274, 278
tumour necrosis factor alpha,
        121
tuna, 226, 274
turkey, 99
turmeric, 100, 210

ulcerative colitis, 164, 166, 167,
        168
ulcerative proctitis, 164
ulcers, gastrointestinal
    best first steps, 174
    bleeding, 176
    causes of, 173
    diet &, 175–6
    doctors &, 174–5
    instant relief for, 175
    introduction to, 173
    medications causing, 30, 32,
        34, 173, 201
    medications for, 174–5
    surgery for, 176
Ulcyte, 175
unsaturated fats, 195
uric acid, 192, 193, 194, 195
ustekinumab, 288

valaciclovir, 245
Valium, 109
Valpro, 184
valproate, 184
varicella zoster virus, 244, 245,
        246
vegan diet, 19
Vegemite, 194
vegetables, 94
    body pain &, 125
    face and mouth pain &, 145,
        146
    gastrointestinal pain &, 156,
        158, 163, 175
    joint pain &, 209, 210
    nerve pain &, 249
    pain-fighting shopping list
        for, 98, 99

pelvic pain &, 264, 278
psoriasis &, 289
sneaking in more, 104–5
weight loss &, 94, 101, 185
venlafaxine, 32, 85, 184, 231,
        235
venting, 42
verapamil, 179
video games, 86
visualisation, 81, 138, 185
vitamin A, 288
vitamin B, 249, 278
vitamin C, 134, 195, 210
vitamin D, 19, 287
vitamin E, 274, 283
vitamin supplements, 142, 167
vulnerability, 23
vulvodynia, 279–81

walking, 19, 26, 36, 59, 60, 63–4,
        93, 110, 111, 129, 167, 171,
        187, 203, 225–6
walking meditation, 82
walking poles, 66
walking sticks, 193, 205, 209
wall push-ups, 69–70
wall squat (exercise), 299, 323
wall stretch (exercise), 303
walnuts, 98, 204, 209, 226, 242
warfarin, 34
water aerobics, 129, 206, 209,
        257
water consumption
    burning mouth syndrome &,
        141
    cramps &, 67
    gout &, 194
    haemorrhoids &, 157, 159
    heartburn &, 162
    IBS &, 172
    importance of, 91, 105, 125
    lupus &, 134
    PMS &, 278
    sinusitis &, 149
    sunburn &, 284
    tension headaches &, 187
    vulvodynia &, 281
    weight-loss &, 105
    see also dehydration
watermelons, 98
weather pain trigger, 89, 93
weight gain, 97
weight loss
    exercise &, 59, 63
    joint pain &, 194–5, 203, 209
    leg and foot pain &, 222, 229
    pain relief &, 100–5, 162, 185
    psoriasis &, 289
wellbeing, 26
wellness, 138–9
wellness centres, 52
'what ifs', 21–2
wheat products, 93
whiplash injuries, 117

whole grains, 94, 97, 99, 101,
        125, 146, 156, 158, 163, 185,
        194, 203, 209, 226, 249,
        264, 274, 278
wide hands (exercise), 313
willow bark, 32
windburn, 283
wine, 92, 99
women
    arthritis &, 200, 206
    burning mouth syndrome &,
        140
    carpal tunnel syndrome &, 251
    chronic pelvic pain &, 33
    CRPS &, 234
    endometriosis &, 261–5, 266,
        271
    gout &, 192
    IBS &, 169
    interstitial cystitis &, 266
    menstrual cramps &, 30, 34,
        67, 93, 271–4
    migraines &, 183
    pain medications &, 29
    pain tolerance &, 29
    PMS &, 275–8
    TMD &, 150
    trigeminal neuralgia &, 247
    vulvodynia &, 279–81
work environment, 92
work hours, 163
working with pain, 19
wrist extension (exercise), 304
wrist flexion (exercise), 305

Xylocaine ointment, 280

Yasmin, 276
Yaz, 276
yeast infections, 279, 280
yellow squash, 105
YMCAs, 74
yoga, 14, 171
    back pain &, 61, 110
    breathing techniques &, 70
    fibromyalgia &, 130
    head pain &, 185, 187
    introduction to, 75
    muscle and tendon soreness
        &, 256
    mystery pain &, 232
    pelvic pain &, 270, 278
yogurt, 176, 194

Zantac, 161
zolmitriptan, 183
Zoloft, 33
zolpidem, 35, 232
Zomig, 183
zopiclone, 35, 232
Zostavax, 245
Zostrix, 242, 249
Zoton, 162, 175
zucchini, 104